Ecosocial Work in Community Practice

This book focuses on ecosocial work within the context of community practice. It aims to provide insights on understanding key issues, concepts and debates surrounding the mainstreaming of ecosocial work for sustainable community development. Divided into three parts, the first part of the book focuses on ecosocial work and ecosocial change around water, the ecology of coastal communities experiencing climate change, and environmental degradation. The second part includes chapters on ecosocial change and community practice in other kinds of bioregions. Finally, the third part primarily focuses on pedagogical approaches for teaching ecosocial work. This book was originally published as a special issue of the *Journal of Community Practice*.

Komalsingh Rambaree is an associate professor of social work at the University of Gävle, Sweden. He has been involved in several community work projects with youth and adolescents, as well as with coastal communities in Mauritius and some other Western Indian Ocean countries. He is currently engaged in teaching, learning, and researching issues related to ecosocial/green social work, international social work, adolescent and youth development, and computer assisted qualitative data analysis with ATLAS-ti.

Meredith C. F. Powers is an associate professor in the department of social work at UNC Greensboro, USA. Her applied scholarship includes climate justice, climate migration, ecosocial worldviews, and eco-therapy. She is the Founding Director of the Climate Justice Program of IFSW and of the Green/EcoSocial Work Collaborative Network.

Richard J. Smith is a native of Michigan. He currently serves as a core advisor for the International Ecocity Standards project of Ecocity Builders, Inc. In Detroit, he serves on the Hope Village Steering Committee and the Urban Learning and Leadership Collaborative. Smith's research has been published in the *Journal of Urban Affairs*, *Journal of Policy Practice*, *International Journal of Social Welfare*, *Social Work*, *Urban Studies*, and others.

Ecosocial Work in Community Practice

Embracing Ecosocial Worldviews and Promoting Sustainability

Edited by
Komalsingh Rambaree, Meredith C. F. Powers and Richard J. Smith

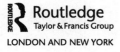
LONDON AND NEW YORK

First published 2023
by Routledge
4 Park Square, Milton Park, Abingdon, Oxon OX14 4RN

and by Routledge
605 Third Avenue, New York, NY 10158

Routledge is an imprint of the Taylor & Francis Group, an informa business

Chapters 1 and 4–19 © 2023 Taylor & Francis
Chapter 2 © 2019 Jessica H. Jönsson. Originally published as Open Access.
Chapter 3 © 2019 Komalsingh Rambaree, Stefan Sjöberg, and Päivi Turunen. Originally published as Open Access.

With the exception of Chapters 2 and 3, no part of this book may be reprinted or reproduced or utilised in any form or by any electronic, mechanical, or other means, now known or hereafter invented, including photocopying and recording, or in any information storage or retrieval system, without permission in writing from the publishers. For details on the rights for Chapters 2 and 3, please see the chapters' Open Access footnotes.

Trademark notice: Product or corporate names may be trademarks or registered trademarks and are used only for identification and explanation without intent to infringe.

British Library Cataloguing in Publication Data
A catalogue record for this book is available from the British Library

ISBN13: 978-1-032-38906-6 (hbk)
ISBN13: 978-1-032-38907-3 (pbk)
ISBN13: 978-1-003-34739-2 (ebk)

DOI: 10.4324/9781003347392

Typeset in Minion Pro
by Newgen Publishing UK

Publisher's Note
The publisher accepts responsibility for any inconsistencies that may have arisen during the conversion of this book from journal articles to book chapters, namely the inclusion of journal terminology.

Disclaimer
Every effort has been made to contact copyright holders for their permission to reprint material in this book. The publishers would be grateful to hear from any copyright holder who is not here acknowledged and will undertake to rectify any errors or omissions in future editions of this book.

Contents

Citation Information	vii
Notes on Contributors	x

1   Ecosocial work and social change in community practice   **1**
Komalsingh Rambaree, Meredith C. F. Powers, and Richard J. Smith

PART I
Socio-Ecological Problems, Policies, and Interventions Related to Coastal Ecosystems   9

2   Overfishing, social problems, and ecosocial sustainability in Senegalese fishing communities   **11**
Jessica H. Jönsson

3   Ecosocial change and community resilience: The case of "Bönan" in glocal transition   **29**
Komalsingh Rambaree, Stefan Sjöberg, and Päivi Turunen

4   "Todo ha sido a pulmón": Community organizing after disaster in Puerto Rico   **47**
R. Anna Hayward, Zachary Morris, Yamirelis Otero Ramos, and Alejandro Silva Díaz

5   An intersectionality-based analysis of high seas policy making stagnation and equity in United Nations negotiations   **58**
Jessica L. Decker Sparks and Shannon M. Sliva

PART II
Ecological Injustices from the Legacy of Colonialism   77

6   Collective survival strategies and anti-colonial practice in ecosocial work   **79**
Finn McLafferty Bell, Mary Kate Dennis, and Amy Krings

7   Indigenous perspectives for strengthening social responses to global environmental changes: A response to the social work grand challenge on environmental change   **96**
Shanondora Billiot, Ramona Beltrán, Danica Brown, Felicia M. Mitchell, and Angela Fernandez

vi CONTENTS

8 "Let's talk about the real issue": Localized perceptions of environment and
implications for ecosocial work practice 117
Joonmo Kang, Vanessa D. Fabbre, and Christine C. Ekenga

9 Urban flooding, social equity, and "backyard" green infrastructure:
An area for multidisciplinary practice 134
Lisa Reyes Mason, Kelsey N. Ellis, and Jon M. Hathaway

10 Clean and green organizing in urban neighborhoods: Measuring perceived
and objective outcomes 151
Nicole Mattocks, Megan Meyer, Karen M. Hopkins, and Amy Cohen-Callow

PART III
**Contradictions, Connections, and Challenges between the Global and
Local Communities** 169

11 Local–global linkages: Challenges in organizing functional communities for
ecosocial justice 171
Joel Izlar

12 "Mining is like a search and destroy mission": The case of Silver City 190
August Kvam and Jennifer Willett

13 Amassing rural power in the fight against fracking in Maryland:
A report from the field 206
Kathleen H. Powell, Ann Bristow, and Francis L. Precht

14 The future of environmental social work: Looking to community initiatives
for models of prevention 216
Samantha Teixeira, John Mathias, and Amy Krings

15 Green grey hairs: A life course perspective on environmental engagement 232
Mary Kate Dennis and Paul Stock

16 Preparing social workers for ecosocial work practice and community building 248
Meredith C. F. Powers, Cathryne Schmitz, and Micalagh Beckwith Moritz

17 Integrating youth participation and ecosocial work: New possibilities to
advance environmental and social justice 262
Tania Schusler, Amy Krings, and Melissa Hernández

18 Social work students' perspective on environmental justice: Gaps and
challenges for preparing students 278
Jessica L. Decker Sparks, Katie Massey Combs, and Jennifer Yu

19 Nature and social work pedagogy: How U.S. social work educators are
integrating issues of the natural environment into their teaching 289
Jon Hudson

Index 305

Citation Information

The chapters in this book were originally published in the *Journal of Community Practice*, volume 27, issue 3–4 (2019). When citing this material, please use the original page numbering for each article, as follows:

Chapter 1

Ecosocial work and social change in community practice
Komalsingh Rambaree, Meredith C. F. Powers, and Richard J. Smith
Journal of Community Practice, volume 27, issue 3–4 (2019), pp. 205–212

Chapter 2

Overfishing, social problems, and ecosocial sustainability in Senegalese fishing communities
Jessica H. Jönsson
Journal of Community Practice, volume 27, issue 3–4 (2019), pp. 213–230

Chapter 3

Ecosocial change and community resilience: The case of "Bönan" in glocal transition
Komalsingh Rambaree, Stefan Sjöberg, and Päivi Turunen
Journal of Community Practice, volume 27, issue 3–4 (2019), pp. 231–248

Chapter 4

"Todo ha sido a pulmón": Community organizing after disaster in Puerto Rico
R. Anna Hayward, Zachary Morris, Yamirelis Otero Ramos, and Alejandro Silva Díaz
Journal of Community Practice, volume 27, issue 3–4 (2019), pp. 249–259

Chapter 5

An intersectionality-based analysis of high seas policy making stagnation and equity in United Nations negotiations
Jessica L. Decker Sparks and Shannon M. Sliva
Journal of Community Practice, volume 27, issue 3–4 (2019), pp. 260–278

Chapter 6

Collective survival strategies and anti-colonial practice in ecosocial work
Finn McLafferty Bell, Mary Kate Dennis, and Amy Krings
Journal of Community Practice, volume 27, issue 3–4 (2019), pp. 279–295

Chapter 7

Indigenous perspectives for strengthening social responses to global environmental changes: A response to the social work grand challenge on environmental change
Shanondora Billiot, Ramona Beltrán, Danica Brown, Felicia M. Mitchell, and Angela Fernandez
Journal of Community Practice, volume 27, issue 3–4 (2019), pp. 296–316

Chapter 8

"Let's talk about the real issue": Localized perceptions of environment and implications for ecosocial work practice
Joonmo Kang, Vanessa D. Fabbre, and Christine C. Ekenga
Journal of Community Practice, volume 27, issue 3–4 (2019), pp. 317–333

Chapter 9

Urban flooding, social equity, and "backyard" green infrastructure: An area for multidisciplinary practice
Lisa Reyes Mason, Kelsey N. Ellis, and Jon M. Hathaway
Journal of Community Practice, volume 27, issue 3–4 (2019), pp. 334–350

Chapter 10

Clean and green organizing in urban neighborhoods: Measuring perceived and objective outcomes
Nicole Mattocks, Megan Meyer, Karen M. Hopkins, and Amy Cohen-Callow
Journal of Community Practice, volume 27, issue 3–4 (2019), pp. 351–368

Chapter 11

Local–global linkages: Challenges in organizing functional communities for ecosocial justice
Joel Izlar
Journal of Community Practice, volume 27, issue 3–4 (2019), pp. 369–387

Chapter 12

"Mining is like a search and destroy mission": The case of Silver City
August Kvam and Jennifer Willett
Journal of Community Practice, volume 27, issue 3–4 (2019), pp. 388–403

Chapter 13

Amassing rural power in the fight against fracking in Maryland: A report from the field
Kathleen H. Powell, Ann Bristow, and Francis L. Precht
Journal of Community Practice, volume 27, issue 3–4 (2019), pp. 404–413

Chapter 14

The future of environmental social work: Looking to community initiatives for models of prevention
Samantha Teixeira, John Mathias, and Amy Krings
Journal of Community Practice, volume 27, issue 3–4 (2019), pp. 414–429

Chapter 15

Green grey hairs: A life course perspective on environmental engagement
Mary Kate Dennis and Paul Stock
Journal of Community Practice, volume 27, issue 3–4 (2019), pp. 430–445

Chapter 16

Preparing social workers for ecosocial work practice and community building
Meredith Powers, Cathryne Schmitz, and Micalagh Beckwith Moritz
Journal of Community Practice, volume 27, issue 3–4 (2019), pp. 446–459

Chapter 17

Integrating youth participation and ecosocial work: New possibilities to advance environmental and social justice
Tania Schusler, Amy Krings, and Melissa Hernández
Journal of Community Practice, volume 27, issue 3–4 (2019), pp. 460–475

Chapter 18

Social work students' perspective on environmental justice: Gaps and challenges for preparing students
Jessica L. Decker Sparks, Katie Massey Combs, and Jennifer Yu
Journal of Community Practice, volume 27, issue 3–4 (2019), pp. 476–486

Chapter 19

Nature and social work pedagogy: How U.S. social work educators are integrating issues of the natural environment into their teaching
Jon Hudson
Journal of Community Practice, volume 27, issue 3–4 (2019), pp. 487–502

For any permission-related enquiries please visit:
www.tandfonline.com/page/help/permissions

Notes on Contributors

Micalagh Beckwith Moritz, The Sycamore House, Episcopal Service Corps, Harrisburg, Pennsylvania, USA.

Finn McLafferty Bell, School of Social Work, College of Literature, Science, and the Arts, University of Michigan, Ann Arbor, USA.

Ramona Beltrán, Social Work, University of Denver, Denver, Colorado, USA.

Shanondora Billiot, School of Social Work, University of Illinois Urbana-Champaign, Urbana, Illinois, USA.

Ann Bristow, Frostburg State University, Frostburg, Maryland, USA

Danica Brown, School of Social Work, Portland State University, Portland, OR, USA

Amy Cohen-Callow, University of Maryland, Baltimore, MD, USA.

Katie Massey Combs, Center for Conservation Medicine, Graduate School of Social Work, University of Denver, Colorado, USA.

Jessica L. Decker Sparks, Rights Lab, University of Nottingham, Nottingham, UK.

Mary Kate Dennis, Faculty of Social Work, University of Manitoba, Winnipeg, Manitoba, Canada.

Alejandro Silva Díaz, Mentes Puertorriqueñas en Acción, San Juan, Puerto Rico.

Christine C. Ekenga, Brown School at Washington University in St. Louis, St Louis, Missouri, USA.

Kelsey N. Ellis, Department of Geography, University of Tennessee, Knoxville, Tennessee, USA.

Vanessa D. Fabbre, Brown School at Washington University in St. Louis, St Louis, Missouri, USA.

Angela Fernandez, School of Social Work, University of Washington, Seattle, Washington, USA.

Jon M. Hathaway, Department of Civil and Environmental Engineering, University of Tennessee, Knoxville, USA.

R. Anna Hayward, Stony Brook University School of Social Welfare, Stony Brook, NY, USA.

NOTES ON CONTRIBUTORS

Melissa Hernández, Institute of Environmental Sustainability, Loyola University Chicago, Chicago, Illinois, USA.

Karen M. Hopkins, University of Maryland, Baltimore, MD, USA.

Jon Hudson, Department of Social Work, University of Wisconsin, Oshkosh, Oshkosh, Wisconsin, USA.

Joel Izlar, Social Work, University of Georgia, Athens, GA, USA.

Jessica H. Jönsson, School of Law, Psychology and Social Work, Örebro University, Örebro, Sweden.

Joonmo Kang, Brown School at Washington University in St. Louis, St Louis, Missouri, USA.

Amy Krings, School of Social Work, Loyola University Chicago, Chicago, IL, USA.

August Kvam, School of Social Work, University of Nevada, Reno, Nevada, USA.

Lisa Reyes Mason, Graduate School of Social Work, University of Denver, Denver, USA.

John Mathias, College of Social Work, Florida State University, Tallahassee, USA.

Nicole Mattocks, University of Maryland, Baltimore, MD, USA.

Megan Meyer, University of Maryland, Baltimore, MD, USA.

Felicia M. Mitchell, School of Social Work, Arizona State University, Phoenix, Arizona, USA.

Zachary Morris, Stony Brook University School of Social Welfare, Stony Brook, NY, USA.

Kathleen H. Powell, Department of Social Work, Frostburg State University, Frostburg, Maryland, USA.

Meredith C. F. Powers, Social Work Department, University of North Carolina at Greensboro, NC, USA.

Francis L. Precht, Frostburg State University, Frostburg, Maryland, USA.

Komalsingh Rambaree, Department of Social Work and Criminology, University of Gävle, Sweden.

Yamirelis Otero Ramos, Stony Brook University School of Social Welfare, Stony Brook, NY, USA.

Cathryne Schmitz, Social Work, University of North Carolina at Greensboro School of Health and Human Sciences, North Carolina, USA.

Tania Schusler, Institute of Environmental Sustainability, Loyola University Chicago, Chicago, Illinois, USA.

Stefan Sjöberg, Department of Social Work & Criminology, University of Gävle, Gävle, Sweden.

Shannon M. Sliva, Graduate School of Social Work, University of Denver, Denver, Colorado, USA.

Richard J. Smith, Core Advisor, International Ecocity Standards Project, Ecocity Builders, Inc., USA.

Paul Stock, Sociology and the Environmental Studies Program, University of Kansas, Lawrence, KS, USA.

Päivi Turunen, Department of Social Work & Criminology, University of Gävle, Gävle, Sweden.

Samantha Teixeira, School of Social Work, Boston College, Chestnut Hill, MA, USA.

Jennifer Willett, School of Social Work, University of Nevada, Reno, Nevada, USA.

Jennifer Yu, Wildlife Center of Virginia, Waynesboro, Virginia, USA.

Ecosocial work and social change in community practice

Komalsingh Rambaree, Meredith C. F. Powers, and Richard J. Smith

This special issue entitled, "Ecosocial Work and Social Change in Community Practice," focuses on an array of contexts, policies, practices, and challenges as well as successes related to an emerging vision for ecosocial work. Ecosocial work *is* social work, with all its depth and breadth, but it approaches the analysis of social problems, issues, and concerns with an ecosocial paradigm or lens, rather than an anthropocentric lens (Matthies & Närhi, 2016). Thus, ecosocial work is not a specialty within social work, rather all social work can, and we argue *should*, be ecosocial work.

The ecosocial lens recognizes the interconnectedness of all life in our ecosystem, and thus, the fair and sustainable use of resources to promote these relationships and the well-being of all. This lens requires us to critically examine and question modern societal structures, values, beliefs, practices, and ways of life that lead to social and ecological injustices through over-consumerism, materialism, anthropocentrism, oppression, and exploitation of people and planet (Boetto, 2017; Coates, 2003; Matthies, Närhi, & Ward, 2001).

From this perspective, ecosocial work is inclusive of structural social work in addressing the social structures causing social problems. It, therefore, pays particular attention to the socio-economic and political structures of a society/community; and, above all, it highlights how neo-liberalization increases inequality and vulnerability in certain communities (Matthies & Närhi, 2016). Ecosocial work encompasses green social work, interprofessional green care practices that bring people into contact with nature, and degrowth perspectives (Boetto, 2017; D'Alisa, Demaria, & Kallis, 2014; Dominelli, 2012; Ramsay & Boddy, 2017; Powers & Rinkel, 2018). We recognize that there is debate around some terms and concepts and the authors in this special issue may have various ways of presenting ecosocial work. As editors, we concur with a general consensus that *environmental justice* is more anthropocentric as it focuses on the impact on human populations and disparities created as a result of climate change, environmental degradation, and policies related to environmental management (e.g., fishing policies, disaster recovery). *Ecological justice*, on the other hand articulates a broader, ecosocial vision of justice – justice for the ecosystem as a whole with the understanding that humans are only one part of this ecosystem. If the ecosystem collapses, humans may not survive.

Ecosocial work is applicable at all levels of practice (e.g., micro, mezzo, macro) (see Rinkel & Powers, 2018); for purposes of this special issue, we focus on its application in community practice. The *Journal of Community Practice* is a fitting home for this special issue because it is the official journal of the Association for Community Organization and Social Action (ACOSA). This year, ACOSA changed the words represented by letters "SA" from "Social Administration" to "Social Action." This distinguishes us better by emphasizing that social work is not just about "administering" social programs, but about actually bringing people together to engage in social action to create social change that enhances the well-being of society. Thus, it is fitting that we have a special issue devoted to Ecosocial Work and Social Change, because this extends the vision of macro practice from society to the ecosystem, and offers a way forward for lasting and effective change. For example, ecosocial work includes interventions toward meeting the United

Nations' Sustainable Development Goals, protecting people and the planet, and ensuring prosperity for all, including future generations (Smith, 2013; Smith & Rey, 2018).

The field of community practice encompasses activities as diverse as community organizing, prevention activities, policy advocacy, and organizing functional communities (Weil, Reisch, & Ohmer, 2012). Community – as a network of people based on geography, needs and concerns, and/or having a collective identity – is central to social work practice in many countries (Sjöberg, Rambaree, & Jojo, 2015). In particular, professional social work originates from community work practice, alongside individual casework practice (Payne & Campling, 2005). Community development can be conceptualized as an outcome, a process, and a practice that promotes collective actions based on the needs and concerns of a community. Development is not exclusively linked to any one economic model (e.g., post-industrial growth economic perspective, degrowth approach). Social workers who practice within the interdisciplinary realm of community development are educated and trained to pay particular attention to the needs and concerns of the most vulnerable and disenfranchised members of a community. However, if social workers conceptualize community from an anthropocentric lens, it may exclude relationships with companion species and other aspects of the natural environment. Social workers using the ecosocial lens (sometimes identifying themselves as ecosocial workers), on the other hand, focus not only on the social, cultural, economic, and political aspects, but also on the relationships with the biophysical aspects of a community (Phillips & Pittman, 2009). Thus, the ecosocial lens is a holistic framework for promoting sustainable community development (Matthies et al., 2001).

We situate this special issue on ecosocial work in the context of community practice and social change, and we acknowledge it is part of a bigger, complex context, with historical and current conversations. This special issue aims to answer questions such as, how do we (re)center or (de)center from an anthropocentric lens to an ecosocial lens within social work? And, through the ecosocial lens, how can we separate our work toward sustainable community development from the typically accepted, post-industrial growth model, looking instead at degrowth perspectives as a path to a sustainable future? And, how do we mainstream ecosocial work in the profession? Within these queries, this special issue presents several themes. While these themes emerged, we also acknowledge that they are overlapping and interconnected with other themes, and not discrete. First, several articles focus on ecosocial work and ecosocial change around water, in particular, the ecology of coastal communities experiencing climate change and environmental degradation. The next section includes articles about ecosocial change and community practice in other kinds of bioregions. Finally, another set of articles primarily focus on pedagogical approaches for teaching ecosocial work. Below, we present brief summaries of the articles with editorial commentary as they relate to ecosocial work and our overarching questions for this special issue.

Ecosocial work, ecosocial change, water, and coastal communities

The ecosystem is the most natural and basic community for all living and non-living organisms, and it provides essential relationships and services for the well-being of all. Today, there is growing evidence that neoliberal capitalism, an outgrowth of colonialism, is among the root causes for climate change and other anthropogenic disturbances that are damaging ecosystem resources (Dellasala & Goldstein, 2018; Klein, 2014). Neoliberal capitalism is also at the source of conflicts related to the distribution and governance of ecosystem resources and services in various geographical communities (e.g., coastal communities). In particular, the pursuit of capital accumulation/profit has led to structural changes at national and international levels. This causes the overexploitation of local and global ecosystem resources by a small minority of individuals from the global community that are affecting livelihoods and causing socio-ecological vulnerabilities and injustices in local communities in various parts of the world.

Coastal communities are particularly vulnerable to climate change and anthropogenic disturbances (e.g., eutrophication, pollution, desertification, biodiversity depletion). Often, such communities consist of a diverse group of stakeholders that range from wealthy investors, hoteliers, and fishing businesses to the chronically poor artisanal fishers. The investors and businesses who earn their livelihoods through extractive activities and exploitation of coastal ecosystem resources and services create severe ecological injustices, such as the disproportionate burden of socio-ecological impacts experienced by traditional farmers and fishermen within a coastal community. Effective community organizing, and advocacy for ecosocial policies and governance of coastal ecosystems are vital for communities to thrive and become sustainable.

In this special issue, the first set of articles analyze and discuss socio-ecological problems, policies, and interventions related to coastal ecosystem resources. For instance, in "Overfishing, Social Problems and Ecosocial Sustainability in Senegalese Fishing Communities," Jönsson adopts a postcolonial perspective to examine the case on how the European Union's (EU) fishing agreement with the Senegalese government is causing the destruction of traditional sustainable living conditions and lifestyles of Senegalese fishing communities. In a similar manner, Rambaree, Sjöberg and Turunen present the case of a local fishing community in Sweden being affected by anthropogenic disturbances caused by industrialization and neoliberal policies and practices in their article entitled, "Ecosocial Change and Community Resilience: The Case of "Bönan" in Glocal Transition." In the article, "'Todo Ha Sido a Pulmón': Community Organizing after Disaster in Puerto Rico," Hayward, Morris, and Ramos present a case study on a coastal community organization and lessons for ecosocial work interventions after a natural disaster. The authors argue for ecosocial work practice within the interdisciplinary arena of professions and through community-led efforts for building community resilience and strategies to respond to environmental vulnerabilities. Additionally, other contributors to this special issue focus on analyzing political structures and policies affecting governance and exploitation of coastal ecosystem resources. Finally, in "An Intersectionality-Based Policy Analysis (IBPA) of High Seas Policy Making Stagnation and Equity in United Nations Negotiations," Sparks and Silva present a policy analysis to argue that the power structures within the United Nations are disproportionately affecting the exploitative marine activities and creating social and ecological injustices.

Ecological injustices from the legacy of colonialism

Climate change and environmental degradation is not limited to coastal communities but also impacts urban and rural communities in deserts, plains, mountains, and forests. In this special issue, the injustices from the legacy of colonialism are addressed extending themes from Lavoie (2012) regarding the conflicts between community organizing for social change and the constraints in operating in nation-building environments that emphasize social control. For example, Bell, Denis, and Krings offer "Collective Survival Strategies and Anti-Colonial Practice in Ecosocial Work." This piece rejects the premise that climate change is "new" and connects environmental damage to a broader history of colonialism. They provide hope that using indigenous knowledge in a decolonizing process can not only be a collective survival strategy, but also a climate resilience strategy. This theme is extended in "Indigenous Perspectives for Strengthening Social Responses to Global Environmental Changes: A Response to the Social Work Grand Challenge on Environmental Change" by Billiot, Beltrán, Brown, Mitchell, and Fernandez. For example, they note that indigenous knowledge can be used in an intervention for collective trauma by using storytelling and community mobilization. Likewise, in order to reflect ecosocial work values, climate resilience needs to respect sovereignty of indigenous people and their lands.

The colonial structures that limit autonomy of local communities also impact settler populations, involuntary migrants, and others. In "'Let's Talk About the Real Issue': Localized Perceptions of Environment and Implications for Ecosocial Work Practice," Kang, Fabbre, and Ekenga provide a case study of North St. Louis, Missouri, US. They find that some residents of this low-income, African-American neighborhood said that the real issue was violence and racism. While respondents report being less concerned about global climate change, they did connect immediate environmental threats, like basement flooding, to a structure of racism, in that one resident felt bamboozled because she was not informed that her home was in a flood zone. The theme of backyard flooding in low-income neighborhoods is also addressed in Mason, Ellis, and Hathaway's article called, "Urban Flooding, Social Equity, and "Backyard" Green Infrastructure: An Area for Multidisciplinary Practice." In a survey of 234 residents, they find that few interviewees knew about ways to use green infrastructure to prevent flooding, but indicated that they were interested in learning more. The authors propose utilizing social networks to educate households about these climate change mitigation practices to close the trust and information gap. Urban communities are also considered in "Clean and Green Organizing in Urban Neighborhoods: Measuring Perceived and Objective Outcomes," an article by Mattocks, Meyer, Hopkins, and Cohen-Callow. The authors find that urban residents have a conflicted set of attitudes toward greening efforts in their neighborhoods because they believe that what constitutes a "clean" social order to promote a feeling of safety is one devoid of vegetation. The authors propose more popular education about the benefits of urban greening.

Contradictions, connections, and challenges between the global and local communities

Other articles in this special issue touch on contradictions between the global and the local communities in other ways. For example, Izlar writes about glocalism in, "Local-Global Linkages: Challenges in Organizing Functional Communities for Ecosocial Justice." While much of the community organizing literature focuses on geographic communities, a functional community is one that has a shared concern or identity, but may not live in proximity. In this article, he presents a case study on e-waste recycling to show how this distributed network of interests in a functional community can make ecosocial change. In contrast, other studies show how contradictions between capital and community are not overcome. For example, in Kvam and Willett's "'Mining is like a Search and Destroy Mission': The Case of Silver City," residents of a mining town feel powerless because state law impedes their ability to make change. In this case, they observe a mining corporation's attempt to provide community benefits, such as a restored water tower that none of the respondents in the study said the community wanted. In contrast, Powell, Bristow, and Precht present a case study of effective state level organizing to shut down fracking in "Amassing Rural Power in the Fight against Fracking: A Maryland Case Study." They use geographic data and coalition building to harness state power for ecosocial change. In the contribution from Teixera, Mathias and Krings entitled, "The Future of Environmental Social Work: Looking to Community Initiatives for Models of Prevention." In this article, they examine environmental justice campaigns and community initiatives in Warren County, North Carolina, US; Flint, Michigan, US; and Kerala, India to provide recommendations on how to mitigate harm from human caused environmental degradation and prepare for a sustainable future. Additionally, Dennis and Stock provide a retrospective of the lifetime of several activists who have combined social and environmental activism in "Green Grey Hairs: A Life Course Perspective on Environmental Engagement." They conclude that intergenerational relationships are not new and offer hope to connect to a new generation of ecosocial change makers.

Ecosocial work pedagogy

While there is not one pedagogical approach for ecosocial work, several models are presented in these articles. The ecosocial lens elicits pedagogical approaches that are multifaceted, interdisciplinary, and expand ways that we may co-create a decolonizing pedagogy that is intrinsically linked to local and/or indigenous knowledge and ecological justice. A critical ecosocial work perspective questions modern societal structures (e.g., economic models), values, beliefs, and ways of life, and pays particular attention to the socio-economic, political structures, and geospatial issues of both community and society. Thus, any pedagogical approach must promote becoming aware of one's worldview or lens, and promote the ecosocial lens and critically examine the anthropocentric lens (Rinkel & Mataira, 2018).

Several global factors have moved the ecosocial lens forward within our profession, including, the Global Agenda for Social Work and Social Development (International Federation of Social Workers, International Association of Schools of Social Work, & International Council on Social Welfare, 2012), eliciting pedagogical conversations and resources (see Gray, Coates, & Hetherington, 2012; Dominelli, 2018; Krings, Victor, Mathias, & Perron, 2018; Mason & Rigg, 2019; Powers & Rinkel, 2018). Within the European context, for example, Matthies, Stamm, Hirvilammi, and Närhi (2019) present 50 interesting examples of ecosocial initiatives at community level in Finland, Italy, Germany, Belgium, and the UK. The authors provide concrete examples on how social workers operating at community level can engage in sustainability transition of societies through ecosocial work. Additionally, in national arenas, the ecosocial lens is also becoming more discussed and embraced. For example, the American Academy of Social Work and Social Welfare included in its Twelve Grand Challenges for Social Work (Kemp, Mason, & Palinka, 2015) the question "How can social work create social responses to a changing environment?" Also, in 2015 in the US, the Council on Social Work Education (CSWE) added *environmental justice* to its third competency: "Advance human rights and social, economic, and environmental justice" and as a component in the fifth competency of "Policy Engagement." While some of the contributors to this special issue worked with CSWE to make this change, we also acknowledge that embedding it is just one way to move this conversation forward, and we must move beyond embedding to promote the full embrace of an ecosocial lens across the global profession at large. We also acknowledge that some social work professionals and organizations have always or have already shifted to embrace the ecosocial lens, and we look to them for guidance.

Several articles in this special issue focus on promoting ecosocial work through our pedagogical approaches. These articles include various settings, audiences, and strategies in formal classrooms, field internships, study abroad courses, conferences, and in popular education. First, Powers, Schmitz, and Beckwith Moritz, in their article "Preparing Social Workers for Ecosocial Practice and Community Change," note the pedagogical approaches of the infusion model and the integration model (Boetto, 2017). Each of these models is elaborated through examples from the authors' own experiences. Both models are seen as necessary in advancing the ecosocial lens within the profession, and social work educators, as well as students, are leaders in this work. Next, Schusler, Krings, and Hernández offer an article about popular education with indigenous youth and youth of color entitled "Integrating Youth Participation and Ecosocial Work: New Possibilities to Advance Environmental and Social Justice." When provided the opportunity, youth articulate a vision of a just future that is unique to their shared identities, connected to place and land, and respects self-determination. They made a commitment to future collaboration and movement building based on authentic communication, loving acceptance, and solidarity. For these youth, social justice is inseparable from environmental issues.

In an article entitled, "Social Work Students' Perspective on Environmental Justice: Gaps and Challenges for Preparing Students," Decker-Sparks, Combs, and Yu report on how prepared 14 social work students feel they are for doing environmental justice work. While the students in the study report that environmental justice is a relevant issue, they report having difficulty connecting it to social work clients and report feeling overwhelmed by the magnitude of the situation. Part of this, they say, comes from their own detachment, but also having trouble understanding the feedback loops in the ecosystem. The authors recommend engaging other disciplines but also to have activities in social work classrooms that develop concrete ways of connecting the environment to social work.

The debate around terms and concepts such as environmental justice and ecological justice is articulated in the contribution by Hudson entitled, "Nature and Social Work Pedagogy: How U.S. Social Work Educators are Integrating Issues of The Natural Environment Into Their Teaching." Hudson interviewed 16 social work educators about their relationship to the natural environment. He finds that his respondents mostly agreed that theory courses were the best place to teach about the natural environment, but there were few materials to use. Respondents were particularly interested in sustainability and food systems. Hudson is careful to distinguish environmental justice (i.e., human-centered) from ecological justice and finds that some of the social workers he interviewed were beginning to focus on issues of ecological justice.

Conclusion

We acknowledge the global, historical and current conversation in which we situate this special issue. We are pleased to offer it as one of the many emerging scholarly resources that are increasingly available as we address the global ecological crisis as a profession. The aims of this special issue were to explore how to de-center from an anthropocentric lens to an ecosocial lens within social work, decouple sustainable development from the post-industrial growth model and embrace a degrowth approach, and mainstream ecosocial work in the profession, and specifically within our pedagogical approaches. With these overarching aims for this special issue, we were pleased to have such a broad range of topics covered within the articles.

Indeed, some articles were so unique in their cutting edge content, that we had to overcome struggles to get the best reviewers.

Several articles connect ecosocial work to the detrimental legacy of colonization; however, we hope that future ecosocial work scholarship explicitly critiques growth as an ideology and articulates a vision of prosperity without growth. Additionally, this special issue provides a few models and examples that schools of social work may use to promote an ecosocial lens and teach about the environment so that social workers can better respond to the changing environment. Articles in this special issue also point us toward degrowth as a strategy for restorative practices to better realize ecological justice.

Despite the breadth of the articles in this special issue, we note that there are several limitations that we hope future research and scholarship on ecosocial work will address. First, the most prominent limitation of this special issue is that almost all of our articles are primarily by authors from and about places in the US. And, although we do have content from Bönan, Sweden; Coastal Senegal; a University Program in Belize, and Kerala, India, we had hoped to receive more submissions that better represent the global ecosocial community practice that exists. We also note that future ecosocial work scholarship should address the controversial values and interventions around mere limits to population growth without considering the limits of economic growth. Finally, more ecosocial work scholarship that critically appraises ineffective environmental practices (e.g., greenwashing) are also warranted. While the articles in this special issue covered, to varying degrees, some aspects of the aims of this special issue, future scholarship could further explore these topics in greater depth.

We hope that this special issue intrigues, enlightens, inspires, and elicits conversations as we move forward in our collective efforts to address the ecological crisis through ecosocial work and community practice.

References

Boetto, H. (2017). A transformative eco-social model: Challenging modernist assumptions in social work. *British Journal of Social Work*, *47*(1), 48–67. doi:10.1093/bjsw/bcw149

Coates, J. (2003). Exploring the roots of the environmental crisis: Opportunity for social transformation. *Critical Social Work*, *3*(1), 44–66. https://ojs.uwindsor.ca/index.php/csw/article/view/5631

D'Alisa, G., Demaria, F., & Kallis, G. (2014). *Degrowth: A vocabulary for a new era*. London, UK: Routledge.

Dominelli, L. (2012). *Green social work: From environmental crises to environmental justice*. Malden, MA: Polity.

Dominelli, L. (2018). *The Routledge handbook of green social work*. London, UK: Routledge.

Gray, M., Coates, J., & Hetherington, T. (Eds.). (2012). *Environmental social work*. London, UK: Routledge.

International Federation of Social Workers, International Association of Schools of Social Work, & International Council on Social Welfare. (2012). The global agenda for social work and social development: Commitment to action. *Journal of Social Work Education*, *48*(4), 837–843. doi:10.1080/10437797.2012.10662225

Kemp, S., Mason, L. R., & Palinka, L. (2015). *Create social responses to a changing environment*. Retrieved from http://grandchallengesforsocialwork.org/grand-challenges-initiative/12-challenges/create-social-responses-to-a-changing-environment/

Krings, A., Victor, B. G., Mathias, J., & Perron, B. E. (2018). Environmental social work in the disciplinary literature, 1991–2015. *International Social Work*. Advance online publication. doi:10.1177/0020872818788397

Lavoie, C. (2012). Race, power and social action in neighborhood community organizing: Reproducing and resisting the social construction of the other. *Journal of Community Practice*, *20*(3), 241–259. doi:10.1080/10705422.2012.700277

Mason, L. R., & Rigg, J. (2019). Climate change, social justice: Making the case for community inclusion. In L. R. Mason & J. Rigg (Eds.), *People and climate change: Vulnerability, adaptation, and social justice* (pp. 3–19). New York, NY: Oxford.

Matthies, A.-L., & Närhi, K. (Eds.). (2016). *The Ecosocial Transition of Societies: The contribution of social work and social policy.* London, UK: Routledge.

Matthies, A.-L., Närhi, K., & Ward, D. (Eds.). (2001). *The eco-social approach in social work.* Jyväskylä, Finland: Sophi Publishers.

Matthies, A.-L., Stamm, I., Hirvilammi, T., & Närhi, K. (2019). Ecosocial innovations and their capacity to integrate ecological, economic and social sustainability transition. *Sustainability, 11*(7), 2107. doi:10.3390/su11072107

Payne, M., & Campling, J. (2005). *The origins of social work: Continuity and change.* London, UK: Palgrave.

Phillips, R., & Pittman, R. (2009). *Introduction to community development.* London, UK: Routledge.

Powers, M., & Rinkel, M. (Eds.). (2018). *Social work promoting community and environmental sustainability: A workbook for social work practitioners and educators* (Vol. 2). Rheinfelden, Switzerland: International Federation of Social Work (IFSW). Retrieved from https://www.ifsw.org/product/books/social-work-promoting-community-and-environmental-sustainability-volume-2/

Ramsay, S., & Boddy, J. (2017). Environmental social work: A concept analysis. *The British Journal of Social Work, 47*(1), 68–86. doi:10.1093/bjsw/bcw078

Rinkel, M., & Mataira, P. (2018). Developing critical self-awareness to incorporate sustainability into worldviews. In M. Rinkel & M. Powers (Eds.), *Social work promoting community and environmental sustainability: A workbook for social work practitioners and educators* (Vol. 2). Rheinfelden, Switzerland: International Federation of Social Work (IFSW).

Sjöberg, S., Rambaree, K., & Jojo, B. (2015). Collective empowerment: a comparative study of community work in Mumbai and Stockholm. *International Journal of Social Welfare, 24*(4), 364–375. doi:10.1111/ijsw.12137

Smith, R. J. (2013). A social worker's report from the United Nations Conference on Sustainable Development (Rio + 20). *Social Work, 58*(4), 369–372. doi:10.1093/sw/swt032

Smith, R. J., & Rey, S. J. (2018). Spatial approaches to measure subnational inequality: Implications for Sustainable Development Goals. *Development Policy Review, 36*(S2), O657–O675. doi:10.1111/dpr.12363

Weil, M., Reisch, M., & Ohmer, M. L. (2012). *The handbook of community practice.* London, UK: SAGE.

Komalsingh Rambaree

Meredith C. F. Powers

Richard J. Smith

Part I

Socio-Ecological Problems, Policies, and Interventions Related to Coastal Ecosystems

ⓐ OPEN ACCESS

Overfishing, social problems, and ecosocial sustainability in Senegalese fishing communities

Jessica H. Jönsson

ABSTRACT
This study explores living conditions of people in Senegalese fishing communities in relation to environmental change and unregulated fishing by foreign boats, weakening local opportunities and increasing forced migration of youth, creating problems for the future development of local fishery communities. It employs a postcolonial perspective and analyzes data collected through interviews with individuals from Senegalese fishing communities, social workers and relevant documents. The results show local reactions based on alliances between social workers and local community members to overfishing and the need for national and global structural changes. It is argued that EU's fishing agreements with Senegalese government is one of the reasons behind youths' forced migration to EU countries and that the betterment of the living conditions of fishery communities in Senegal requires not only already emerging alliances between social workers and local community members, but also national and global structural changes to protect Africa's fishing communities and local fisheries.

Introduction

Climate change and ecosocial transformations represent some of the most challenging issues facing global social work today. Climate change has led to the destruction of traditional living conditions in local communities, increasing social exclusion and marginalization, conflicts, wars and forced migration at local and global levels (Dominelli, 2012; Gray, Coates, & Hetherington, 2013; Kamali, 2015). Such environmental changes affected local communities in the coastal areas of West African countries, such as Senegal, Liberia, Sierra Leone and Cape Verde that are mainly dependent on natural resources, such as fishing, for their living (Food and Agriculture Organization [FAO], 2018a; Tvedten & Hersoug, 1992). As much as 40 percent of the ocean is heavily affected by pollution, depleted fisheries, loss of coastal homes and other human activities (United Nations Development Programme [UNDP], 2018). Along African western coasts, overfishing and declining fishing stocks

---

This is an Open Access article distributed under the terms of the Creative Commons Attribution-NonCommercial-NoDerivatives License (http://creativecommons.org/licenses/by-nc-nd/4.0/), which permits non-commercial re-use, distribution, and reproduction in any medium, provided the original work is properly cited, and is not altered, transformed, or built upon in any way.

have led to local exploitations of marine resources, which have impoverished the marine ecosystem (Ndour et al., 2014) and created economic and social problems leading to increasing poverty and forced migration (Alder & Sumaila, 2004; Jönsson & Kamali, 2012). Besides, such countries' fishing sector is drawn into a competitive industrial system through neoliberal structural adjustments, which harms and threatens the traditional fishing of local fishers and excludes them of being a competitor on equal terms in such an uncontrolled market. This has led to increasing poverty, unemployment, social stress, and declining health and well-being for local communities. Many people are forced to leave such communities in hope of being able to find jobs and take care of their families in other areas and countries, including those successfully reaching Europe (Alder & Sumaila, 2004; Jönsson & Kamali, 2012; Mbaye, 2014; Sall & Morand, 2008).

This study explores the consequences of current transformations of the position of local people in Senegalese fishing communities in relation to overfishing, environmental change, the weakening of local communities and forced migration. It employs a critical postcolonial perspective and analyzes data collected through interviews with individuals from local Senegalese fishing communities, social workers and other civil actors. Further, it explores the roles and contributions of community practice for achieving environmental and social community sustainability. The following research questions have guided the study: *What are local peoples' experiences from overfishing and declining fishing stocks, depletion of local marine resources and ecosystems in Senegalese fishing communities? How does the local community respond to overfishing and environmental crisis in the Senegalese fishing communities? What are the future challenges for social work in meeting the current changes in local Senegalese fishing communities?*

Methods

Since the main objective of the study is to examine the situation of local people in fishing communities and how environmental and socioeconomic changes have impact on livelihoods and local opportunities, the study has a qualitative methodological approach. The study is based on 14 interviews conducted with individuals from local Senegalese fishing communities (five men and two women), social workers (two men and one woman) and other civil actors (three men and one woman), from coastal areas. Six interviews were conducted in 2010 and eight interviews were completed in 2015. The interviews have been supplemented by data collected from electronic documents and articles about local fishing communities in Senegal. The interviewees have been contacted initially through key informants in African NGO organizations in Europe. This provided the researcher with further contacts with other Senegalese informants who are living in European countries and in Senegal. Five of the interviewees are coming from fishing communities of the coastal areas in western Senegal (now living as migrants in European countries) and the other nine interviewees are living in fishing communities of western Senegal, in coastal areas which have been subjected to over-fishing for decades. Finding those with enough knowledge and individual experiences concerning local fishing communities has not been easy. I had to use a snowball method which includes the risk of gathering information from a network of friends or members of the same family.

The collected material was analyzed using a qualitative content analysis (Downe-Wamboldt, 1992; Graneheim & Lundman, 2004) to identify relevant themes and categories. Given the political and global content of the study, a *critical* content analysis was used in analyzing the empirical material (Johnson, Mathis, & Short, 2016). Critical content analysis helps to explore discursive power relations in unequal contexts (Botelho & Rudman, 2009) and helps to generate the latent content of interviews conducted with former colonized people and the way they are defining their own situation and the context to which they are referring. This required a combination of deductive and inductive approaches to the analysis of the data described by Mayring (2000). This has been done by applying a postcolonial perspective in order to generate relevant themes for answering the research questions. The following two main themes have been generated through the analysis of data: *Hunger, social problems and forced migration*, and *Responses and resistance*. Given the fact that Senegal is a former colonized country, the postcolonial perspective is considered relevant and necessary to understand the current situation and being able to analyze what people are telling about their everyday lives in a postcolonial world. This perspective has also helped to reduce the methodological biases influenced by unequal discursive power/knowledge relations in the process of research (Olsson, 2007) and the role of researcher in taking an advocacy role (Lindeman, 2007) representing a non-colonized country. Although interviewees' narratives are affected by the position of the interviewer within existing structural power relations, including ethnic differences between researcher and the interviewees, this does not mean that white scholars cannot do research across differences. However, we have to be aware of and challenge white privileges and question how such privilege may shape research experiences (Andersen, 1993). Such differences in power relations and using methods of conducting research across differences, which examine the living conditions of people and the conditions and circumstances that shape their experiences, requires the researcher's reflexivity and critical awareness (Andersen, 1993; Temple & Edwards, 2002).

Theoretical framework and research context

Ecosocial transformations and sustainability in a neoliberal world order

Environmental and social crises do not exist in a vacuum, but rather within a global neoliberal socioeconomic and political environment supporting an uncontrolled global market with the main aim of maximizing its economic revenues (Ferguson, Ioakimidis, & Lavalette, 2018; Kamali, 2015). A way of understanding environmental change and the destruction of local communities is to consider a capitalism world system, which since the vein of colonialism and its aftermaths globalized the capitalist market and system (Wallerstein, 2017). Therefore, the matter of climate change and its local and human consequences cannot be properly addressed if the very roots of its problem, namely capitalism and the neoliberal economy are not critically analyzed, counteracted, and changed (Parr, 2013). As suggested by Naomi Klein (2014, p. 21) it is a question of capitalism vs. the climate:

> ... our economic system and our planetary system are now at war. Or, more accurately, our economy is at war with many forms of life on earth, including human life. What the climate needs to avoid collapse is a contraction in humanity's use of resources; what our economic model demands to avoid collapse is unfettered expansion. Only one of these sets of rules can be changed, and it's not the laws of nature.

In the case of Senegal, as for many other postcolonial nations in the Global South, neoliberal global development policies have been accompanied with increasing poverty and inequality, environmental degradation and climate change, civil war and ethnic conflict, forced migration, and the weakening of local communities. The triumph of neoliberal globalization, which started in the 1980s, structural adjustment policies forced on the country by the World Bank and the International Monetary Fund [IMF] led to destructive consequences for many African countries unable to meet the increasing needs of people who have lost their traditional livelihoods and are forced to move to urban areas or neighboring countries in search of better opportunities (Sarr, 2005; Sewpaul, 2013). Public and social services in postcolonial West Africa have gone through substantial changes influenced by postcolonial state building, globalization, uneven development, structural adjustment programs, and the inapplicability of the colonial models, which have accompanied restrictions to employment, increased poverty and social problems and growing marginalization of many groups (Sarr, 2005). Besides, and may be as a result of such changes, many such countries have been harmed by ethnic conflicts and "small wars" in the region (Kamali, 2015).

Many African countries are not only suffering from the neoliberal reforms launched by their own, often corrupted, states in cooperation with Western global organizations, but also from the unequal "agreements" forced on them. For example, agreements between the European Union (EU) and many African countries have resulted in the destruction of traditional life for many people in local communities, in various forms of exploitation of local resources, and have created economic and social problems in those countries (Alder & Sumaila, 2004; Gegout, 2016; Jönsson & Kamali, 2012). Such interventions have in many cases negative consequences for local fishery communities and destroys their traditional living conditions. In cases, such efforts of "development", as defined by the World Bank and the IMF and would be achieved by the neoliberal structural adjustment, have led to the destruction of local communities, increasing poverty, separation of families, and forced migration (Adepoju, 2003; Jönsson & Kamali, 2012).

The failure of development policies, which do not lead to changing and improving structural inequalities and generate development in local communities, have resulted in critical approaches and concepts of sustainability. Based on a process of neoliberal globalization, the concept of sustainable development is mainly based on technocratic and capitalist Western ideology of development (Adams, 1995). After more than 50 years since the influential article of Garrett Hardin (1968) "The Tragedy of the Commons" was published, foreign destructive interventions in commons, has forced local people, who made their livings of small-scale fishery, to leave their communities in hope of better life chances somewhere else. As Ostrom, Burger, Field, Norgaard, and Policansky (1999) put it, previous generations complained that change was taking place faster and faster and population growth, economic development, capital and labor mobility, and technological change push us past environmental thresholds before we know it. However, past lessons are less and less applicable to current problems. Today, sustainable development is part of the idea of "green capitalism", which encourages consumerism as the path to development (Bruno & Karliner, 2002). This is mainly based on a neoliberal ideology and a West-centric understanding of development, which do not target structural inequalities and promote social justice (Dominelli, 2012; Ferguson et al., 2018; Kamali, 2015).

Critical analyses are needed to unveil the underlying mechanisms behind a seemingly neutral globalization project and consider the relationship between colonialism, development and (neoliberal) globalization (McMichael, 2012). Likewise, the global profession of social work needs developing a critical position toward the ideology of global neoliberalism and its local practices. This should influence practices of social work in our postcolonial world.

Some academics argue that the "green revolution", which concerns land-based issues of sustainable development, should also include a "blue revolution" which would mean considering the question of the world's seas and oceans and its related food production, such as fishing (Soluri, 2011; Somayaji & Coelho, 2017). Although, there are shortcomings in "The 2030

Agenda", the Sustainable Development Goals (SDGs) and related ongoing international and national processes, which depends on the UN's ambitions of "getting onboard" as many countries as possible, the Agenda and its goals are relevant to the fisheries and aquaculture sector (FAO, 2018a). The commitment to leave no one behind in fisheries and aquaculture is a call to focus action and cooperation on efforts that will help to achieve the core ambitions of the 2030 Agenda for the benefit of fish workers, their families and their communities, for food and socioeconomic security (Lynch et al., 2017). The Agenda contains 17 Sustainable Development Goals, among those, the protection of the coastal ecosystems. Goal 14: Conserve and sustainability use the oceans, seas and marine resources for sustainable development, is a recognition of ecosocial problems of coastal areas and the need for action.

Ecosocial problems and social work

International organizations of social work (International Federation of Social Workers [IFSW], International Association of Schools of Social Work [IASSW], & International Council on Social Welfare [ICSW]) have put forward a Global Agenda which, emphasizes the need for greater international cooperation around development issues, for acknowledging the global roots of local problems and the need for global actions. As it is stated in the Global Agenda (IFSW, IASSW, & ICSW, 2012, p. 2) "We recognize that the past and present political, economic, cultural and social orders, shaped in specific contexts, have unequal consequences for global, national and local communities and have negative impacts on people" and therefore "feel compelled to advocate for a new world order which makes a reality of respect for human rights and dignity and a different structure of human relationships". In this respect, social work globally should "commit ourselves to supporting, influencing and enabling structures and systems that positively address the root causes of oppression and inequality". The Global Agenda emphasizes working toward environmental sustainability, strengthening recognition of the importance of human relationships and is closely related to the universal mission of social work based on its codes of ethics and the global definition of social work (IFSW, 2014). This is an important step to counteract when social work becomes a support for a neoliberal global development instead of being the agent of social change and social justice (Ferguson et al., 2018). As suggested by Gray and Webb (2013, p. 8):

> In endorsing a critical social work agenda, a challenge for these international social work organizations would be to declare openly their opposition to the malign tendencies of neoliberalism and the destructive nature of state capitalism. Indeed, rather than vainly offering up sanguine diets of "Global Social Work" through best-practice models, the International Federations of Social Workers should be

launching militant agendas, such as "In Defence of Equality: Social work Against Neoliberal Capitalism".

Since the 1990s, there has been growing awareness about the role of social work with environmental issues. New approaches of "Green social work", "Environmental Social work" or "Ecological social work" have been developed in order deepen the understanding of the relationship between human communities, their physical environment and ecosystems (e.g. Dominelli, 2012; Gray et al., 2013; McKinnon & Alston, 2016). Dominelli (2012) describe the necessity of green social work in terms of addressing social inequalities, changing socio-economic conditions and developments rooted in neoliberalism and environmental degradation that impact disadvantaged communities. She urges social workers to support people in protecting the environment, obtain environmental justice, and to mobilize people in various partnerships and alliances that promote people's and the earth's well-being.

Research context: social work in Senegal

Senegal was a French colony and the French reforms after the Second World War were aimed at developing the proper labor force in colonies and so influenced social policy in Senegal. Social work was therefore a part of colonial policies and programs for the country. The first team of social workers was addressed in 1955 as a part of the colonial social affairs cabinet (Sarr, 2005). The first two decades after gaining independence in 1960, the Senegalese government restructured the social work intervention to help the most vulnerable groups, such as the disabled, widows and orphans. However, the structural adjustment policies forced on the country by the World Bank and the IMF in 1980s and further neoliberalization of the country not only led to the achievement of the goals of "development" of the country, but also reinforced the country's structural and social problems (Sarr, 2005). Growing socioeconomic gaps has led to increasing social problems, armed conflicts, growing number of children living on the street, AIDS and forced migration. The failure of the state in establish a coherent social policy which would help the most vulnerable in society led to the establishment of a new policy of "mutual care" which put in reality the most burden of the social care on civil society and NGOs. This was called "traditional solidarity". Such policies of indigenization of welfare practices based on cooperation and social support networks that respond to social need and promote community well-being, which have been institutionalized in Southern African communities for many centuries (Patel, Kaseke, & Midgley, 2012) have also been practiced in the post-war and post-colonial Senegal (Sarr, 2005). However, the indigenous system is not as strong or effective as before (Apt, 2002), partly because many people have migrated to the cities (Patel et al., 2012). There are several NGOs engaging in providing services to people in Senegal, such as Islamic associations and NGOs. They are organized according to their main field of activity: schooling, socio-cultural activities and (reproductive) healthcare (Renders, 2002). However, participation of people in different private and NGO projects is low since the extent of social problems and social exclusions and the weaknesses of the NGOs in providing substantial help and services (Dorsner, 2004).

The shortcomings of the NGOs to provide services to a growing number of marginalized people combined with the lack of effective social policy has led to growing social problems. Social work in Senegal is harmed by adopting Western models that have led to the erosion of traditional solidarities and local support systems, and their substitution with professional interventions through formal government and non-government services (Dominelli, 2012; Gray, 2016; Sewpaul, 2006). Recent decades of overfishing of the Senegalese shores has added to the problem of the destruction of local communities and their support systems.

Results

This section of the paper is based on the analysis of the conducted interviews and relevant documents which help to generate an understanding of the main objective of the study and its research questions. In the first part, the local peoples' experiences from and consequences of overfishing and declining fishing stocks will be elaborated on.

Analyzing the documents, such as those presented by Greenpeace (2017a) shows that West African waters are attractive for foreign fishing operations because they are amongst the most fertile in the world. Foreign fishing fleets have moved into the waters of the coast of West Africa, areas already subjected to overfishing for many years. According to Greenpeace European unit (2019), the European vessels have the capacity to catch between two and three times more than the sustainable level, which provides Europe with most of the subsidies and biggest share of fishing opportunities. By destroying the fish stocks, these foreign industries are now threatening the livelihoods of local fisherman and their families in Senegal. Documents presented by the Food and Agriculture Organization of the United Nations (FAO), show that Senegal is an example of a trend across the world, in which 90% of fisheries are fully fished or facing collapse (FAO, 2018b). Decades of overfishing have exploited artisanal fishing industries, which nations like Senegal have long relied on to for food- and socioeconomic security. Worse yet, this is happening at a time when climate change is reducing the amount of food grown own land (FAO, 2016). This transformation in Senegal is a violation of the earlier mentioned UN Sustainable Development Goal 14, which refers to *Life Below Water* and people depending on marine and coastal biodiversity for their livelihoods (UNDP, 2018).

The following concerns local peoples' experiences from and consequences of overfishing and declining fishing stocks, depletion of local marine resources and ecosystems in Senegalese fishing communities.

Overfishing leads to hunger, social problems, and forced migration

Interviewees from local Senegalese fishing communities have told me about difficulties of getting fish. They have to sail far from the shore to have any chance of catching fish. In addition, the huge foreign ships in many cases destroy the local fishers fishing nets. The villagers feel angry, frustrated and powerless. A young man, Goundo originally from a fishing village in Dakar says:

> … people have been fishing for generations, my father was a fisherman, my grand-father began teaching me how to fish. This situation now … has put fishermen out of work. We fear that, in the future, there will be no fishermen left here. That is why many have fled to the Sea towards Europe … .

The worsening living conditions of people in costal fishery areas has been a narrative appearing in almost all interviews, irrespective of gender of the interviewees. As Fatou, a woman from a fishing family, says:

> It is not like before, everything has been harder, fishing, working, living. We have to work much harder now to get fish, to make living, it is hard, I feel sad for my children, my family, everybody who are living here, everybody has huge problems to make living.

The current situation creates local social problems, such as unemployment, poverty, lack of health and educational opportunities, frustration and social tensions between local populations losing their traditional ways of income and livelihood. As all the interviewees point out, decreasing employment opportunities in many West African countries force young people to emigrate to large cities, where work is hard to find, or to leave for neighboring countries, and Europe further afield (see also Cross, 2013). Senegalese social workers witness the deteriorating living conditions for people in these areas as one of social workers interviewed in this study, Moustapha, with experience from working in local fishing communities in Senegal says:

> … families do not have any resources and income to afford their children's education and healthcare and are living under inhuman conditions, which depends on foreign exploitation of these people's and areas resources. This leads to destructive consequences for people's livelihoods and force some to become involved in other activities in their struggle for survival; activities like crime or simply leaving their traditional villages.

People in the coastal areas of Senegal, particularly the increasing majority of young people suffer from the lack of employment opportunities, which is leading to forced migration (Adepoju, 2003; Cross, 2009). Historically, fishing communities in many African countries are known as being relatively immobile with sustainable living conditions. This fact has however changed dramatically since the appearance of new international fishing actors in their waters. As mentioned earlier, decreasing fishing opportunity influences many aspects of local communities' sustainable lifestyles and living conditions, forcing many youth to emigrate in search of employment opportunities. Many young West Africans end up as "illegal migrants" in other countries (Cross, 2009; Jönsson & Kamali, 2012; Sall & Morand, 2008). However, migration to Europe is for many a very costly and dangerous process, with major risks for migrants' lives. The desperate endeavors of many people to tackle poverty and the destruction of their traditional life chances force them to move to both urban areas in major West African cities and to Europe. This creates a new market, which even creates a new function for the old fishing boats. As one of the interviewees, a young man from Senegal, Saliou, says:

> The fishing boats of the local communities formerly used for fishing now is used to transport people to Europe, even if the boats are old and not secure for taking so many people onboard that is why some of them are not reaching European coasts.

The migration journey to Europe is considered as one of the ultimate rescue mission for many young people from fishing communities in West Africa. As Muhammed says:

> There is not much to do here, there is no job, no income, no security, no future, for me or for my family, I have to leave. Even in our large cities there is nothing for us, but many be going to Europe would save me from problems, getting job, income and could help my family here.

Many find it the only way out of an increasing poverty in their local communities which leave them unprotected and poor. A phenomenon mentioned by several research participants is that many families "agreed" to send young members on the dangerous journey to Europe in order for the youngsters to obtain a job in Europe and send money back to their families, as Mamoudo says:

> I have to make this journey since my parents, my brothers and sisters, the entire family are dependent on me being able to send them some money for their living. Travelling to Europe is a costly business, is dangerous and I have to make it, the family give me some money, they sell their belongings for me to be able to reach Europe and take care of them … .it is not a choice, it is a duty and we have no other way … . I have tried everything … nothing more to do.

Mamoudo's narrative is not unique and others tell more or less the same reason for their decision to emigrate to Europe. The oppressive international engagement in fishing industry in West African waters has more or less destroyed may traditional lifestyles of fishing communities and do not leave many other options than forced migration. However, although some youth succeed to overcome the dangers of migration and leave their deprived communities, many are left behind and have to deal with the local problems and challenges to their (un)sustainable lives.

Responses and resistance in Senegal's fishing communities

Local communities are responding to overfishing and the environmental crisis in Senegal. Communities react in different ways. Local organizations, such as NGOs and religious associations together with social workers, try to combat the local consequences of recent destructive developments in fishing communities, such as increasing poverty and disintegration of communities. One example is what is called the "crisis of youth" because of many youth leaving the community. Social workers together with other civil social actors in the area try to hinder young men from emigrating. The emigration of young men influences the demographic sustainability of such fishing communities, as Emanuelle Bouilly's study in Thiaroye-sur-Mer, a suburb of Dakar which is traditionally a fishing community, have shown. Even mothers who initially encouraged their sons to board the boats to Europe, after the death of many migrants are now trying to discourage this kind of family-based mobility (Bouilly, 2008). According to social workers, migration to both urban areas and neighboring countries as well as to European countries, where many of them end up as "illegal" migrants, is not a free choice, but an action for survival which is forced on many people who otherwise would not leave their local communities, families and their homes. As Fatima, a local social worker says:

> We have tried together with local villagers, religious groups and NGOs to conduct meetings in order to convince people to stay and work for the improvement of everybody's' living conditions, otherwise they are not going to have any community left if everybody who is strong and can work leaves.

Some local social workers are organizing these meetings and are have discussions with villagers. However, this seems to be, as Fatima says, a "race against the clock". Another woman, Khadi, who works in a local NGO says:

> There is no support from nowhere, not government or any other organizations, beside a few people here who work hard to change such a misery. We cannot force people to stay when there is not much to do here, no fishing, no work, no nothing. Government should take some responsibility, but I know they don't, they think only about their own pockets.

Such understanding of the role of government in supporting international engagement in overfishing in those areas is witness to the role of many postcolonial governments in West African countries. Former colonial powers and their new global organizations, such as the EU, are still trying to keep their colonial advantages by forcing "fishing agreements" on such countries.

The local communities' experiences with the Fisheries Partnership Agreement are that they are destructive for local communities. As one of the interviewees, Abdou, puts it.

> Many foreign countries, including the EU, think of their own interests and not what we, people in this local community who are living of fisheries, need for their livings. They want our fish not our development, for then they are not going to get our fish as easily as they do now. There are people in Senegal who gets benefit of such agreements but not families in need and who live of fishery.

Besides, the working conditions for social workers are increasingly worsening in fishing communities. This is mainly based on the increasing influence of foreign fishery companies and international organizations' agreements with weakening states which are retreating from their responsibilities for the wellbeing of people. Therefore, many social work activities are organized by NGOs and religious groups almost without any support from the government. However, the weakening of the traditional solidarity bonds in such communities, which mainly depend on increasing poverty, create difficulties for social worker. This forces many social workers to leave and those staying behind are working under difficult conditions. According to social worker Moustapha:

> Social workers are very few and many of the educated social workers, who should stay in our countries to work with huge social problems of people who need them, are moving to urban areas or to Western countries in search of better work opportunities.

This is a serious problem for many African countries in need of a strong profession of educated social workers. However, the shortage of economic resources for many African nation-states, combined with corruption and cooperation with international actors whose interests do not coincide with those of the local communities, hinder the development of the social work profession (Sarr, 2005). Many agricultural and fishery agreements between the EU and costal African contracts have destructive consequences for local communities. This stems from the lack of a sustainable perspective on the part of the EU and the severe corruption of many African countries and governments (Jönsson & Kamali, 2012). This makes the resistance to destructive consequences of contracts between Senegal government, EU and other international agents and companies very difficult. There will be huge challenges in changing such a destructive and unsustainable development in fishing communities.

However, there are examples of fishers who have organized themselves to protect fishing areas and demonstrated against foreign investment – and overfishing and for development alternatives like sustainable fishing practices. Such demonstrations appeared since 2011 and resulted in some cases in changing laws in order to limit foreign fishing in Senegalese waters

(Greenpeace, 2014; Valo, 2014). This has led to the emergence of alliances between actors of civil society and social workers in helping families with limited opportunity to pursue their traditional fishing activities. There have also been reactions from international non-governmental organizations (INGOs), such as Greenpeace. As one example, in 2017, the Greenpeace ship Esperanza sailed to West Africa to "document the beauties of these rich waters, and bear witness to a growing threat to food security from decades of overfishing" (Greenpeace, 2017b, p. 1). It was called "the expedition of hope":

> West African waters are a treasure we need to protect. Globally, seas are being emptied and livelihood and food security are threatened by overfishing. We sail in West Africa to unite the region for a better management of shared fish resources. Now it is time to act.

This was welcomed by many local fishermen desperate to combat this problem.

Future challenges for social work in Senegalese fishing communities

This research provides further evidence from fishing communities that neoliberal globalization is behind the worsening of living conditions in non-Western countries (see also Jönsson & Kamali, 2012; Kamali, 2015). As argued in this paper, Senegalese local fishermen are suffering from an uncontrolled global market in which foreign vessels are emptying Senegalese coastal waters from fish, which was used as way of living and making fish a profitable commodity in the capitalist global market. The Commons are using up their livelihood and "sustainable development" turns to be empty declarations. Although the protests of local fishermen showed that local mobilizations and protests can create limitations for foreign vessels, the powerful agents and their local supporters are continuing the exploitation of Senegalese waters and deteriorating commons living conditions. As argued in this paper, one of the limitations for the international social work organizations is that they have not declared openly their opposition to neoliberal politics (Gray & Webb, 2013). Social work needs documents in which the role of globalization of an uncontrolled neoliberal market and policies is more explicitly stated and in which social work is declared as a global anticapitalistic and anticolonial movement for social change and social justice. Such documents should be given support by powerful international organizations, such as the UN and EU and other organizations aiming at improving sustainable development. Given increasing neoliberal globalization and European protectionism, social work could take a more active role in global transformations which are taking place in countries of the Global South, such as West African countries. European social workers and social work unions could make alliances with local social workers, civil actors and anticapitalistic social movements both globally and in West African countries in order to reinforce local resistance and engagement for change in fishing communities. Since local social problems, such as those of Senegalese fishing communities have global roots, the movements and actions against such problems should also be globally organized and supported.

Social work has many opportunities to counteract the devastating consequences of neoliberal globalization by cooperating with local community organizations and agents, national and international organizations engaged in realization of a sustainable development. The declaration of human rights (UDHR) (United Nations, 1948) and principles of social justice as emphasized in the recently adopted Global Social Work Statement of Ethical Principles [GSWSEP] (IASSW, 2018) provide guidance. The UN resolution, "Transforming our World: The 2030 Agenda for Sustainable Development" (United Nations, 2015), could make a ground for further action and measures for the protection of coastal ecosystems in West Africa. Deepening cooperation of international social work associations (IFSW, IASSW, ICSW) with the UN is needed to change the destructive trends of neoliberal globalization and its consequences for local fishing communities. This partnership should involve governments as well as people living in poverty, marginalized groups, civil society and indigenous and local communities, such as Senegalese fishing communities. Social work as a global movement could address the need for taking care of our seas and oceans as part of a "blue revolution" for combining the need of increasing global human food production and sustainability in fisheries (Soluri, 2011; Somayaji & Coelho, 2017).

Conclusion

Destruction of fishing communities' traditional sustainable living conditions and lifestyles is far from being a local problem. The EU and other powerful countries play a decisive role in such a destructive change of local communities in West Africa which force many youths of leaving their communities and migrate to EU countries. This is problematic for the EU politicians who complain about increasing migration and suggests that they are not aware of the role of EU actors and policy in creating hardship in and driving migration from West Africa. Local communities are subjected to powerful global forces, such as the EU, national postcolonial governments in cooperation with international governments and organizations and powerful multinational companies. Such a powerful alliance creating unbearable problems for many local people, cannot be counteracted only by local actors, who are fighting an unequal struggle. Social work could play a central role for a global mobilization for change in this area. Such mobilization needs cooperation and alliance with local and global actors and awareness of the shortcomings of the international organizations' declarations and actions. In the same vein, we need a critical perspective on the ongoing colonizing processes that reproduce inappropriate social work approaches based on Western models.

New horizons are needed for an inclusive and anticolonial social work practice responding appropriately to local concerns, such as those in West African societies, while critically aware of the impact of international development policies on local communities (Jönsson, 2016). Local social work could be supported by national structural reforms to eliminate overfishing in coastal areas. Cooperation between the international social work associations (IFSW, IASSW, ICSW) with the UN, in realization of the declaration of human rights and an equality-based sustainable development should include people in fishing communities. Although local communities are drained of their young population, who in many cases seek their future in European countries, there are many locals who are working to make fishing communities a better place for the young generation. This, however, needs international solidarity and national governments to pay attention to a local and human catastrophe not only targeting many of such communities but also the future sustainability of food production. The crisis of the oceans transports serious consequences for the rest of the world in terms of biodiversity loss, livelihoods, fresh water, clean air, rain, and protection against climate change. Commitments for international action to protect Africa's fishing communities and local fisheries are urgently required.

Acknowledgments

Much appreciation is owed to the men and women from coastal areas and local fishing communities in Senegal, for their generosity in sharing their knowledge and experiences. Many thanks to the social workers and actors of nongovernmental organizations for participating in the study. Thanks also to key informants in African organizations in Europe for their assistance and willingness in finding contacts with interviewees and research participants.

Disclosure statement

No potential conflict of interest was reported by the author.

References

Adams, W. M. (1995). Green development theory? Environmentalism and sustainable development. In J. Crush (Ed.), *Power of development* (pp. 87–99). New York, NY: Routledge.

Adepoju, A. (2003). Migration in West Africa. *Development, 46*(3), 37–41. doi:10.1177/10116370030463006

Alder, J., & Sumaila, U. R. (2004). Western Africa: A fish basket of Europe past and present. *The Journal of Environment & Development, 13*(2), 156–178. doi:10.1177/1070496504266092

Andersen, M. L. (1993). Studying across difference: Race, class, and gender in qualitative research. In J. H. Stanfield & R. M. Dennis (Eds.), *Race and ethnicity in research methods* (pp. 39–52). London, England: SAGE Publications Inc.

Apt, N. A. (2002). Aging and the changing role of the family and the community: An African perspective. *International Social Security Review, 55*(1), 39–47. doi:10.1111/1468-246X.00113

Botelho, M. J., & Rudman, M. K. (2009). *Critical multicultural analysis of children's literature: Mirrors, windows, and doors.* New York, NY: Routledge.

Bouilly, E. (2008). Les enjeux féminins de la migration masculine: Le collectif des femmes pour la lutte contre l'immigration clandestine de Thiaroye-sur-Mer [Women and the male migrants in Thiaroye-sur-Mer, Senegal]. *Politique Africaine, 1*(109), 16–31. doi:10.3917/polaf.109.0016

Bruno, K., & Karliner, J. (2002). *The corporate takeover of sustainable development.* Oakland, CA: Food First Books.

Cross, H. (2009). The EU migration regime and West African clandestine migrants. *Journal of Contemporary European Research, 5*(2), 171–187.

Cross, H. (2013). Labour and underdevelopment? Migration, dispossession and accumulation in West Africa and Europe. *Review of African Political Economy, 40*(136), 202–218. doi:10.1080/03056244.2013.794727

Dominelli, L. (2012). *Green social work: From environmental crises to environmental justice.* Cambridge, England: Polity Press.

Dorsner, C. (2004). Social exclusion and participation in community development projects: Evidence from Senegal. *Social Policy and Administration, 38*(4), 366–382. doi:10.1111/j.1467-9515.2004.00396.x

Downe-Wamboldt, B. (1992). Content analysis: Method, applications, and issues. *Health Care for Women International, 13*(3), 313–321. doi:10.1080/07399339209516006

Ferguson, I., Ioakimidis, V., & Lavalette, M. (2018). *Global social work in a political context: Radical perspectives.* Bristol, England: Policy Press.

Food and Agriculture Organization of the United Nations. (2016). *The state of food and agriculture: Climate change agriculture and food security.* Retrieved from http://www.fao.org/3/a-i6030e.pdf

Food and Agriculture Organization of the United Nations. (2018a). *The state of world fisheries and aquaculture: Meeting the sustainable goals.* Retrieved from http://www.fao.org/3/i9540en/i9540en.pdf

Food and Agriculture Organization of the United Nations. (2018b). *General situation of world fish stocks.* Retrieved from http://www.fao.org/newsroom/common/ecg/1000505/en/stocks.pdf

Gegout, C. (2016). Unethical power Europe? Something fishy about EU trade and development policies. *Third World Quarterly, 37*(12), 2192–2210. doi:10.1080/01436597.2016.1176855

Graneheim, U. H., & Lundman, B. (2004). Qualitative content analysis in nursing research: Concepts, procedures and measures to achieve trustworthiness. *Nurse Education Today, 24* (2), 105–112. doi:10.1016/j.nedt.2003.10.001

Gray, M. (Ed.). (2016). *The handbook of social work and social development in Africa.* London, England: Routledge.

Gray, M., Coates, J., & Hetherington, T. (Eds.). (2013). *Environmental social work.* London, England: Routledge.

Gray, M., & Webb, S. (2013). *The new politics of social work.* Basingstoke, England: Palgrave Macmillan.

Greenpeace. (2014) *Russian fishing trawler arrested as local fishermen in Senegal protest foreign industrial fleets.* Retrieved from https://www.greenpeace.org/usa/news/russian-fishing-trawler-arrested-as-local-fishermen-in-senegal-protest-foreign-industrial-fleets/

Greenpeace. (2017a). *Exploitations of West Africa's coasts.* Retrieved from https://www.green peace.org/archive-africa/en/campaigns/Defending-Our-Oceans-Hub/

Greenpeace. (2017b). *The cost of ocean destruction: Report from Greenpeace ship tour of West African fisheries.* Retrieved from https://storage.googleapis.com/planet4-africa-stateless /2018/10/154ab281-154ab281-the.cost_.of_.ocean_.destruction.pdf

Greenpeace. (2019). *Countdown 2020 – will the EU deliver its promise of healthy seas and shift to low-impact fishing?* Retrieved from https://www.greenpeace.org/archive-eu-unit/en/cam paigns/oceans/

Hardin, G. (1968). The tragedy of the Commons. *Science, 162*(3859), 1243–1248.

International Association of Schools of Social Work. (2018). *Global social work statement of ethical principles.* Retrieved from https://www.iassw-aiets.org/wp-content/uploads/2018/04/ Global-Social-Work-Statement-of-Ethical-Principles-IASSW-27-April-2018-1.pdf

International Federation of Social Workers. (2014). *Global definition of social work.* Retrieved from https://www.ifsw.org/what-is-social-work/global-definition-of-social-work/

International Federation of Social Workers, International Association of Schools of Social Work, & International Council on Social Welfare. (2012). *The global agenda for social work and social development: Commitment to action.* Retrieved from http://cdn.ifsw.org/assets/ globalagenda2012.pdf

Johnson, H., Mathis, J., & Short, K. G. (2016). *Critical content analysis of children's and young adult literature: Reframing perspective.* New York, NY: Routledge.

Jönsson, J. H. (2016). Poverty alleviation, development, and social work practice in West Africa: A focus on Senegal. In M. Gray (Ed.), *The handbook of social work and social development in Africa* (pp. 243–255). London, England: Routledge.

Jönsson, J. H., & Kamali, M. (2012). Fishing for development: A question for social work. *International Social Work, 55*(4), 504–521. doi:10.1177/0020872812436625

Kamali, M. (2015). *War, violence and social justice: Theories for social work.* London, England: Routledge.

Klein, N. (2014). *This changes everything: Capitalism vs. the climate.* New York, NY: Simon & Schuster.

Lindeman, N. (2007). Creating knowledge for advocacy: The discourse of research at a conservation organization. *Technical Communication Quarterly, 16*(4), 431–451. doi:10.1080/10572250701370056

Lynch, A. J., Cowx, I. G., Fluet-Chouinard, E., Glaser, S. M., Phang, T. D., Beard, S. D., & Youn, S. (2017). Inland fisheries - invisible but integral to the UN sustainable development Agenda for ending poverty by 2030. *Global Environmental Change, 47*, 167–173. doi:10.1016/j.gloenvcha.2017.10.005

Mayring, P. (2000). Qualitative content analysis. *Forum: Qualitative Social Research, 1*(2), 1–10.

Mbaye, L. M. (2014). "Barcelona or die": Understanding illegal migration from Senegal. *Journal of Migration, 3*(21), 2–19. doi:10.1186/s40176-014-0021-8

McKinnon, J., & Alston, M. (Eds.). (2016). *Ecological social work: Towards sustainability.* New York, NY: Palgrave.

McMichael, P. (2012). *Development and social change: A global perspective* (5th ed.). London, England: SAGE Publications Inc.

Ndour, I., Le Loc'h, F., Kantoussan, J., Thiaw, M., Diadhiou, H. D., & Ecoutin, J. M. (2014). Changes in the trophic structure, abundance and species diversity of exploited fish assemblages in the artisanal fisheries of the northern coast, Senegal, West Africa. *African Journal of Marine Science, 36*(3), 361–368. doi:10.2989/1814232X.2014.950696

Olsson, M. (2007). Power/knowledge: The discursive construction of an author. *The Library Quarterly: Information, Community, Policy, 77*(2), 219–240. doi:10.1086/517845

Ostrom, E., Burger, J., Field, C. B., Norgaard, R. B., & Policansky, D. (1999). Revisiting the commons: Local lessons, global challenges. *Science, 284*(5412), 278–282. doi:10.1126/science.284.5412.278

Parr, A. (2013). *The wrath of capital: Neoliberalism and climate change politics.* New York, NY: Columbia University Press.

Patel, L., Kaseke, E., & Midgley, J. (2012). Indigenous welfare and community-based social development: Lessons from African innovations. *Journal of Community Practice, 20*(1–2), 12–13. doi:10.1080/10705422.2012.644217

Renders, M. (2002). An ambiguous adventure: Muslim organisations and the discourse of 'development' in Senegal. *Journal of Religion in Africa, 32*(1), 61–82. doi:10.1163/15700660260048474

Sall, A., & Morand, P. (2008). Pêche artisanale et emigration des jeunes Africains par voie piroguière [Small-scale fisheries and seaborne emigration of young Africans]. *Politique Africaine, 109*(1), 32–41. doi:10.3917/polaf.109.0032

Sarr, F. (2005). Changes in social policy and the social services in Senegal. In I. Ferguson, M. Lavalette, & E. Whitmore (Eds.), *Globalisation, global justice and social work* (pp. 55–65). London, England: Routledge.

Sewpaul, V. (2006). The global local dialect: Challenges for African scholarship and social work in a post-colonial world. *British Journal of Social Work, 36*(3), 419–434. doi:10.1093/bjsw/bcl003

Sewpaul, V. (2013). Neoliberalism and social work in South Africa. *Critical and Radical Social Work, 1*(1), 15–30. doi:10.1332/204986013X665947

Soluri, J. (2011). Something fishy: Chile's blue revolution, commodity diseases, and the problem of sustainability. *Latin American Research Review, 46*(2), 55–78.

Somayaji, G., & Coelho, J. P. (2017). Fissures of a blue revolution: The Ramponkars' response to mechanised fishing in Goa. *Social Change, 47*(2), 200–213. doi:10.1177/0049085717696392

Temple, B., & Edwards, R. (2002). Interpreters/translators and cross-language research: reflexivity and border crossings. *International Journal of Qualitative Methods, 1*(2), 1–12. doi:10.1177/160940690200100201

Tvedten, I, & Hersoug, B. (1992). *Fishing for development: small-scale fisheries in africa.* Uppsala, Sweden: The Scandinavian Institute of African Studies.

United Nations. (1948). *United Nations declaration of human rights.* New York, NY: Author. Retrieved from https://www.ohchr.org/EN/UDHR/Documents/UDHR_Translations/eng.pdf

United Nations. (2015). *Transforming our world: The 2030 agenda for sustainable development.* New York, NY: Author. Retrieved from https://sustainabledevelopment.un.org/content/documents/21252030%20Agenda%20for%20Sustainable%20Development%20web.pdf

United Nations Development Programme. (2018). *Goal 14: Life below water.* Retrieved from http://www.undp.org/content/undp/en/home/sustainable-development-goals/goal-14-life-below-water.html

Valo, M. (2014, February 18). Senegal fears its fish may be off the menu for local consumption. *The Guardian.* Retrieved from https://www.theguardian.com/world/2014/feb/18/overfishing-factory-joal-senegal

Wallerstein, I. (2017). *The world-system and Africa.* New York, NY: Diasporic Africa Press.

🔓 OPEN ACCESS

Ecosocial change and community resilience: The case of "Bönan" in glocal transition

Komalsingh Rambaree ⓘ, Stefan Sjöberg, and Päivi Turunen

ABSTRACT
The aim of this article was to identify and discuss ecosocial changes and community resilience mechanisms in a coastal fishing community of Sweden – Bönan. Data were collected through eight semi-structured interviews and field observations. An abductive thematic analysis was used to analyze data and background literature. The findings showed that Bönan has been exposed to a combination of ecosocial changes that have transformed the community, and therefore required community resilience interventions. This article concludes that social workers need to take an active part in ecosocial work for enhancing community resilience.

A core aspect of neoliberalism is the deregulation of the economy in order to create a free flow of capital, goods, and labor across national boundaries for ultimately seeking cheaper resources in maximizing profit and efficiency (Harvey, 2005; Heron, 2008). In particular, neoliberal globalization is connected to the term "glocalization" through which global processes are linked with local effects (Livholts & Bryant, 2017; Robertson, 1992). Within the process of glocalization, both global and local factors, therefore, interact and change living conditions of a community where the inhabitants not only see themselves as part of the local environment but the global planet (Persson & Erlandsson, 2014). While neoliberalism represents opportunities for the global market economy, it also acts as a destructive force that brings negative ecosocial changes and challenges to glocal communities. In this study, community is broadly defined as an entity – with geographic boundaries and shared fate that is composed of built, natural, social, cultural, and economic environments that influence one another in complex ways (Norris et al., 2008). Coastal communities are referred to as those communities that reside along coastal zones and/or have a particular interest in coastal ecosystem resources and services. Coastal communities usually consist of a wide range of community members such as fishers, traders and hoteliers.

This is an Open Access article distributed under the terms of the Creative Commons Attribution-NonCommercial-NoDerivatives License (http://creativecommons.org/licenses/by-nc-nd/4.0/), which permits non-commercial re-use, distribution, and reproduction in any medium, provided the original work is properly cited, and is not altered, transformed, or built upon in any way.

Many communities throughout the world are facing anthropogenic disturbances (Campanini & Lombard, 2018; Dominelli, 2018; Rinkel & Powers, 2017; Wilson, 2012), commonly referred to those human induced changes that have negative impact on the environment (Wilson, 2012). In this connection, there is an urgent call for social workers to develop and strengthen ecosocial work interventions in creating social responses to environmental changes (Kemp & Palinkas, 2015; Matthies, Närhi, & Ward, 2001). Ecosocial work is that specific branch in social work that, besides of the social aspects, analyzes the human-nature interactions in enhancing and promoting the well-being of all. In this endeavor, community resilience – the adaptive capacity of the community to effectively deal with disturbances – is a vital component of ecosocial work in community practice.

Within this context, this article aims to identify and discuss the ecosocial changes affecting Bönan (a fishing community in Sweden) and the resilience mechanisms that have helped the community through the process of glocal transition. The fishing community from Bönan represents an interesting case study on a tiny fishing community that has been exposed to glocal ecosocial disturbances, but also makes an example of community resilience. Following the World War II, the community Bönan faced several problems related to anthropogenic disturbances from industrialization and urbanization. The structural changes and ecological disturbances started affecting the social and living conditions of the community. Despite structural and ecological crises, after some years Bönan has been regenerated and is now an attractive location for property development and new settlers. The case study of Bönan, therefore, enables a deeper understanding of both structural and lived experiences of people from Bönan, through which roles and implications for ecosocial work in community practice are highlighted. With reference to the case study of Bönan, the following research questions are answered in this article: (a) What have been the major ecosocial changes in this particular coastal community? (b) How did the coastal community manage to build its resilience? (c) What implications for ecosocial work in community practice can be drawn from this case study?

Conceptual and theoretical framework

During the past few years, there has been a revival of ecosocial thinking within social work (Ramsay & Boddy, 2017). An ecosocial perspective within social work emphasizes that human beings are social and organic, intrinsically embedded in mutually dependent relationships within the larger ecosystem (Hoff & Pollack, 1993). In this sense, ecosocial work goes beyond structural social work by putting the emphasis on sustainability and nature (Närhi & Matthies, 2016). An ecosocial perspective particularly reiterates the argument that there is a strong link between bio-physical environmental problems and social problems, social inequalities, and social change at the global and local levels (Matthies et al., 2001; Rambaree, 2013; Rambaree & Ahmadi, 2017).

Within the ecosocial perspective, community resilience is considered as an important aspect for community practice. Resilience is commonly defined as the adaptive capacity of a system to recover from a disturbance. A resilience perspective focuses on adjustments that sustain and enhance the capacity of ecosocial systems to cope with, adapt to, and shape change and learn to live with uncertainty and shock (Folke, 2006). According to the Stockholm Resilience Centre (2015), resilience begins with the belief that humans and nature are strongly coupled to the point that they should be conceived of as one socio-ecological system. From this perspective, community resilience is conceptualized as the process of adaptation in dealing with ecosocial changes in the community. In particular, Magis (2010, p. 401) defines community resilience as the "existence, development and engagement of community resources by community members to thrive in an environment characterized by change, uncertainty, unpredictability, and surprise". In a similar manner, Pfefferbaum and Klomp (2013, p. 279) explain that community resilience "emerges from collective activity in which individuals join in efforts that foster response and recovery for the whole". An important aspect of community resilience is the community's capacity to handle processes of transition.

Within this context, transition theory provides a suitable perspective through which the process of community resilience can be better understood. Transition theory focuses on the human-environment interactions over space and time within the process of ecosocial change (Wilson, 2012). The strength of transition theory lies in its ability to trace community resilience pathways through an emphasis on power relations in understanding vulnerabilities, and the overlapping nature of processes of ecosocial change (ibid). In this article, transition theory is primarily used to describe the resilience pathways of Bönan in building its community capitals, both historically and in recent times.

Community capitals are defined as types of community-based resources that are capable of producing additional resources through investment (Emery & Flora, 2006). One conceptual framework of community capitals includes seven forms of community resources (i.e., cultural, natural, human, social, financial, political, and built) and provides better understanding of how communities work (Anglin, 2015). Community capitals are therefore essential aspects to focus on in studying ecosocial changes and conditions of community development within a specific community. A focus on community capitals allows researchers to have a structured understanding of collective action and social mobilization mechanisms in enhancing community resilience and responses to anthropogenic disturbances.

Based on the literature review, a theoretical and conceptual framework, as depicted in Figure 1, was used in undertaking this study. The study had a point of departure in the transition theory that considers the experiences of a local community to ecosocial changes within the context of glocalization in order to consider the implications of ecosocial work. In this endeavor, certain

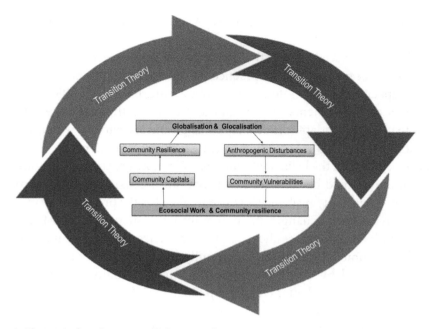

Figure 1. Theoretical and conceptual framework.

central concepts derived from the literature review such as anthropogenic disturbances, community vulnerabilities, community resilience and community capitals, are considered as the framework for this study.

Method

This case study is based on a hermeneutic qualitative approach that focuses on the interpretations of how inhabitants of a local coastal community – Bönan – in Sweden describe their lived experiences of ecosocial changes. Data were collected through eight semi-structured interviews with key informants from the Bönan community. In order to gather views and materials from a diverse population, key informants were purposefully chosen as follows: three community leaders, two fishermen, two social workers and one representative from maritime services (pilot station) based in Bönan. Out of the eight interviewees, seven were above 60-years old and four of them were females. The key informants were identified by reviewing the literature on Bönan and through snowball technique. The most crucial criterion in the purposeful selection of the interviewees was that informants were required to have own lived experiences of how Bönan has changed over the last five decades, since the study questions required answers on ecosocial changes over that long-term period. The interview guide had several central questions, such as; how the informants would describe the ecosocial changes in the community; the reasons, causes, and impact of such changes on sociocultural lives and livelihoods; how they foresee the future of Bönan as a coastal community.

The interviews were held during the months of May and August 2018. Each interview lasted for an average duration of about an hour. During two field study visits to Bönan, the research team made observational notes, took photos, and collected background literature to supplement the interview data. The researchers reflected together on the impressions from the field and the interesting aspects noticed in the case study. All this was to gather knowledge about the community and to get a contextual basis that was of use in the concrete interview sessions. In addition, the key informant interview data were supported with shorter interviews with two local residents about the life in Bönan today, as well as publications related to ecosocial issues regarding Bönan. For the collection, semi-structured interview questions were designed based on a review of the literature that were used in developing the theoretical/conceptual framework of this study. In particular, the literature review and the theoretical/conceptual framework were focused on transition theory, ecosocial changes and community resilience associated with the context of Bönan. Historical studies, scientific reports, and contemporary information about Bönan and similar coastal communities in Sweden from the Internet, were utilized as background literature to support the interview data and the discussion of the findings. The discussion of the findings, therefore, includes analysis of the background literature.

All interviews were recorded using digital audio devices with the informed consent of the research participants. The research team carefully followed social research ethical guidelines and considerations as outlined by the Swedish Research Council (2018). Prior to the interviews, a literature review in designing a theoretical/conceptual framework for this study was undertaken with the help of ATLAS-ti V.8.2 (a computer-aided qualitative data analysis software, ATLAS.ti Scientific Software Development GmbH, 2017). Key concepts from the literature were selected and organized as a theoretical and conceptual framework (Refer to Figure 1) for gathering and analyzing data. Gathered data, in digital audio recording format, together with field notes and background literature were input in and analyzed with ATLAS.ti V.8.2., and an abductive thematic network analysis was adopted.

The abductive approach is a pragmatic way of undertaking social investigation through the use of abductive reasoning for making exploratory inferences from empirical findings with reference to the theoretical framework based on background literature (Haig, 2008; Rambaree & Faxelid, 2013). The theoretical framework that guides data collection are subjected to further development/changes based on empirical findings from the field. Such an approach incorporates back and forth movement between theory and evidence during the analytical process of the gathered data. While listening to the recorded interviews the researchers selected quotations (in audio format) that were pertinent to the conceptual and theoretical framework of the study. These quotations were codified using keywords or phrases to provide meaning and were then grouped and linked as themes based on the conceptual framework (Attride-Stirling, 2001; Clarke & Braun, 2013) using the network function and platform within ATLAS.ti. Drawing from the gathered background literature and the theoretical framework, the following themes were used in the analysis of the findings: 1) structural and ecosocial changes, 2) community resilience and community capital, and 3) role of social work in community practice.

Findings and discussion

Historical context of the coastal fishing community, Bönan

Bönan is a small locality situated 13 km northeast of the city of Gävle in the eastern part of Sweden. It lies within the coastal zone of the Gästrikland province at the Baltic Sea coastline (Refer to Figure 2). The Baltic Sea is a marginal sea of the Atlantic Ocean covering a surface area of about 415 000 square kilometers, and is enclosed by the nine countries – Sweden, Finland, Russia, Estonia, Latvia, Lithuania, Poland, Germany, and Denmark (Swedish Agency for Marine and Water Management, 2013). Historically, this sea has been an arena of economic, political and environmental conflicts between several different countries.

In 1491, the Port of Gävle obtained the rights to become a cargo harbor and, from the 17th century onward, began receiving regular cargo shipments from various parts of Europe (Port of Gävle, n.d.). Consequently, the area located next to the harbor – Bönan – became a strategic part of the port and maritime center of Gävle. Around 1840, a lighthouse was built in Bönan to support the growing number of iron shipments from the Port of Gävle. According to the officer from maritime services, Bönan is still one of the three main strategic maritime pilot stations in Sweden. In fact, during the 19th century, Gävle was the largest city in the northern part of Sweden and one of the five biggest cities in the country. As a result of the trading boom, many traders in Gävle became wealthy (Port of Gävle, n.d.).

During the early period of the 18th century, some fishermen moved from the Gävle city to Bönan. Later, other individuals, including small-scale traders and business owners, joined them. By the 19th century, Bönan had established itself as a community composed mainly of fishing families. Some respondents recalled certain key inhabitants from that period, such as a doctor, a shoemaker, and pilots working for the maritime services. Most respondents highlighted that Bönan had good civic engagement among its community members. These community members also started to organize the area by building infrastructure and hosting socio-cultural events in the locality. Established at the beginning of the 19th century, a popular hotel/bar, a grocery shop, an open dancefloor, and a village swimming pool became regular meeting places for some community

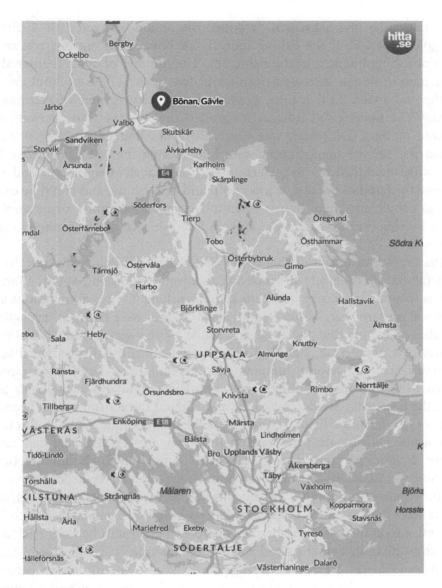

Figure 2. Map of Bönan.

members. At that time, steamboats were the main mode of public transportation between Bönan and the city of Gävle. According to some informants, families of fishermen had to row their boats to Gävle city so they could sell their catch. In 1843, the community members built the chapel of Bönan which is still in use today. They also had a primary school that opened in 1866, but it was closed in 1965. During those days, community members also founded a solidarity fund for funerals (known as *Begravningskassa* in Swedish). The fishermen proudly proclaimed the contributions of their parents and grandparents in establishing the Bönan community.

In particular, the fishermen described the period between 1930-1950s as the golden period of the fishing industry in Bönan. During this era, commercial fishing boomed in the Baltic Sea. The number of boats registered to fishermen in Bönan increased from about five in the 1740s to about twenty by the mid-1940s. At that time, there were about 30 registered fishermen in Bönan. The interviewed fishermen reported that, during those periods, the income of those fishermen was nearly 30 times that of workers in other industries. Several smokehouses were built during the 1940s to smoke the fish, which included herring. Herring was an important source of food and income for families because it was cheap and nourishing, and could be easily sold to people outside of Bönan. Even today, Bönan is known for its smoked Baltic herring (known as *Bönaböckling* in Swedish) that can be found in some places.

The long-term ecosocial changes of Bönan and the Baltic Sea have to do with industrialization and urbanization following the Second World War, as well as with the increasing pollution and overfishing. Chemical munitions and chemical warfare agents from World War II, which were dumped throughout the Baltic Sea, affected the flora and fauna of the sea surrounding Bönan (Szarejko & Namieśnik, 2009). Moreover, fertilizer runoff from coastal agricultural fields, and sewage dumping from pipelines and cruise ships, rapidly increased the dioxins and other persistent organic pollutants in the Baltic Sea.

In the late 1990s, Sweden raised the alarm about the consumption of certain types of fish from the Baltic Sea due to the high level of dioxins found in their fatty acids. Dioxins are persistent organic pollutants (POPs) that can cause severe long-term impacts on ecosystems and human health (Helsinki Commission, 2004). In 2002, the European Union adopted regulations concerning the human consumption of Baltic herring. However, Finland, Sweden, and Latvia have been granted some exemptions to these regulations due to the cultural importance of Baltic herring, the perceived health benefits related to fish consumption, and the need to protect fishermen's livelihoods in these countries (Pihlajamäki, Sarkki, & Haapasaari, 2018). The discussion between authorities and fishermen in Sweden regarding the balance of health benefits from eating fish and the risks related to overconsumption is still ongoing. In 2011, the Swedish Food Agency (as referred to in Swedish Radio News, 2012, p. 1) reported that only 15% of the Swedish population was aware of the nutritional advice to limit their intake of Baltic fish. Many Swedes still like to eat herring, and smoked herring is an integral part of Bönan's cultural identity.

In addition, the Chernobyl disaster in April 1986 created further burdens on the coastal communities in Gästrikland, including Bönan. Bönan suffered radioactive pollution following rainfall from toxic clouds of radioactive iodine and cesium-137. Consequently, elk and boar hunting, as well as wild mushroom and wild berry picking from the forest (popular/cultural activities for many people in Sweden) were banned in the region because of radioactive pollution. Today,

Bönan is regarded as a locality which is in the process of being regenerated as an attractive housing area. The marine conditions of the Baltic Sea are being closely monitored and some improvements are being noticed (Swedish Agency for Marine and Water Management, 2013). Figure 3 shows a picture of one part of the fishing area of Bönan as it looks today.

Theme 1: structural and ecosocial changes

According to most informants, Bönan underwent several drastic ecosocial changes beginning in the 1950s. The fishermen reported that overfishing in the Baltic Sea by boats from several different countries began affecting their fish catch during those periods. However, one informant stated, " … human beings are greedy … the fishermen's boats – they all had big salmon nets." She continued by saying that "they never thought they could fish all the salmon out … there was an overflow of fish, people did not worry and they thought that they could go on forever and ever."

In a similar vein, marine scientists have reported a decrease in fish biomass and a marked decline in fish catch that started in the mid-1940s in the Baltic Sea (Persson, 2010; Thurow, 1997). In addition, the Baltic cod stock collapsed in the late 1980s; since then, the Baltic herring and sprat have been the main commercial catch species in terms of volume in the Baltic Sea (Pihlajamäki et al., 2018). It is commonly known that fisheries have a direct impact on the environment through the removal of biomass and indirectly affect the ecosystem by altering conditions within the food web (Persson, 2010).

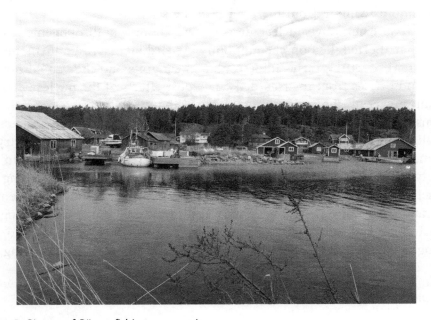

Figure 3. Picture of Bönan fishing community.

Sweden is still among the top-ranked overfishing nations in the Baltic Sea because it has one of the highest rates of fishing above that advised by scientists (Esteban & Carpenter, 2014). According to the interviewed fishermen, the effects of globalization in Bönan are readily apparent. They reported that outside of Bönan there are nowadays around 25 international fishing vessels – including those from Denmark, Finland, Norway, Spain, and Baltic countries – competing with each other for fish. The fishermen pointed out that today almost all of the herring caught in the open waters outside Bönan are transported in long-distance trucks to southern Sweden, Denmark and even to Spain to be powdered and processed into fish pellets/meal. These fish pellets/meal are then transported again by long-distance trucks to the north-western part of Norway to feed the salmon in fisheries. Finally, the salmon are exported all around the world, including to Sweden and, of course, also to Bönan. In addition, the fish pellets are transported to Finland and Russia as animal feed for the fur industry.

The decline in the number of fish caught in the Baltic Sea has also been linked to eutrophication resulting from World War II, industrialization, and rapid urbanization around the coastal areas of the region. The Baltic Sea has been considered as one of the most polluted seas in the world. For instance, an 89-year-old female interviewee mentioned that, during the 1950s, nobody in Bönan had indoor toilets and it was very common for people to pitch their kitchen refuse into the sea. She also stated that "during those days, people were not so environmentally conscious ... nobody gave a thought to what was happening." One of the fishermen talked about the situation in the 1970s and reported that "the sea was very polluted ... sometimes I could see sewage and condoms coming from the river into the sea."

The 1986 Chernobyl nuclear disaster was another anthropogenic disturbance that affected the Bönan community. According to a respondent, people were afraid of letting their children play in sandpits and they could not eat fruits and berries from their gardens. The post-effects of the nuclear disaster had an impact on the socio-cultural lives of the inhabitants.

This combination of assorted ecological changes within the process of globalization is a large contributor to the decline of the fishing industry in Bönan. In fact, only a couple of older fishermen remain in business in the locality today. Many of the younger generation of fishermen left fishing for other industry work in the nearby town of Sandviken and many of the new generation of young people have moved away from Bönan. The ecological disturbances and structural changes brought by globalization altered the demographical profile of Bönan. One respondent reported the following:

" ... there used to be buses coming from Sandvik (a steel company in Sandviken) to pick up employees, as there were many workers available here."

The interviewed fishermen from Bönan could not see any prospects for herring fishing for human consumption and one of them remarked that "it's something from the past now ... it's not possible [to fish] for a living any longer. We can never compete with the industrial globalized way of fishing." Further reflecting on this issue, the other fisher reported that the only possible option would be to "prohibit trawling of small fishes. That is the only thing that might work." In the interviews with the fishermen, it is evident that the deregulated access of big international trailing boats to trawl small fish has severely impacted both local small-scale fishing and the community's economy. The fishermen argued for sustainability measures through the reintroduction of the EU's prohibition on the fishing of herring for non-human consumption. Between 1977 and 1998, the direct fishing and landing of herring for purposes other than human consumption were prohibited in the EU based on overexploitation and declining herring stocks (Pihlajamäki et al., 2018).

Theme 2: community resilience and community capital

As a community, Bönan required adjusting to and coping with the adversity of anthropogenic disturbances in the Baltic Sea. In the 1950s, people who continued to reside in Bönan began working in non-fishing industries and found employment outside the local area. The steel, wood, and paper processing industries in the nearby areas attracted young people from Bönan. The port of Gävle, which was expanded closer to Bönan during the 1960s, is referred to as an example of strong community capital (i.e., built capital) for enhancing the community's resilience by some of the interviewees. The port of Gävle is now one of the largest terminals for the trade of petroleum and chemicals in Sweden. The interviewee working for the maritime services stated that there has been no major incident – such as a boat collision or oil spill – in this part of Sweden. Given that there is always a risk for such incidents, there is high vigilance and extra care in supporting the ships' movement in this particular region. Based in Bönan, the maritime center, with its pilot boats, was also regarded as community capital by a number of interviewees.

Beginning in the early 2000s, community members enhanced their community capitals through a regional community development organization called Norrlandet.se (www.norrlandet.se). Norrlandet.se functions as an umbrella organization with cooperation between public bodies (such as municipal authorities) and local community associations (known as *Bygdeföreningen* in Swedish). The interviews showed that there was no community work carried out by social services. However, a former head of social services from the municipality of Gävle living in the neighborhood fishing community joined the community organization movement after his retirement, and this lead to collaborative community work in Bönan. According to most of the interviewees, the organization mainly works towards the regeneration of the area by trying to influence politicians and local policy makers. Some interviewees opined that

Norrlandet.se plays a vital role in community development activities through cultural, social, economic, political, infrastructural, and environmental initiatives. One of the interviewees highlighted their upcoming projects regarding social mobilization in the local community areas and stated, " … we will soon launch our book on our affiliated community organizations and the locality".

Through bridging and bonding of social capital, community members have played a vital role in addressing and influencing decision makers regarding the recent infrastructure processes that led to the expansion of roads, recreational facilities, and utilities such as water, heating and internet services in Bönan. Norrlandet.se is also involved in the promotion of tourism activities, such as international sailing competitions, and in providing information on, and marketing smoked herring from Bönan. According to some of the interviewees, community members are working towards the foundation of a secure elderly home with built-in assistance and facilities (known as *Trygghetsboende* in Swedish) that would allow the seniors from the region to continue to live in the community.

One of the interviewees made the following statement, which is linked to community capital in the analysis of the findings:

> " … all associations joined together … thanks to this (collective mobilization) we got better facilities and connections (water, sewage, and optic fiber) … we play a very important role in addressing community concerns and issues with the municipality and to organize all the people here … "

Over the last few years, the number of inhabitants in Bönan has increased from 273 in 2003 to 901 in 2017 (Statistiska centralbyrån, 2017). A vital contributor to this growth has been community development measures undertaken by the municipal authorities, such as investments in new roads, municipal water, and sewer pipes, and modern internet cables. According to almost all interviewees, real estate prices in Bönan have drastically increased over the past few years because of the improved infrastructure, and closeness of the locality to the sea and the city of Gävle. In fact, a number of interviewees reported that Bönan is attracting wealthy people, such as hockey players and celebrities from the region. People are beginning to reinvest in local micro-businesses, such as restaurants and cafes. The informants described how Bönan has undergone a process of community transition. The area is gradually becoming gentrified. Infrastructural development is typically only an option for those who have money. Gentrification is often accompanied by increased housing costs and a decrease in traditional cultural and social ties (Smith, Lehning, & Kim, 2013). This is illustrated by a quotation from a social worker from the region who observed, "I have the impression that there are more upper layers of society living there nowadays." In a similar way one of the interviewed fishermen sighed, "Well, that's other people. More wealthy kinds of people are settling down here." Several informants stressed that common people can no longer afford the continuously growing housing prices in the attractive seaside location of Bönan.

Theme 3: role of social work in community practice

Interviews and field observations indicate that formal social work in Bönan was discussed in neither ecosocial nor in community work terms. Community work was mainly left to local organization initiatives, such as those undertaken by Norrlandet.se. Social workers had only individual tasks and cases focused on the clinical and social care of individuals, families and elderly. For instance, a retired social worker stated that social work in Sweden: "has become clinical, instrumental, and evidence-orientated".

However, in the city of Gävle, some examples of community work carried out by professional social workers (referred as field social workers within the municipality of Gävle) could be identified (Hansson, Lundgren, & Sjöberg, 2018; Sjöberg & Turunen, 2018). Interestingly, the retired head of social services from the municipality of Gävle had taken a leading role in re-organizing community activities in Bönan. He has played a central role by enhancing community development and community resilience on a regional level in and around Bönan. In an interview, he mentioned that he was probably chosen to lead community development initiatives because of his previous knowledge and skills as the leader of social services and because he had good knowledge of the localities in Gävle.

Implications for ecosocial work in community practice

This study highlights the fact that the process of glocalization does not only concern the global economy and technology, but also ecosocial aspects of small coastal communities – such as Bönan. Policies and practices based on neoliberal ideologies of exploitation of fishing and nature globally can bring drastic glocal ecosocial changes to the wellbeing of local communities. This study presents specific findings on how external forces – such as the deregulated global fishing industry and market-driven increase of housing prices – are transforming a picturesque coastal community towards gentrification. In the case of Bönan, social workers were not involved in the transition of Bönan and its community development. However, in the times of environmental changes, social workers have a vital role to play in the impact assessment of diverse types of ecosocial changes in the community.

Sustainable community development requires social workers to start critically analyzing environmental disturbances from ecosocial perspectives and to enhance community resilience through capacity building, collective empowerment, social mobilization, and the promotion of social cohesion and living conditions within communities (Sjöberg, Rambaree, & Jojo, 2015;

Sjöberg & Turunen, 2018). In addition, social workers can identify mechanisms through which community capitals may be built, enhanced, and used for sustaining livelihoods and wellbeing for all without harming the ecosystem and causing gentrification. They could engage in community work with the aim to bring about ecosocial changes that integrate equality, opportunity, and responsibility in the fair distribution of ecosystem resources and services (Gamble & Hoff, 2013; Rambaree & Rock, 2018).

In this endeavor, community-based social workers need to organize multidisciplinary teams and involve themselves in multi-sectorial collaboration in dealing with ecosocial changes. Community capital building, networking, and alliances with other social actors have a pivotal role in a social change-oriented community work practice for sustainability. The work by the former head of social services is an example of how professional social workers could engage in ecosocial community work. There is a need for professional skills and competences in the community capital building of a resilience process. Together with the stakeholders in community, social workers can take active part in ecosocial impact assessment based on successful participatory models (Harley & Scandrett, 2019; Penha-Lopes & Henfrey, 2019), and plan appropriate interventions such as ecosocial awareness creation, social mobilization, advocacy, lobbying, community capacity building for resilience, and community-based conflict resolutions.

Community-based social workers in Gävle city help to coordinate community collaborative groups, and they are a link from the community to political bodies in the city and pose issues about identified needs in the community (Sjöberg & Turunen, 2018; Turunen, 2004, 2009). Such community work, combined with an ecosocial perspective that is lacking today, needs to be established in communities such as Bönan. Based on how they already work in Gävle city, community-based social workers could then start to interact with inhabitants, identify common problems and needs, organize meetings to stimulate increased awareness around ecosocial issues, help to organize community activities and contribute to community capacity building and social mobilization with demands for constructive ecosocial change. A concrete intervention would be to mobilize together with other coastal communities to advocate and act as pressure group for the regulation of the large-scale fishing industry for the protection of the coastal ecosystem.

Conclusion

This study found that Bönan used to be a vibrant fishing community during the 18th century until 1950s. Respondents described how structural changes and anthropogenic disturbances resulting from the processes of globalization lead to ecosocial changes in Bönan – glocally. In particular, research findings revealed that the community resilience process was mainly driven by collaborative community development work between the local municipal and local community organizations. The findings also highlighted that social workers that were working in Bönan were not directly involved in community development, or in protecting the community and its people from anthropogenic disturbances in promoting the wellbeing for all. To ensure community resilience by enhancing the capabilities of people and community capitals, social work needs to take nature into consideration. Therefore, this article argues that there is a need for social workers to take an active part in ecosocial work for critically analyzing existing ecosocial challenges and promoting sustainable development.

The latest environmental crisis – a result of the extremely warm and dry summer of 2018 – startled the entirety of Swedish society when forests caught fire, streams dried up, and the level of available ground water diminished. These events disturbed not only the ecological balance, but also the self-image of security, which is often taken for granted in Sweden. This study therefore supports the claim that social workers around the world need to "be the change" in the community (Rinkel & Powers, 2017) by incorporating environmental aspects into practice.

Acknowledgments

We would like to acknowledge the contribution of respondents who participated in this study.

Disclosure statement

No potential conflict of interest was reported by the authors.

ORCID

Komalsingh Rambaree http://orcid.org/0000-0003-0886-7402

References

Anglin, A. E. (2015). Facilitating community change: The community capitals framework, its relevance to community psychology practice, and its application in a Georgia community. *Global Journal of Community Psychology Practice*, 6(2), 1–15. doi:10.7728/0602201504

ATLAS.ti Scientific Software Development GmbH. (2017). *ATLAS-ti version 8.2*. Retrieved from https://atlasti.com/product/v8-windows/

Attride-Stirling, J. (2001). Thematic networks: an analytic tool for qualitative research. *Qualitative Research*, 1(3), 385–405. doi:10.1177/146879410100100307

Campanini, A., & Lombard, A. (2018). International association of schools of social work (IASSW): Promoting environmental and community sustainability. *International Journal of Social Work*, 61(4), 486–489. doi:10.1177/0020872818770563

Clarke, V., & Braun, V. (2013). *Successful qualitative research: A practical guide for beginners*. London, UK: Sage.

Dominelli, L. (Ed.). (2018). *The Routledge handbook of green social work*. London, UK: Routledge.

Emery, M., & Flora, C. (2006). Spiraling-up: Mapping community transformation with community capitals framework. *Community Development, 37*(1), 19–35. doi:10.1080/15575330609490152

Esteban, A., & Carpenter, G. (2014). *Landing the blame: Overfishing in the Baltic Sea Uncovering the countries most responsible for overfishing in EU waters.* Retrieved from https://neweconomics.org/uploads/files/6b367a20b86e868eb1_s3m6bxiqe.pdf

Folke, C. (2006). Resilience: The emergence of a perspective for social–ecological systems analyses. *Global Environmental Change, 16*, 253–267. doi:10.1016/j.gloenvcha.2006.04.002

Gamble, D. N., & Hoff, M. D. (2013). Sustainable community development. In M. Weil, M. Reisch, & M. L. Ohmer (Eds.), *Handbook for community practice* (2nd ed., pp. 215–232). Thousand Oaks, CA: Sage.

Haig, B. D. (2008). Scientific method, abduction, and clinical reasoning. *Journal of Clinical Psychology, 64*, 1013–1018. doi:10.1002/jclp.20505

Hansson, M., Lundgren, I., & Sjöberg, S. (2018). Fältarbete i utsatta bostadsområden [Field work in vulnerable neighborhoods]. In S. Sjöberg & P. Turunen (Eds.), *Samhällsarbete – aktörer, arenor och perspektiv* [Community work - Actors, arenas and perspectives] (pp. 139–158). Lund, Sweden: Studentlitteratur.

Harley, A., & Scandrett, E. (Eds.). (2019). *Environmental justice, popular struggle and community development.* Bristol, UK: Polity Press.

Harvey, D. (2005). *A brief history of neoliberalism.* New York, NY: Oxford University Press.

Helsinki Commission. (2004). *Baltic marine environment protection commission.* Retrieved from http://www.helcom.fi/Lists/Publications/Dioxins%20in%20the%20Baltic%20Sea.pdf

Heron, T. (2008). Globalization, neoliberalism and the exercise of human agency. *International Journal of Politics, Culture, and Society, 20*(1), 85–101. doi:10.1177/0160597614544958

Hoff, M., & Pollack, R. (1993). Social dimensions of the environmental crisis: Challenges for social work. *Social Work, 38*(2), 204–221.

Kemp, S. P., & Palinkas, L. A., (with Wong, M., Wagner, K., Mason, L. R., Chi, I., Nurius, P., Floersch, J., & Rechkemmer, A.). (2015). *Strengthening the social response to the human impacts of environmental change* (Grand Challenges for Social Work Initiative Working Paper No. 5). Cleveland: American Academy of Social Work and Social Welfare. Retrieved from https://aaswsw.org/wp-content/uploads/2015/03/Social-Work-and-Global-Environmental-Change-3.24.15.pdf

Livholts, M., & Bryant, L. (Eds.). (2017). *Social work in a glocalized world.* London, UK: Routledge.

Magis, K. (2010). Community resilience: An indicator of social sustainability. *Society & Natural Resources, 23*(5), 401–416. doi:10.1080/08941920903305674

Matthies, A., Närhi, K., & Ward, D. (Eds.). (2001). *The eco-social approach in social work.* Jyväskylä, Finland: Sophi Publishers.

Närhi, K., & Matthies, A. (2016). The ecosocial approach in social work as a framework for structural social work. *International Social Work, 61*(4), 490–502. doi:10.1177/0020872816644663

Norris, H. F., Stevens, P. S., Pfefferbaum, B., Wyche, K., Pfefferbaum, B., Wyche, Æ. K. F., & Pfefferbaum, R. L. (2008). Community resilience as a metaphor, theory, set of capacities, and strategy for disaster readiness and strategy for disaster readiness. *American Journal of Community Psychology, 41*(1–2), 127–150. doi:10.1007/s10464-007-9156-6

Penha-Lopes, G., & Henfrey, T. (Eds.). (2019). *Reshaping the future: How communities are catalysing social, economic and ecological transformation in Europe.* Brussels: ECOLISE. Retrieved from https://www.ecolise.eu/wp-content/uploads/2016/02/Status-Report-on-Community-led-Action-on-Sustainability-Climate-Change-in-Europe-2019.pdf

Persson, D., & Erlandsson, L.-K. (2014). Ecopation: Connecting sustainability, glocalisation and well-being. *Journal of Occupational Science, 21*(1), 12–24. doi:10.1080/14427591.2013.867561

Persson, L. (2010). Sweden's fisheries catches in the Baltic Sea (1950–2007). In P. Rossing, S. Booth, & D. Zeller (Eds.), *Total marine fisheries extractions by country in the Baltic Sea: 1950-present* (pp. 225–263). Fisheries Centre Research Reports 18 (1). Vancouver, BC: Fisheries Centre, University of British Columbia, Canada.

Pfefferbaum, R. L., & Klomp, R. W. (2013). Community resilience, disasters, and the public's health. In F. G. Murphy (Ed.), *Community engagement, organization, and development for public health practice* (pp. 275–298). New York, NY: Springer.

Pihlajamäki, M., Sarkki, S., & Haapasaari, P. (2018). Food security and safety in fisheries governance – A case study on Baltic herring. *Marine Policy, 97*(1), 211–219. doi:10.1016/j.marpol.2018.06.003

Port of Gävle. (n.d.). *History*. Retrieved from https://gavlehamn.se/historia

Rambaree, K. (2013). Social work and sustainable development: Local voices from Mauritius. *Australian Social Work, 66*(2), 261–276. doi:10.1080/0312407X.2013.784793

Rambaree, K., & Ahmadi, F. (2017). Ecosocial work for sustainable development: Implications for social work education, practice and research. In A. Fagerström & G. M. Cunningham (Eds.), *A good life for all: Essays on sustainability celebrating 60 years of making life better* (pp. 71–94). Mjölby, Sweden: Atremi AB.

Rambaree, K., & Faxelid, E. (2013). Considering abductive thematic network analysis with ATLAS.ti 6.2. In N. Sappleton (Ed.), *Advancing research methods with new media technologies* (pp. 170–186). Hershey, PA: IGI Global.

Rambaree, K., & Rock, L. (2018). Green social work within integrated coastal zone management: Mauritius and Barbados. In L. Dominelli (Ed.), *The Routledge handbook of green social work* (pp. 242–253). London, UK: Routledge.

Ramsay, S., & Boddy, J. (2017). Environmental social work: A concept analysis. *The British Journal of Social Work, 47*(1), 68–86. doi:10.1093/bjsw/bcw078

Rinkel, M., & Powers, M. (Eds.). (2017). *Social work promoting community and environmental sustainability: A workbook for global social workers and educators.* Berne, Switzerland: IFSW.

Robertson, R. (1992). *Globalization: Social theory and global culture.* London, UK: Sage.

Sjöberg, S., Rambaree, K., & Jojo, B. (2015). Collective empowerment: A comparative study of community work in Mumbai and Stockholm. *International Journal of Social Welfare, 24* (4), 364–375. doi:10.1111/ijsw.12137

Sjöberg, S., & Turunen, P. (2018). *Samhällsarbete: Aktörer, arenor och perspektiv* [Community Work - Actors, Arenas and Perspectives]. Lund, Sweden: Studentlitteratur.

Smith, R. J., Lehning, A., & Kim, K. (2013). Aging in place in gentrifying neighborhoods: Implications for physical and mental health. *The Gerontologist, 58*(1), 26–35. doi:10.1093/geront/gnx105

Statistiska centralbyrån. (2017). *Tätorter; arealer, befolkning* [*Densely built-up areas; Areas, population*]. Retrieved from https://www.scb.se/hitta-statistik/statistik-efter-amne/miljo/markanvandning/tatorter/

Stockholm Resilience Centre. (2015). *What is resilience? An introduction to a popular yet often misunderstood concept.* Retrieved from http://stockholmresilience.org/research/research-news/2015-02-19-what-is-resilience.html

Swedish Agency for Marine and Water Management. (2013). *The Baltic Sea – Our common treasure: Economics of saving the sea: The maritime and water authority's report 2013* (Report No. 4). Retrieved from https://stockholmresilience.org/download/18.4531be2013c d58e844853b/BalticSTERN_The+Baltic+Sea+-+Our+Common+Treasure.+Economics+of +Saving+the+Sea_0314.pdf

Swedish Radio News. (2012, October 12). *Swedes ignoring toxic fish advice.* Retrieved from https://sverigesradio.se/sida/artikel.aspx?programid=2054&artikel=5306915

Swedish Research Council. (2018). *Rules and guidelines for research*. Retrieved from http://www.codex.vr.se/en/forskninghumsam.shtml

Szarejko, A., & Namieśnik, J. (2009). The Baltic Sea as a dumping site of chemical munitions and chemical warfare agents. *Chemistry and Ecology, 25*(1), 13–26. doi:10.1080/02757540802657177

Thurow, F. (1997). Estimation of total fish biomass in the Baltic sea during the 20th century. *ICES Journal of Marine Sciences, 54*, 444–461. doi:10.1006/jmsc.1996.0195

Turunen, P. (2004). *Samhällsarbete i Norden: diskurser och praktiker i omvandling* [Community Work in Scandinavia: Discourses and Practices in Transformation]. Växjö, Sweden: Växjö University Press.

Turunen, P. (2009). Nordic community work in transition: A change toward diversity and reflexivity. In G. Hutchinson (Ed.), *Community work in the Nordic countries: New trends* (pp. 38–63). Oslo, Norway: Universitetsforlaget.

Wilson, G. (2012). *Community resilience and environmental transitions*. London, UK: Routledge.

"Todo ha sido a pulmón": Community organizing after disaster in Puerto Rico

R. Anna Hayward ⓘ, Zachary Morris ⓘ, Yamirelis Otero Ramos, and Alejandro Silva Díaz

ABSTRACT
In this Notes from the Field, we highlight the work of community based organizations that filled essential gaps in the disaster recovery efforts in Puerto Rico for communities that were heavily damaged by Hurricane Maria yet received little formal government aid. We describe community mobilizing and organizing efforts and identify key lessons for eco-social work practice. As disaster risk increases with climate change, community led efforts are likely to prove vital for the effective protection of the most vulnerable population groups.

Introduction

On September 20th, 2017 the U.S. territory of Puerto Rico was severely impacted by Hurricane Maria, a major Category 4 storm. The widespread destruction, including the downing of the electricity grid, the transportation network, and the water supply, resulted in approximately 135,000 Puerto Ricans relocating off of the archipelago (Hinojosa, Román, & Meléndez, 2018). Tragically, an estimated 4,600 people lost their lives in the disaster (Kishore et al., 2018) – a number substantially larger than the mortality count provided by the government which initially reported 64 lives lost but was later revised to 1,427 (Puerto Rican Government, 2018a). A more recent study suggests that in the 5 months following the hurricane the excess mortality rate attributable to Maria was between 2,658 and 3,290 persons, representing a higher risk of death for all citizens, but up to 45% higher for older males, and those in low SES municipalities (Santos-Burgoa et al., 2018). The unreliability of the official mortality figure, which was widely scrutinized in the press, is perhaps emblematic of the larger failures of governance that occurred in the preparation and response to the storm. A recently released FEMA report assessing the agency's preparation for the hurricane indicates that the government widely underestimated the human impacts of the cyclone (Federal Emergency Management Agency [FEMA], 2018, p. 9). Only 37 percent of municipal governments reported that their emergency response plans worked adequately (Puerto Rican Government, 2018a).

Puerto Ricans were highly susceptible to the storm's impact due to a combination of geographic, economic, and political factors. Puerto Rico has a history of environmental injustice and degradation, including the unregulated construction on the coast line and the 18 Superfund sites on the island (Dietrich, Garriga-López, & Garriga-López, 2017; U. S. Environmental Protection Agency, 2017), that limited protection from the storm and exacerbated the risks to public health (Brown et al., 2018). Adding to the disaster risk, moreover, was the under-developed social welfare system that failed to meet the basic social welfare needs of large segments of the population before the hurricane, let alone afterwards (Morris, Hayward, & Otero, 2018).

In this *Notes from the Field*, we highlight the work of one community based non-profit organization that filled essential gaps in the disaster recovery efforts in Puerto Rico for highly vulnerable communities. Specifically, we present a case study of this organization's response to two adjacent communities that were heavily damaged by Hurricane Maria yet received little formal government aid. We describe community mobilizing and organizing efforts and identify key lessons for eco-social work practice. We ultimately argue that the necessity of effective community interventions is particularly salient for the most marginalized population groups who are often disenfranchised politically and thus receive less governmental relief.

Background

Ecosocial work practice & disaster response

Social workers have long played an important role in disaster recovery – aiding in community organizing, relief efforts, and psychological and mental health interventions in the aftermath of disasters (Mathbor, 2007). Over the past decade disaster intervention in social work has emerged as a specialized area of practice (Alston, Hazeleger, & Hargreaves, 2019). "Eco-social work" or "green social work" have also emerged as areas of practice concerned with responding to the effects of climate change on vulnerable population groups across the globe (Besthorn & Hudson, 2017; Dominelli, 2018). The American Academy of Social Work and Social Welfare (AASWSW) identified *Create Social Responses to a Changing Environment* as one of 12 Grand Challenges for the next decade. This challenge focuses on social work interventions related to disaster preparation and response including the biopsychosocial, interpersonal, and mental health impacts of climate impacts such as severe weather events (Kemp et al., 2015). Specific goals for this challenge include community-based adaptation and resilience building, disaster mitigation, and specific training on disaster preparedness and response for social workers (Kemp et al., 2015). Social workers are uniquely trained in engagement, advocacy, and strengths based practice – key skills for responding to the structural, health, mental health, and concrete needs of communities in the aftermath of natural disasters (Tiong Tan & Yuen, 2013). Social work scholars have identified roles for social work in environmental concerns (Miller, Hayward, & Shaw, 2012), in response to climate change (Hetherington & Boddy, 2013;Peeters, 2012), and in preparing for climate change and disaster response in the particularly vulnerable small island nations (Joseph, 2017). However, social work practitioners and organizers are not always at the forefront of these efforts.

Lessons from community response and resilience during other natural disasters can inform this work both in the U.S. and internationally. Culture and resources may create conflict between "outside" aid and local community efforts; for example, following the 2009 tsunami in American Samoa, outside aid had more of a destabilizing effect than local community efforts because of misunderstandings about community resources, needs, and capacities (Binder & Baker, 2017). In the US, social capital, social cohesion and SES of neighborhoods have been identified as the strongest predictors of vulnerability to climate shocks, losses following disaster, and lower resilience from subsequent events (Cagney, Sterrett, Benz, & Tompson, 2016; Kim & Marcouiller, 2016) pointing to a need to address environmental justice in social work practice. Despite an increased understanding of social workers' role in building community resilience in response to an expanded person-in-environment framework (e.g., Molyneux, 2010; Ungar, 2002) and the development of ecosocial work as a practice that directly addresses climate change impacts on vulnerable communities (Hetherington & Boddy, 2013), an ecosocial work role has yet to be elaborated and formalized in post-disaster scenarios. By understanding the community response to a climate related event such as Hurricane Maria, we can begin to further articulate social work's role both inside and outside of formal governmental and non-profit organizations.

Governmental and community responses to disaster relief

Disaster relief is arguably the most essential service provided by governments and thus community driven efforts are typically viewed as supplemental to government led initiatives. Dauber (2013) argues that disaster relief was the original form of social welfare aid provided to the American republic and thus set an important legal and political precedent in the targeting of relief. Governments may, however, be at a particular disadvantage in their response to disasters due to incentive and information problems (see, Coyne & Lemke, 2011). Because disasters are rare events and preparedness can be costly, politicians may lack an incentive to invest in disaster readiness. Moreover, since disaster events often have unpredictable consequences and bring forth complexities in readying a response, governmental authorities often lack the requisite information to respond effectively. Both incentive and information problems are likely to have contributed to the failed governmental response following Hurricane Maria (FEMA, 2018; Puerto Rican Government, 2018a).

Given that government efforts at disaster relief often fall short, much contemporary disaster scholarship has highlighted the role of community efforts as vital for response and recovery (Grube & Storr, 2014; Vallance & Carlton, 2015). Community response to disaster relief can be defined as the collective response of any non-governmental group capable of collective action in response to the human and environmental impacts of a disaster (see, Vallance & Carlton, 2015). Coyne and Lemke (2011) characterize disaster recovery in the U.S. as "polycentric" in that decision making during recovery is dispersed across organizations, including governmental and non-governmental authorities. Grube and Storr (2014) demonstrate how a community was able to "self-govern" following Hurricane Katrina among a similarly failed governmental recovery effort. With the limitations of a governmental response to disaster relief in Puerto Rico, clarifying the processes in which community initiatives "self-govern" in diverse contexts can be important for developing future disaster preparedness strategies (see, Banerjee & Gillespie, 1994). Following Maria, for example, previously organized research groups serving vulnerable communities were able to mobilize resources and provide assistance, building on established relationships and providing needed aid (Brown et al., 2018).

Description of Mentes Puertorriqueñas en Acción, inc

Mentes Puertorriqueñas en Acción, Inc. (MPA) is a 501c3 non- profit organization with a mission to empower a network of young change agents to generate effective and inclusive initiatives for Puerto Rico. Since its formal inception in 2009, the organization has engaged in a number of programs directed in inserting youth in civic engagement efforts through volunteerism, internships, discussions and exposure. Although Over the past 10 years, 266 students have participated in their programs, and over 1,100 have participated in their workshops or events. Although MPA is not a social service organization, of the full- time team of 5 employees, there is one social worker on staff. After the hurricane, MPA focused their efforts on hurricane response, mobilizing volunteers, and adapting their internship program to a disaster response internship initiative for 18 college students. Mainly funded by private donations and foundations such as the Banco Popular Foundation, Fundación Ángel Ramos, Fundación Comunitaria de PR, and Friends of Puerto Rico, and housed in Banco Popular's Social Innovation and Collaboration Community co-working space, the organization operates mainly in the metropolitan area, although their projects and events serve the wider main Island.

The communities of Villa Calma & Villa del Sol

Villa Calma and Villa del Sol are situated within the municipality of Toa Baja about 20 km outside of metropolitan San Juan, the capital city of Puerto Rico. The two communities are surrounded by a series of canals, some of which cross the community and are regulated by La Plata Lake dam in the neighboring municipality of Toa Alta. The communities were both flooded during the storm when La Plata Lake dam was opened (standard procedure when the dam reaches overflowing level at 51.3M) (Puerto Rican Government, 2018b). In a study done by the Puerto Rico Aqueduct and Sewer Authority (PRASA), the infrastructure's vulnerability to climate change was evaluated and extreme precipitation and water overflow were not indicated as a risk associated with storms and hurricanes (Autoridad de Acueductos y Alcantarillados, 2014). This contrasts with the actual damage caused in the Villa Calma community as a direct result of the La Plata Lake dam opening. Thus the agency overseeing the dam operation may not have anticipated the flooding that occurred after Maria.

While the two communities share the same geography and are physically situated across a dividing main road from each other, they have distinct characteristics that impact their ability to respond to climate shocks such as hurricanes. Villa Calma is a more established community, incorporated over 50 years ago of over 300 homes, where homeowners do not own the land on which there homes are situated. Villa Calma is consists of approximately 40% older adults (over age 65) along with young families and single people living in multi-generational homes. During the hurricane, Villa Calma flooded up to the 2nd floor of the residences and many fled to shelter during the storm. Villa del Sol is a newer cooperative community, established in 2009 with 175 partners, with a collective ownership model, formerly a settler community comprised primarily of immigrants from the Dominican Republic (at least 80% are immigrants). Both communities share geographical boundaries with the canals and precarious land ownership status. Limited information is available on the demographic make-up of these two communities, but both have limited resources and are considered low socioeconomic status (SES) neighborhoods.

Methodology

To understand the community response in these two communities we employed an exploratory case study methodology using a holistic single-case design (Yin, 2003). Descriptive case study methodology was appropriate in this case because the focus was on one larger issue (community response to the hurricane) and one bounded system (in this case, community based agency and adjacent communities) was selected to explore the issue (Creswell, 2007). Our primary research questions were: (1) How did the community organization respond and mobilize volunteers in the immediate aftermath of the hurricane?

(2) How did community leaders respond to the disaster both immediately following the disaster and in the year that followed?

This exploratory case study was determined exempt from IRB supervision by the authors' University Institutional Review Board. We completed informal interviews with a total of 4 individuals: representatives from MPA (n = 1), Villa del Sol (n = 2), and Villa Calma (n = 1) both over the phone and during in person meetings in Puerto Rico on August 2018 (almost a year after Hurricane Maria made landfall on September 20, 2017). Our sample was limited in scope and based on snowball sampling after initial contact with MPA's Executive Director. Community leaders were interviewed in their community settings, both during walking tours of the area and in informal meeting spaces (a leader's home and a community center). Interviews were conducted in English and Spanish by a native speaking research assistant, transcribed and then analyzed using case description technique (Yin, 2003) focusing on the particular context and "story" of the year following the storm. Three of the authors also toured the affected area.

Case study

Community mobilization

Immediately following the storm MPA organized the #EnAcción initiative, the first effort to specifically mobilize communities in a post-disaster scenario. This initiative grew organically, and evolved to adapt MPA's traditional programs to recovery efforts. As of August, 2018, 439 volunteers had been engaged on 26 brigades and trainings, investing 2,947 work hours in the Villas del Sol and Villa Calma communities.

MPA began organizing volunteers within 10 days of the hurricane. Despite the lack of connectivity, the use of internet and cell phone technology was crucial to these efforts. Email, SMS and social media (especially Facebook) were key in reaching out to potential volunteers and community leaders, as well as AM radio appearances. Initially, a Google form was created and distributed via MPA's Facebook page, which had 8,340 followers the night before the hurricane. While data about email forwards and other word of mouth are not available, the Facebook post was viewed by 13,258 users, and the initial recruitment was sent to 319 contacts via email. Respondents to the Google form were asked to provide contact information and a total of 848 unique respondents were logged and contacted.

One key factor in the coordination and collaboration process was the availability of spaces where word of mouth could flow quickly and easily: the Social Innovation and Collaboration Community co-working space, where MPA operates from, became the leading non-profit disaster response operating center by housing 120 NGOs. Because this space had higher resiliency factors (power, water, internet connectivity, etc.), MPA and other entities were could more easily communicate with communities, identify immediate needs, and leverage resources to facilitate their work in the community.

Internet and phone service was slower to be restored in the most heavily damaged areas, thus communication with authorities was quite difficult and only occurred through personal connections. However, organization and mobilization locally started immediately, before power and phone service were restored. In the community setting, organization and mobilization happened more immediately and before power and internet service were restored. One community leader from Villa Calma described having 16 friends and family staying in the second floor of her elevated home located adjacent to one of the flooded canals. As the flood water subsided and internet was available in places, residents were mobilized locally and tasks were distributed by ability, at the same time, contacts were made to outside organizations for help. It was clear from the outset that governmental support would not be forthcoming:

> The mayor recognized the importance of our work within the communities. He knew that the municipality was bankrupt, so he raised his hands ("señal de rendición") because he couldn't do anything. – M., Villa Calma

Thus community members mobilized informally on the ground, first checking on family members and neighbors in the community and then organizing a more organized response.

Community response following the hurricane

A recurring theme both during the mobilization stage and during the community response to the storm was that assistance from governmental organizations or other groups was not expected or anticipated. As one community leader in Villa de Sol stated *"We did not receive help from the big organizations, "todo ha sido a pulmón."* in other words, the community had to do everything on their own.

Both the community organization (MPA) and informal and formal leaders within the two communities responded almost immediately to the needs of affected community members. In our interviews with community leaders, it was clear that no immediate governmental help was expected to appear – community leaders and residents had to provide for basic needs of residents immediately following the storm and up until almost a year later.

> We were lucky that there were leaders in the communities that took care of things, found the resources and distributed them through the communities. The government did not provide anything – they didn't have anything to offer. Everything we received came from non-profits, churches that came with resources and food. – M., Villa Calma

No psychological services were reported to have been provided either immediately after the hurricane or in the year since. The first focus was on concrete needs such as food, water, housing, and clearing of dangerous structures. In Villa Calma, this was achieved with a team effort moving from house to house:

> Some [of the community members] would clean down stairs and the streets and houses while others, and the ones that did not have the strength to do hard labor, would focus on cooking and feeding everyone. Each day they would clean a different house and "poquito a poquito" ["little by little"] we finished cleaning the entire community. Help from volunteers was also important. We came together and began to work. – M., Villa Calma

Accessing food and water, including accessing donated food and supplies was a challenge both in the immediate aftermath of the storm and even weeks later. Food provided in shelter services was inadequate:

> I had 16 people from my community with me at the shelter and the experience was horrible. They would give us a carton milk and a small cereal box for everyone. That was all we would get until 8pm – M., Villa Calma

As a result, community leaders prioritized developing community kitchens, often out of their own homes. A major role for community leaders on the ground was contacting non-profits via the internet and phone and acting as a spokesperson for the community this began immediately after the storm and continued with attempts to secure funding from FEMA. The inadequacy and inconsistency of FEMA funding was a major concern for community leaders and residents:

> People did not have titles for their homes so that meant they did not receive anything from FEMA. There was also no uniformity in the process. Two different people had the same amount of damages and would not receive the same help ($200 vs. $10,000). The amount of aid people would get would depend on the inspector you were assigned to. – M., Villa Calma

An important post-disaster benefit, once some recovery funds were secured, was the use of these funds to provide employment via construction contracts. These contracts were seen as a positive benefit in the post-disaster context and as a "win-win situation because you are making income while helping your community which empowers the community and creates sustainability," as stated by a community leader in Villa del Sol who also added "If you want to help the communities give them the resources directly."

Finally, an additional role emerged for MPA in assisting the fledgling community organization in Villa del Solas a fiscal sponsor. This allows the community to receive funds from donors who expect a tax-compliance structure. The MPA is now mentoring the community group to reach a level of compliance so that they can eventually solicit funds without the need of a fiscal sponsor intermediary.

Discussion

At the time of our visit to Puerto Rico, almost a year after Hurricane Maria, many communities in Puerto Rico were still in a recovery mode. This descriptive case study provides insight into community response to the disaster and lessons for ecosocial work practice in post disaster scenarios. The relationship between social and environmental justice serves as the basis for social work interventions in communities affected by climate change (Hetherington & Boddy, 2013) and community building and organizing remain core social work practices for addressing these concerns. Disaster preparation and response plans should be integrated in all community work, with a thorough understanding of the unique needs of different communities – even those in close physical proximity may have different populations, needs, and resources. Moreover, providing centralized work spaces and prioritizing the maintenance of infrastructure during disaster events could be an important lesson for future disaster responses. With this approach eco-social work can work with and in communities to build "community resilience" to disaster risks (Case, 2016).

This case study highlighted the need for interdisciplinary social work practice including collaboration with other aid organizations (for food, water, medical care), legal assistance (especially around housing and FEMA guidance), and communities less affected by the disaster (for volunteers and other assistance). In our observations we also noted a dearth of psychological services for both disaster victims and those in supportive role. This suggests disparities in access to mental health first aid and other mental health responses. Our case study further demonstrated that absent effective governmental disaster efforts, community initiatives are essential for disaster recovery efforts, particularly for populations who are among the least likely to receive formal support. Strengthening the capacity of local non-governmental organizations, researchers, social workers, and other groups with existing close ties to communities are best positioned to respond to disaster event, as noted in the recent FEMA (2018) report, should thus be seen as a priority in disaster preparedness efforts. With the risk of disaster increasing with climate change, vulnerable populations may expect to rely more often on their mobilized community led efforts, and not their formal governments, to receive the most elementary social and environmental protection.

Disclosure statement

No potential conflict of interest was reported by the authors.

ORCID

R. Anna Hayward ⓘ http://orcid.org/0000-0002-7513-8608
Zachary Morris ⓘ http://orcid.org/0000-0003-3593-3911

References

Alston, M., Hazeleger, T., & Hargreaves, D. (2019). *Social work and disasters: A handbook for practice*. London, UK: Routledge.

Autoridad de Acueductos y Alcantarillados. (2014). *Cambio climático: Estudio de vulnerabilidad-Tarea 2*. Retrieved from https://www.acueductospr.com/INFRAESTRUCTURA/download/CAMBIO%20CLIMATICO/2014-09-23_Estudio%20de%20Vulnerabilidad_Final%20REv.pdf

Banerjee, M. M., & Gillespie, D. F. (1994). Linking disaster preparedness and organizational response effectiveness. *Journal of Community Practice, 1*(3), 129–142. doi:10.1300/J125v01n03_09

Besthorn, F. H., & Hudson, J. (2017). The spiritual dimensions of ecosocial work in the context of global climate change. In B. R. Crisp (Ed.), *The Routledge handbook of religion, spirituality and social work* (pp. 338–346). London, UK: Routledge.

Binder, S. B., & Baker, C. K. (2017). Culture, local capacity, and outside aid: A community perspective on disaster response after the 2009 tsunami in American Sāmoa. *Disasters, 41*(2), 282–305. doi:10.1111/disa.12203

Brown, P., Vega, C. M. V., Murphy, C. B., Welton, M., Torres, H., Rosario, Z., … Meeker, J. D. (2018). Hurricanes and the environmental justice Island: Irma and Maria in Puerto Rico. *Environmental Justice, 11*(4), 148–153. doi:10.1089/env.2018.0003

Cagney, K. A., Sterrett, D., Benz, J., & Tompson, T. (2016). Social resources and community resilience in the wake of Superstorm Sandy. *PLoS One, 11*(8), e0160824. doi:10.1371/journal.pone.0160824

Case, R. A. (2016). Eco-social work and community resilience: Insights from water activism in Canada. *Journal of Social Work, 17*(4), 391–412. doi:10.1177/1468017316644695

Coyne, C., & Lemke, J. (2011). Polycentricity in disaster relief. *Studies in Emergent Orders, 4*, 40–57.

Creswell, J. W. (2007). *Qualitative inquiry & research design: Choosing among five approaches* (2nd ed.). New York, NY: SAGE.

Dauber, M. L. (2013). *The sympathetic state: Disaster relief and the origins of the American welfare state*. Chicago, IL: University of Chicago Press.

Dietrich, A., Garriga-López, M., & Garriga-López, C. (2017). Hurricane Maria exposes Puerto Rico's stark environmental and health inequalities. *Items*. Retrieved from https://items.ssrc.org/hurricane-maria-exposes-puerto-ricos-stark-environmental-and-health-inequalities/

Dominelli, L. (Ed.). (2018). *The Routledge handbook of green social work*. London, UK: Routledge.

Federal Emergency Management Agency. (2018, July). *2017 hurricane seasons FEMA after-action report*. Retrieved from https://www.fema.gov/media-library data/1531743865541d16794d43d3082544435e1471da07880/2017FEMAHurricaneAAR.pdf

Grube, L., & Storr, V. H. (2014). The capacity for self-governance and post-disaster resiliency. *The Review of Austrian Economics, 27*(3), 301–324. doi:10.1007/s11138-013-0210-3

Hetherington, T., & Boddy, J. (2013). Ecosocial work with marginalized populations: Time for action on climate change. In *Environmental social work* (pp. 66–81). London/New York: Routledge.

Hinojosa, J., Román, N., & Meléndez, E. (2018, March). *Puerto Rican post-Maria relocation by states*. Center for Puerto Rican Studies. Hunter College. Retrieved from https://centropr.hunter.cuny.edu/sites/default/files/PDF/Schoolenroll-v4-27-2018.pdf

Joseph, D. D. (2017). Social work models for climate adaptation: The case of small islands in the Caribbean. *Regional Environmental Change, 17*(4), 1117–1126. doi:10.1007/s10113-017-1114-8

Kemp, S. P., Palinkas, L. A., Wong, M., Wagner, K., Reyes Mason, L., Chi, I., … Rechkemmer, A. (2015). *Strengthening the social response to the human impacts of environmental change* (Grand Challenges for Social Work Initiative Working Paper No. 5). Cleveland, OH: American Academy of Social Work and Social Welfare.

Kim, H., & Marcouiller, D. W. (2016). Natural disaster response, community resilience, and economic capacity: A case study of coastal Florida. *Society & Natural Resources, 29*(8), 981–997. doi:10.1080/08941920.2015.1080336

Kishore, N., Marqués, D., Mahmud, A., Kiang, M. V., Rodriguez, I., Fuller, A., ... Maas, L. (2018). Mortality in Puerto Rico after hurricane Maria. *New England Journal of Medicine, 379*, 162–170. doi:10.1056/NEJMsa1803972

Mathbor, G. M. (2007). Enhancement of community preparedness for natural disasters. *International Social Work, 50*(3), 357–369. doi:10.1177/0020872807076049

Miller, S. E., Hayward, R. A., & Shaw, T. V. (2012). Environmental shifts for social work: A principles approach. *International Journal of Social Welfare, 21*(3), 270–277. doi:10.1111/j.1468-2397.2011.00848.x

Molyneux, R. (2010). The practical realities of ecosocial work: A review of the literature. *Critical Social Work, 11*(2), 61–68.

Morris, Z. A., Hayward, R. A., & Otero, Y. (2018). The political determinants of disaster risk: Assessing the unfolding aftermath of hurricane Maria for people with disabilities in Puerto Rico. *Environmental Justice, 11*(2), 89–94. doi:10.1089/env.2017.0043

Peeters, J. (2012). A comment on 'climate change: Social workers' roles and contributions to policy debates and interventions'. *International Journal of Social Welfare, 21*, 105–107. doi:10.1111/j.1468-2397.2011.00847.x

Puerto Rican Government. (2018a, June). *Transformation and innovation in the wake of devastation: Preliminary draft.* Puerto Rico. Retrieved from http://www.p3.pr.gov/assets/pr-draft-recovery-plan-for-comment-july-9-2018.pdf

Puerto Rican Government. (2018b). *Autoridad de acueductos y alcantarillados.* Retrieved from http://www.acueductospr.com/AAARepresas/tabla

Santos-Burgoa, C., Goldman, A., Andrade, E., Barrett, N., Colon-Ramos, U., Edberg, M., ... Zeger, S. (2018). *Ascertainment of the estimated excess mortality from hurricane Maria in Puerto Rico.* Retrieved from https://hsrc.himmelfarb.gwu.edu/sphhs_global_facpubs/288

Tiong Tan, N., & Yuen, F. (2013). Social work, strengths perspective, and disaster management: Roles of social workers and models for intervention. *Journal of Social Work in Disability & Rehabilitation, 12*(1–2), 1–7. doi:10.1080/1536710X.2013.784170

U. S. Environmental Protection Agency. (2017). *National Priorities List (NPL) sites by state.* Retrieved from www.epa.gov/superfund/national-priorities-list-npl-sites-state#PR

Ungar, M. (2002). A deeper, more social ecological social work practice. *Social Service Review, 76*(3), 480–497. doi:10.1086/341185

Vallance, S., & Carlton, S. (2015). First to respond, last to leave: Communities' roles and resilience across the '4Rs'. *International Journal of Disaster Risk Reduction, 14*, 27–36. doi:10.1016/j.ijdrr.2014.10.010

Yin, R. K. (2003). *Case study research: Design & methods* (2nd ed.). Thousand Oaks, CA: SAGE Publications.

An intersectionality-based analysis of high seas policy making stagnation and equity in United Nations negotiations

Jessica L. Decker Sparks ⓘ and Shannon M. Sliva

ABSTRACT
This paper used an intersectionality-based policy analysis to critically dissect systemic power structures within the UN that likely contributed to marine policy making's stagnation. An empirical analysis of UN organ structure and composition in relation to a state's gross domestic product found inequities in representation and leadership between large and small economies and elucidated how a state's economic status influences its ability to participate in international marine policy processes. Without recognition of these power disparities, upcoming negotiations for a new high seas treaty could perpetuate the marginalization of low-income states disproportionately affected by exploitative marine activities' impacts on human security.

The American Academy of Social Work and Social Welfare's Grand Challenges for Social Work call on social workers to "create social responses to a changing environment" by addressing the socioeconomic impacts of environmental challenges with a specific emphasis on "advocacy to elevate public and policy attention to the social and human dimensions of environmental change" (Kemp & Palinkas, 2015, p. 3). However, inequitable governance structures perpetuate the socioeconomic disparities created by environmental changes – threatening achievement of the United Nations' Sustainable Development Goals [SDGs]. As a result, social workers need to move beyond using policy to address environmental inequities and critique the structures used for global governance of shared natural resources. One pertinent example is the governance of the high seas, or the ocean's international waters beyond a singular country's jurisdiction, under the 1982 United Nations Convention on the Law of the Sea [UNCLOS].

One of the ocean's most pressing social-ecological challenges is marine fish stocks' continued decline, with 33.1% of stocks classified as overfished (i.e., fished beyond sustainable levels) in 2015, a 1.4% increase from 2013 (Food and Agriculture Organization (United Nations) [FAO], 2018). These changes are primarily perpetrated by increasing fishing pressures, driven by consumption demands predicated on greater demand for exotic fish products (e.g., sushi), trade globalization, human population growth, and increasing scientific evidence of fish's health and nutritional benefits (FAO, 2018). And, while stocks in developed countries' coastal waters showed some rebounds, these gains were offset by further decreases in developing countries' stocks (FAO, 2018). The persistence of these declines is problematic: Though poorer states lack the capacity to fish on the high seas, and no artisanal or subsistence fishing occurs that far from shore, approximately 54% of low-income, fish-reliant states depend on species that straddle and/or migrate between territorial waters and the high seas (Teh et al., 2016). Of the 10 million tons of fish caught on the high seas, less than 1% contains species found exclusively in the high seas (Sumaila et al., 2015).

Because of this straddling, high seas overfishing impacts reverberate through populations not engaged in the activity. Specifically, high seas overfishing contributes to coastal stock depletions – threatening many of the world's most vulnerable populations. While 3.1 billion people, or more than 40% of the world's population, rely on seafood as their primary protein source, in most coastal developing countries, marine fish constitute more than 50% of dietary protein intake (FAO, 2016). Approximately 90% of small-scale (e.g., subsistence and artisanal), marine capture fishers worldwide (or an estimated 22–26 million impoverished people) live in coastal developing countries where few alternative livelihood activities exist (Teh & Sumaila, 2013). Therefore, high seas governance is a social justice issue of relevance to ecosocial work. This paper offers an Intersectionality-Based Policy Analysis [IBPA] (Hankivsky, 2012) of United Nations [UN] policy-making related to the high seas, including an empirical analysis of committee structures and voting patterns to support this conceptual framework, and an examination of the differential impacts of high seas policymaking on marginalized global populations. The IBPA framework evaluates how intersecting identities and characteristics of a population – here, global states – perpetuate inequities and privileges in policy problems, processes, and responses. It is based on the premise that reducing marginalized populations to a singular identity perpetuates oppression (Hankivsky, 2012). UNCLOS, a macro policy focusing on parties to the convention, ascribes a singular identity to all parties – a member state. This practice inhibits equity by ignoring the plurality of characteristics that formulate each state's identity and how these characteristics interact to influence the state's behaviors and participation in international high seas policy decision-making processes. Considering this intersectionality is also imperative to gaining a more complex understanding of the power relationships between states and how specific characteristics (e.g., major economies) may be more valued, maintaining unequal power distributions throughout the UN system. The paper concludes with recommendations for transforming the problem and the policy process with a focus on equitable outcomes and a discussion of ecosocial work's role in global policymaking.

High seas policy making under the UN convention on the law of the sea (UNCLOS)

Signed in 1982, UNCLOS attempted to create a comprehensive and unified governance regime for Earth's oceans to curb national sovereignty claims (Dieter, 2014). It demarked distinct maritime zones; ascribed national authority (and restrictions) over territorial waters, contiguous zones, and exclusive economic zones; and classified the high seas, " ... all parts of the sea that are not included in the exclusive economic zone, in the territorial sea or in the internal waters of a State, or in the archipelagic waters of an archipelagic State" as international waters beyond national jurisdiction and therefore subject to governance exclusively by UN international and multilateral laws and policies (United Nations (UN), 1982, Part VII, Art. 86, para. 1). Building upon the ideology the high seas were a common-pool resource and thus, access should be open to all states regardless of geography, Article 87 advanced high seas' "freedoms" (United Nations (UN), 2017a).

When states assented to UNCLOS, technology limitations prohibited or limited most high seas activities, including fishing, making strict high seas protections less important in the original negotiations (Visbeck et al., 2014). These technological limitations also constrained the scientific knowledge about the high seas available during negotiations. As technological capacity to exploit high seas resources and scientific understanding simultaneously grew, the scientific community began advocating for new policies to address UNCLOS' deficiencies. Since the 1990s, UN entities have enacted a series of international and regional policies to address UNCLOS' gaps and more consistently apply UNCLOS' regulations to increase the achievement of its objectives.[1] However, these measures are restricted by UNCLOS' superseding authority and have primarily relied on voluntary, non-binding instruments that lack formal enforcement procedures. Benefits of these soft laws can include greater consensus and international cooperation, and easier implementation since they do not depend on each member state's own ratification processes; however, their effectiveness can be hindered by a lack of political will to ensure compliance, which may conflict with the state's economic interests (Visbeck et al., 2014).

On December 24, 2017, the UN adopted a resolution to convene an intergovernmental conference to negotiate a new "internationally legally binding instrument under UNLCOS on the conservation and sustainable use of marine biological diversity of areas beyond national jurisdiction" (UN, 2017a, para. 12). This vote was the culmination of more than a decade of negotiations, and the work of four preparatory meetings convened between 2016 and 2017 to address scientific concerns of inadequate high seas protection and regulation (High Seas Alliance [HSA], 2017). While rhetoric around the length and stagnation of preliminary negotiations focused on tensions between conservation and management for maximum economic and sustainable exploitation, including that espoused by delegates from wealthier states (United Nations (UN), 2017b), less attention was afforded to the underlying power differentials between UN member states.

Building on SDG 14, "Life Below Water," the upcoming internationally binding instrument negotiations present an opportunity to formally institutionalize the SDG's environmental, economic, and social equity aims through more protection oriented high seas regulations (Editorial, 2018). However, socioeconomic and political inequities perpetuated by international policy-making processes, including the recent UNCLOS preparatory meetings, may undermine the SDGs' social justice aims. Scholars have already noted the divergent positions between developed and developing countries in the original UNLCOS negotiations (e.g., Stevenson & Oxman, 1994) and NGOs have critiqued UNCLOS and its subsequent mechanisms for regulatory shortcomings and gaps (e.g., Gjerde, Currie, Wowk, & Sack, 2013). However, many critiques have not considered power differentials potentially entrenched in the UN system, and if existent, how they may influence state engagement or lack thereof in international policy making. The failure to create and implement binding laws more strictly regulating the high seas serves the economic interests of privileged states (i.e., industrialized and large/major economies) while potentially threatening the security of vulnerable states (i.e., small economies, Least Developed Countries [LDCs] and Small Island Developing States [SIDS]). This power dynamic must be understood and remedied to advance greater equity in the new treaty.

Current representations of the problem

UNCLOS and the subsequent UN Straddling Fish Stocks Agreement [UNFSA] established intergovernmental regional fisheries management organizations [RFMOs] as the primary high seas governance mechanism (United Nations (UN), 1995). Any state with a financial or practical interest in the region's fisheries and stock management can be a member of an RFMO, and states can, and do, belong to multiple RFMOs. Existing critiques of UNCLOS and its subsequent multilateral and regional policies have often centered on RFMOs' ineffectiveness in maintaining productive high seas fish stocks. Reasons for this ineffectiveness include diversity and range in directives amongst RFMOs; the production and dissemination of inaccurate catch and by-catch data; member state favoritism; inadequate performance review criteria; a lack of transparency around decision-making processes; enforcement and compliance challenges; exploitation of flag state jurisdiction; inconsistencies in confronting illegal, unreported, and unregulated (IUU) fishing; and political interference suppressing scientific concerns (Dieter, 2014; Gjerde et al., 2013). The use of voluntary and non-binding international and multilateral instruments has failed to address these RFMO problems, primarily because RFMOs can fail to implement recommendations with impunity (Gjerde et al., 2013). Though itself binding, UNCLOS also lacks global compliance mechanisms, instead relying on the right of exclusive jurisdiction for flag states – a mechanism with consistently abused loopholes (Dieter, 2014).

The representation of high seas overfishing resulting from fragmented RFMO governance schemes is important and scientifically justified. However, by constructing the policy problem around the aggregate collection of RFMO party states, it is possible to overlook interactions and power differentials between member states that could influence RFMO effectiveness, and deflect responsibility away from the self-interests of powerful states onto the more collective RFMOs.

Differential impacts

Empirical evidence suggests UNCLOS and RFMOs are failing in their responsibilities to protect and ensure sustainable fish stocks, with high seas fish stocks continuing to decline as a result of overfishing (Cullis-Suzuki & Pauly, 2010). Due to prohibitive costs and technological needs, most high seas fishing is monopolized by commercial vessels unsustainably subsidized by a few wealthy states (e.g., the United States, Russia, and Japan) and 10 states account for more than 60% of high seas fish catch (Sumaila et al., 2015). However, poorer, fish-reliant states will be disproportionately impacted by straddling and/or migrating fish stocks overfished on the high seas (Teh et al., 2016; White & Costello, 2014). Because overfishing's social effects are mediated through economic structures, even if fish stocks collapse, it is likely populations in wealthier states will have access to alternative food and nutrition sources, and comparatively little of the populations in these states rely on fishing as their sole livelihood. However, for the human populations in poorer, fish-reliant states, alternative livelihoods and nutritious food sources are severely limited. The human population is expected to reach 9.6 billion people by 2050, with the majority of this increase anticipated in urban areas of coastal states with pre-existing high food insecurity rates, further pressuring fish stocks that are viewed as an essential resource for poverty alleviation and the attainment of the SDGs (FAO, 2018).

Further, RFMOs are responsible for their funding, leading to notable disparities between organizations (Global Ocean Commission [GOC], 2013). The 11 largest RFMOs (four of which exclusively manage tuna stocks – a species primarily fished and consumed by wealthy states) receive approximately USD \$28 million per year collectively from large repositories such as the European Maritime and Fisheries Fund (funded by EU member states). Even amongst the 11, funds are disproportionately allocated to RFMOs exclusively managing tuna stocks. In 2013, the Inter-American Tropical Tuna Commission [IATTC] received over USD \$6.3 million (the top funded of the 11 largest RFMOs), while the South Pacific Regional Fisheries Management Organization [SPRFMO] received only USD \$706,900 (the least funded of the largest 11 RFMOs) (GOC, 2013). In 2014, Japan, Taiwan/China, and the United States were three of the four largest contributors to the tuna catch, and had a vested interest in contributing funds to tuna RFMOs (Galland, Rogers, & Nickson, 2016). Indeed, there are suggestions the allowable catch limits established by RFMOs are politically influenced through states' donations (Galland et al., 2016).

Current policy responses

After a decade of negotiations (HSA, 2017), UN General Assembly [UNGA] Resolution 69/242 in 2015 called for the creation of an international, legally binding instrument under UNCLOS to enhance biodiversity protection and ensure sustainable high seas' use (United Nations (UN), 2015b). Prior to beginning negotiations in the UNGA though, four preparatory meetings were convened between 2016 and 2017 to draft text for a future treaty, offering an opportunity for economically powerful states (e.g., Russia and the United States) to undermine and dilute language regarding stricter proposed regulations before full treaty negotiations even began. For example, to achieve consensus and appease industrialized states with commercial interests in high seas' resource exploitation, the recommendations were divided into two groups: an A-section, characterized by "convergence" among states; and, a B-section, characterized by "divergence." The primary divisions were about the potential treaty's institutional structures, with developing countries, "calling for an increasingly ambitious and articulated international architecture, with multiple funds and overview and support mechanisms" while developed countries, "were worried about the costs involved, advocating for a light institutional structure" (International Institute for Sustainable Development [IISD], 2017, p. 20).

A SIDS' special case principle including equal engagement, special consideration, and "preferential treatment and access procedures for SIDS and LDCs" and the retention of language from UNFSA about special requirements for SIDS and LDCs and avoiding "disproportionate burdens" was supported by Alliance of Small Island States [AOSIS], the African group, LDCs, and the Pacific Small Island Developing States [PSIDS] (IISD, 2017, p. 9). The United States, Japan, Australia, European Union, Canada, and Switzerland all vocalized opposition. Due to lack of consensus, the special requirements and disproportionate burden language were included in the B-section, and the SIDS special case principle was excluded (IISD, 2017). Moreover, the UNGA was not required to convene an intergovernmental conference for the negotiation of a new binding treaty, and though it did, the draft text provided by the 4th Preparatory Commission was "without prejudice to states' positions during negotiations" (IISD, 2017, p. 4).

The final draft text also suggests industrialized, large economy states may be unwilling to abandon UNCLOS' "freedom of the seas" principle regarding fish commodities. Though the G-77 (i.e., a group of 77 developing states) wanted to include language identifying the potential treaty's overarching objective as "long-term, sustainable use and conservation," the "long-term" descriptor was dropped due to Russia's demands, and instead language about reinforcing effective implementation of UNCLOS was included (IISD, 2017, pp. 6–7). Thus, there should be concerns the new instrument will not significantly depart from previous policy. This divergence between lower and higher income states has also occurred in historical UNCLOS negotiations, such as those concerning the management of seabeds – another resource which poorer states lacked the capacity to exploit – and the common heritage of [hu]mankind (CHM) (See Guntrip, 2003; Nordquist, Rosenne, & Kraska, 2011; Stevenson & Oxman, 1994).

An empirical analysis of UN structure

A 2009 analysis of social-ecological systems approaches in multilateral environmental treaties and negotiations found "questions of power, conflicts, and inequalities" were ignored (Hornborg, 2009, p. 238), serving powerful states' economic interests. Further, historically powerful states have been able to imbue policy development with their self-sovereignty ideology by wielding their economic power (Dreher, Nunnenkamp, & Thiele, 2006). This sub-analysis, conducted within the context of the IBPA framework, explored the likelihood that UN power structures facilitate inequities in marine policy making and other international policy-making processes by providing an empirical analysis of UN organ structure and composition which maps relationships between the economic characteristics of states and their representation in UN organs. The founding hypothesis is that state economic power is a predictor of representation in UN organs, and subsequently, influence on UN policy making, despite the establishing principle that, "The United Nations shall place no restrictions on the eligibility [of member states] ... to participate ... in its principal and subsidiary organs" (United Nations (UN), 1945, Chap. 3, Art. 8).

Methodology

Current and historical UN membership data were procured from official UN websites, including websites for each organ (General Assembly of the United Nations, 2017; International Court of Justice [ICJ], 2017; UN Economic and Social Council, 2017; UN Secretary General, n.d.; UN Security Council, n.d.; United Nations (UN), 2016). Gross domestic product [GDP], LDC, SIDS, and low-income country data was then overlaid upon UN membership data. The list of LDCs and SIDS was retrieved from the UN Office of the High Representative for the Least Developed Countries, Landlocked Developing Countries and Small Island Developing States (2017). [2]Both the GDP rankings for 2016 and the list of low-income countries (i.e., the World Bank's comparable LDC designation) were obtained from the World Bank (2017). The World Bank ranked 185 of the 193 UN member states in 2016. Andorra, Eritrea, North Korea, Libya, Monaco, San Marino, Syria, and Venezuela did not make GDP data available and thus were excluded. The authors divided the list of 185 states into quartiles. Each quartile included 46 states, with the exception of the 2nd quartile (49th to 25th percentile), which included 47 states. Tajikistan, ranked 139th of UN member states, was the 47th state included in the 2nd quartile. GDP was selected as the economic/wealth indicator since it is a measure of market activity frequently used to distinguish economy size and often used in policy making. While it fails to measure human well-being and is limited in its ability to represent informal economic activity, the IBPA analysis was based on a hypothesis that the UN favors highly developed states with large economies despite its founding principle of "sovereign equality" for all member states (UN, 1945, Chap. 1, Art. 2(1)).

Results

Six principal organs comprise the UN system: The General Assembly [UNGA], Security Council [UNSC], International Court of Justice [ICJ], Economic and Social Council [ECOSOC], Trusteeship Council, and the Secretariat. The UNGA is the only organ requiring representation for all UN member states and is divided into five regional groups functioning as voting blocs. With five permanent member states (China, France, Russia, the United Kingdom, and the United States) and 10 additional rotating member states, the UNSC is widely considered the most powerful organ. The UNSC's five permanent member states are also guaranteed representation on the ICJ, comprising one-third of the court's 15 seats, and were the only member states represented on the Trusteeship Council, suspended in 1994. The ECOSOC, which is the primary international body for sustainable development has 54 members. The Secretariat is led by the Secretary-General, elected from one member state.

Of the United Nations Security Council's five permanent members, the United States is ranked first in GDP, China second, the United Kingdom fifth, France sixth, and Russia 12th. While the other 10 UNSC members rotate, 66 UN member states have never served on the council (UNSC, n.d.). Of those 66 members, five were not ranked by GDP. An examination of the remaining 61 states determined only two (3.0%) states are in the upper quartile globally for GDP, while 34 (55.7%) are ranked in the lower quartile (Figure 1). Though 31 of the 47 (66.0%) states classified by the UN as an LDC have served on the UNSC, only 8 of the 27 (21.6%) states classified as a SIDS have served. Only one of the eight states classified as both, Guinea-Bissau, has filled a membership position. Though non-permanent members are selected from each of the five regional groups, states' candidacies for a non-permanent position must first be endorsed by their regional bloc. Once endorsed, they then must be elected by a two-thirds vote in the UNGA. States serve a two-year term and can be re-elected. This system eschews equity for political maneuvering and favoritism. For example, since 1966 when the current regional groups were configured, only 23 (41.8%) of

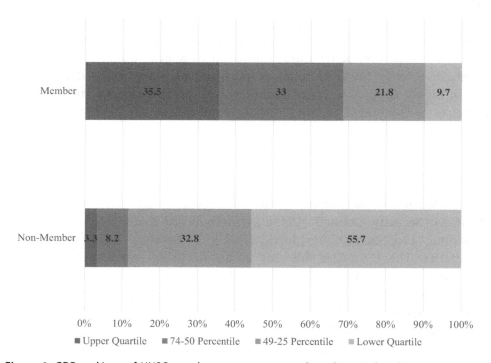

Figure 1. GDP rankings of UNSC members versus non-members, historical and present.

the Asia-Pacific Regional Group's 55 member states have been non-permanent members of the UNSC, with one state – China – serving as a permanent member. Further, 12 of the 23 states have served multiple times, including Japan, which has represented the Asia-Pacific group 10 times since 1966 for a total of 20 years. None of the Asia-Pacific group's SIDS have been represented on the council.

All parties to the Statute of the Court (i.e., all 193 UN member states and some observer states) can nominate a candidate for the International Court of Justice (ICJ), though the state does not advance the candidate. Instead, members of the Permanent Court of Arbitration, who are designated by the state, will propose the nominee. For states that are not members of the Permanent Court of Arbitration, a congruent process is established to propose candidates. To be elected, the nominee must then receive a majority two-thirds vote in concurrent voting in the UNGA and the UNSC. Only 47 of the 193 (24.3%) UN member states have ever been represented on the ICJ, including the five seats continuously held by the UNSC permanent members. Of those 47 members, 26 (55.3%) are ranked in the upper quartile of GDP; whereas, only three (6.4%) are ranked in the lower quartile (Figure 2). Five (10.6%) judges have been appointed from one of the 47 LDCs. In February 2015, Judge Patrick Lipton Robinson from Jamaica was appointed to the court, marking the first time a SIDS was represented. No judges have been appointed from one of the eight states identified as a LDC and SIDS.

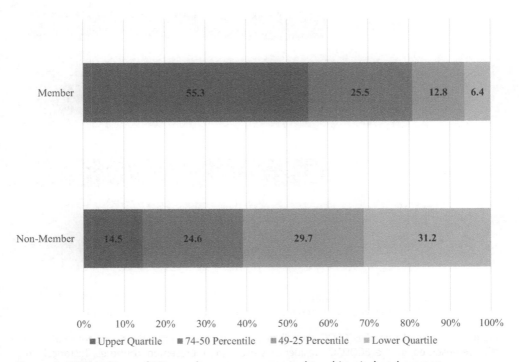

Figure 2. GDP rankings of ICJ members versus non-members, historical and present.

The Economic and Social Council's [ECOSOC] 54 member states are elected for three-year terms by the UNGA. Currently, a set number of seats is allocated to each regional group: African Group (14), Western European and Other States Group (13), Asian Group (11), Latin American and Caribbean Group (10), and Eastern European Group (6). While historical membership data were unavailable, an analysis of the current 54 members determined that only eight LDCs are represented on the ECOSOC, comprising 14.8% of the ECOSOC body and just 17.0% of all LDCs. Half of the African Group's representatives are LDCs. However, when examining GDP rankings, 26 of the 52 (50%) ranked member states are in the upper quartile, while only six (11.5%) are ranked in the lower quartile (Figure 3). Only two of the 54 (3.7%) total members are SIDS, resulting in 5.4% of all SIDS being represented; yet, all five permanent UNSC members are also members of the ECOSOC. None of the eight states classified as both a LDC and SIDS are represented. Historical data on the ECOSOC president indicate that 37 states have been represented. One is unranked by GDP (Venezuela) and one country no longer exists (Yugoslavia). Of the remaining 35 presidential member states, 19 (54.3%) are ranked in the upper quartile for GDP, and zero are ranked in the lower quartile (Figure 3). Three LDCs have been represented, and only one SIDS (Jamaica), which is also classified as a LDC.

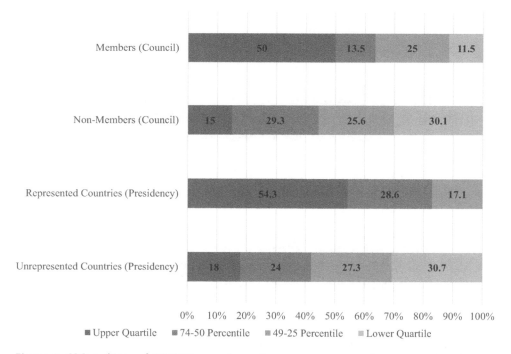

Figure 3. GDP rankings of ECOSOC council members versus non-members, present, and countries represented in the ECOSOC presidency versus non-represented countries, historical and present.

The Secretary-General leads the Secretariat and is "appointed by the General Assembly on the recommendation of the Security Council" (UN Secretary General, n.d., para. 1). The current Secretary-General is from Portugal, and the previous eight Secretary-Generals represented Korea, Ghana, Egypt, Peru, Austria, Myanmar, Sweden, and Norway. Myanmar is the only LDC to produce a Secretary-General, and also has the highest ranked GDP of any LDC, ranking 69th out of the 193 member states. No Secretary-General has been appointed from a SIDS; yet, four out of nine (44.4%) have been appointed from highly developed, Western states.

While every member state is equally represented in the UNGA's body, the body annually elects a president for a one-year term. Candidate nominations rotate between the five regional groups, with the five UNSC permanent members excluded. A total of 71 states have been represented by the presidency, and Argentina is the only state represented twice. Of the 71 presidential member states, three are unaccounted for in GDP rankings, resulting in 68 states for analysis. The UNGA leadership reflects the same dichotomy as other UN organs as 31 states (45.6%) are ranked in the upper quartile for GDP; whereas, five states (7.3%) are ranked in the lower quartile (Figure 4). Only five (10.6%) presidents have been elected from one of the 47 LDCs, and only three (8.1%) from the 37 SIDS. No president has been elected from any of the eight member states classified by the UN as both a LDC and a SIDS. The one vote per country UNGA rule positions less developed states

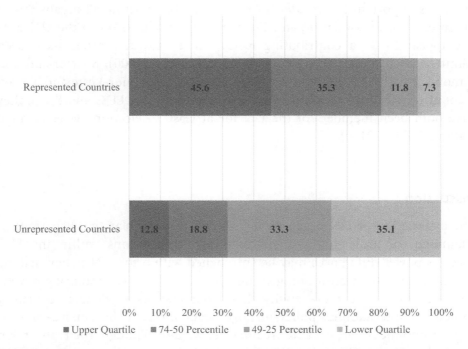

Figure 4. GDP rankings of countries represented versus un-represented in the UNGA presidency.

with small economies as equal members; however, these states may still be positioned as former colonies through the exchange of money and power for votes. In a previous longitudinal analysis of bilateral foreign aid distribution, wealthy, developed states were more likely to give financial aid to their former colonies and to states exhibiting similar voting behaviors in the UNGA (Alesina & Dollar, 2000). While these findings could reflect geopolitical alliances that are highly correlated with former colonial relationships, the authors also expressed concern that poorer states with smaller economies may try to maximize the aid they receive by aligning their votes with their former colonizer's or other developed states' interests (Alesina & Dollar, 2000). If the authors "preferred interpretation" of their findings is correct, "that donors favor their 'friends' in disbursing aid, and an observable manifestation of 'friendship' is the pattern of UN votes" (Alesina & Dollar, 2000, p. 46), there should be considerations that developed states could subvert poorer states' voting power within the UNGA.

Defining economy size by the World Bank's 2016 GDP rankings (2017), the present analysis concluded poorer, less developed states with small economies lack power and are underrepresented in all UN organs, except for the UNGA body, where representation is required. Wealthy, highly developed states, with large economies are overrepresented in all organs, usurp power from poor states and experience few checks on their power due to a monopolization of leadership positions. While the ECOSOC is the most pertinent organ to sustainable development and environmental initiatives, it is important to consider the power structures within all organs due to the interactions between organs. Further, date of admission to the UN does not appear to be a contributing factor, since only five states have been admitted post January 1, 2000: Serbia and Tuvalu (2000), Switzerland and Timor-Leste (2002), and South Sudan (2011). While Timor-Leste and Tuvalu account for two of the eight (25%) states classified as a LDC and SIDS, they have both been members of the UN for at least 15 election cycles (United Nations (UN), 2017c).

Discussion

The exploration of UN organ structure, and in particular the disparities in attainment of leadership and more influential positions within the UN, suggests power differences may be entrenched within the UN policy making system. Due to their positioning within the UN system, economically powerful states may have more ability than poorer states to dictate regulatory content in international policy-making negotiations to be congruent with their economic interests and free-market values. Though their sovereign right, this maneuvering is often for self-gain and at the expense of the common good, which differentially impacts poorer states, and should be an area of concern during the new UNCLOS negotiations.

The analyses also suggest economic power may be used by powerful states to exclude LDCs and SIDS from participating in policy-making processes. Though the UNFSA attempted to increase equity by establishing an assistance fund to aid LDCs and SIDS in implementing the agreement and participating in RFMOs and other regional policy-making processes (UN, 1995), the fund has been depleted on multiple occasions (United Nations (UN), 2015a), and appears to have been depleted since at least October 4, 2016 (Oceans and Law of the Sea in the General Assembly of the United Nations, 2016) – hence poorer states' request for more stable funding in the preparatory meeting. And, at the Eleventh Round of Informal Consultation of States Parties to UNFSA, SIDS efforts to participate in a RFMO – the Western and Central Pacific Fisheries Commission [WCPFC] – were described as being "blocked", despite continued rhetoric about empowering developing states to participate in high seas fisheries management (UN, 2015a). To encourage more developed, large economy states to contribute to a similar fund established under the Port State Measures, it was determined donor states could earmark contributions for specific projects (FAO, 2017). The 2015 UNGA resolution 69/292 agreeing to a new international legally binding instrument under UNCLOS and establishing the preparatory meetings also created a trust fund to assist LDCs in attending the preparatory meetings, but contribution to the trust fund was voluntary (UN, 2015b).

To promote equity in the short term, large economy states should be mandated to contribute to currently voluntary funds to assist LDCs and SIDS participation in policy-making processes and to build their capacity for implementing new regulations and management tools – a request continuously made by LDCs and SIDS (IISD, 2017). These funds could allow LDCs and SIDS to have prolonged and consistent engagement in low-level conference and preparatory meetings where they may have more ability to influence a policy's substantive text, even if they are compelled to vote with powerful countries in the UNGA as previously described, and to build and/or strengthen regional partnerships. To center the interests of LDCs and SIDS, a relative and objective administrative body (e.g., FAO) should have the authority to determine fund distribution, based on standardized indicators of need which also account for relevance and acuity of the policy or action item, rather than allowing developed states to earmark contributed funds based on their own self-interests. This is particularly important when considering financial aid to assist LDCs and SIDS in augmenting capacity with new technologies. Indeed, during the fourth preparatory meeting, AOSIS, Togo, Ghana, PSIDS, and the Caribbean group sought to establish a capacity-building fund to be accessed by SIDS and LDCs citing the need for long-term sustainable funding due to the unsustainable nature of voluntary trust funds

(IISD, 2017). However, the United States, the European Union, Canada, and New Zealand opposed.

The efforts to initiate new negotiations also demonstrated the potential for consortiums of non-governmental members (e.g., High Seas Alliance) to influence international policy making. With deliberate consideration of how these consortiums can be inclusive and equitable, they may present a more leverageable mechanism to create and accelerate new norms within international policy making that can also center underrepresented knowledge in international policy development. Many of these consortiums already feature prominent and reputable environmental organizations – typically from developed countries – that may be perceived as experts by international policy makers based on western standards of scientific merits. However, these organizations can use their privilege to amplify and promote progress made by the consortium's smaller organizations. This may include advancing bottom-up approaches by recognizing and scaling up successful country-specific initiatives into regional and international action.

Further, the new UNCLOS area-based management tools must be designed to equalize fisheries benefits distribution between high and low-income states based on fish dependence and viable alternatives for meeting subsistence and development needs (e.g., food, nutrition, and livelihoods) (Hankivsky, 2012). The establishment of marine protected areas and their level of regulation around restricting catches will likely be one contentious area during treaty negotiations, due to commercial fishing interests. Empirical findings and modeling suggest closing the high seas could reduce inequalities in fisheries benefits distribution by 50% and global annual profitability from fishing (mostly pocketed by industrialized states) will decrease by approximately 1% for every 20% of the high seas closed in the short term, with fishing ultimately becoming more profitable over the long term as stocks rebound (Sumaila et al., 2015; White & Costello, 2014). Additionally, in a study of 46 low-income and fish reliant countries, models suggested 70% of the countries would experience increased catches after closing the high seas (Teh et al., 2016).

Implications for social work

Though marine governance has historically been considered beyond social work's purview, marine degradation resulting from ineffective governance disproportionately threatens marginalized and vulnerable economies, communities, and individuals, making it a social justice issue. Social work's person-in-environment perspective offers a unique and critically needed lens through which to clearly identify the disparate impacts of physical environmental challenges like marine degradation on social development, economic equity, and human rights. Making international marine governance more just will require social work's disruption of entrenched power relations through greater attention to global policymaking and advocacy on behalf of states marginalized within UN power structures.

This challenge has distinct implications for social work educators and scholars as well. Growing curricular offerings in ecosocial work must place increased attention on the social justice implications of the multitude of physical environmental challenges, as well as the global power structures which govern environmental practices. Likewise, scholars of ecosocial work and social policy must extend research on policy impacts to attend more deeply to the policymaking process and its influence on the quality and content of policy solutions. Though the UN is a body of politically appointed representatives, non-governmental advocacy partnerships were influential in convening the renegotiations of UNCLOS. Social work research identifying the disparate impacts of environmental degradation could provide an opportunity for social workers to collaborate within these partnerships, and thus influence the governance of marine ecosystems and other common-pool resources governed by the UN.

Conclusion

Disrupting potential systemic power structures in the UN, particularly in leadership positions, could lead to marginalized states' increased inclusion and representation in policy-making processes. By reducing inequities within the UN and subsequently high seas policy making, potential outcomes may include stabilized and increased financial aid for marginalized states to implement and adopt new regulations and technology; more equitable distribution of marine resources' economic benefits; and, improved transparency and reduced stagnation in high seas policy making. While this analysis was specific to UNCLOS, the statistics about UN organ representation should also be understood in a larger context of social justice and inherent weaknesses in UN structures requiring reforms to more equitably support vulnerable states.[1,2]

Acknowledgments

The authors wish to thank Dr. Jennifer Greenfield for her assistance with the conceptualization of this manuscript.

Notes

1. Food and Agriculture Organization of the United Nations' (FAO) (1993) Agreement to Promote Compliance with International Conservation and Management Measures by Fishing Vessels on the High Seas; (1995) Code of Conduct for Responsible Fisheries;

1. (2002) International Plan of Action to Prevent, Deter and Eliminate Illegal, Unreported and Unregulated Fishing; and (2009) Agreement on Port State Measures to Prevent, Deter, and Eliminate Illegal, Unreported, Unregulated Fishing. United Nations' (1995) Fish Stocks Agreement and (2012) Conference on Sustainable Development.
2. LDCs and SIDS are both designations bestowed by the UN, based on indicators of socioeconomic vulnerabilities. The SIDS designation also considers environmental vulnerabilities resulting from unique island geographies. As such, not all SIDS are also classified as a LDC.

Disclosure statement

No potential conflict of interest was reported by the authors.

ORCID

Jessica L. Decker Sparks ⓘ http://orcid.org/0000-0003-0123-0310

References

Alesina, A., & Dollar, D. (2000). Who gives foreign aid to whom and why? *Journal of Economic Growth, 5*, 33–63. doi:10.1023/A:1009874203400

Cullis-Suzuki, S., & Pauly, D. (2010). Failing the high seas: A global evaluation of regional fisheries management organizations. *Marine Policy, 34*(5), 1036–1042. doi:10.1016/j.marpol.2010.03.002

Dieter, A. (2014). From harbor to high seas: An argument for rethinking fishery management systems and multinational fishing treaties. *Wisconsin International Law Journal, 32*(4), 725–750.

Dreher, A., Nunnenkamp, P., & Thiele, P. (2006). *Does US aid buy UN general assembly votes? A disaggregated analysis* (Working Paper No. 138). Zurich, Switzerland: Swiss Federal Institute of Technology.

Editorial: Protect the high seas from harm. (2018). Discussions on a United Nations treaty to safeguard the open ocean offer an opportunity for scientists. *Nature, 553*, 127–128.

Food and Agriculture Organization of the United Nations. (2016). *The state of world fisheries and aquaculture: Contributing to food security and nutrition for all.* Rome, Italy: FAO.

Food and Agriculture Organization of the United Nations. (2017). *First meeting of the parties to the FAO agreement on port state measures.* Retrieved from http://www.fao.org/3/a-i7909e.pdf

Food and Agriculture Organization of the United Nations. (2018). *The state of world fisheries and aquaculture: Meeting the sustainable development goals.* Rome, Italy: FAO.

Food and Agriculture Organization of the United Nations. (1993). The Agreement to Promote Compliance with International Conservation and Management Meaures by Fishing Vessels on the High Seas, approved on 24 November 1993 By resolution 15/93 of the twenty-seventh session of the fao conference, entered into force 24 april 2003. Retrieved from http://www.fao.org/docrep/meeting/003/x3130m/X3130E00.htm

Galland, G., Rogers, A., & Nickson, A. (2016). *Netting billions: A global valuation of tuna.* Philadelphia, PA: Pew Charitable Trusts.

General Assembly of the United Nations, President of the72nd Session . (2017). *Past presidents.* Retrieved from https://www.un.org/pga/72/past-presidents/

Gjerde, K. M., Currie, D., Wowk, K., & Sack, K. (2013). Ocean in peril: Reforming the management of global ocean living resources in areas beyond natural jurisdiction. *Marine Pollution Bulletin, 74*(2), 540–551. doi:10.1016/j.marpolbul.2013.07.037

Global Ocean Commission. (2013). *Improving accountability and performance in international fisheries management* (Policy options paper No. 9). Oxford, UK: GOC.

Guntrip, E. (2003). The common heritage of mankind: An adequate regime for managing the deep seabed. *Melbourne Journal of International Law, 4*(2), 376.

Hankivsky, O. (Ed.). (2012). *An intersectionality-based policy analysis framework*. Vancouver, BC: Simon Fraser University.

High Seas Alliance. (2017). *UN steps towards an implementing agreement*. Retrieved from http://highseasalliance.org/sites/highseasalliance.org/files/hsa-timeline-update.pdf

Hornborg, A. (2009). Zero-sum challenges in conceptualizing environmental load displacement and ecologically unequal exchange in the world system. *International Journal of Comparative Sociology, 50*(3–4), 237–262. doi:10.1177/0020715209105141

International Court of Justice. (2017). *Members*. Retrieved from https://www.icj-cij.org/en/members

International Institute for Sustainable Development. (2017). *Summary of the 4th session of the preparatory committee on marine biodiversity beyond areas of national jurisdiction*. Retrieved from http://enb.iisd.org/download/pdf/enb25141e.pdf

Kemp, S. P., & Palinkas, L. A. (2015). *Strengthening the social response to the human impacts of environmental change*. Baltimore, MD: AASWSW.

Nordquist, M. H., Rosenne, S., & Kraska, J. (Eds.). (2011). *UNCLOS 1982: A commentary* (Vol. VII). Leiden, Netherlands & Boston, MA: Martinus Nijhoff Publishers.

Oceans and Law of the Sea in the General Assembly of the United Nations. (2016). *Assistance fund under Part VII of the agreement for the implementation of the provisions of the United Nations convention on the law of the sea of 10 December 1982*. Retrieved from https://www.un.org/depts/los/convention_agreements/fishstocktrustfund/fishstocktrustfund.htm

Stevenson, J. R., & Oxman, B. (1994). The future of the United Nations convention on the law of the sea. *The American Journal of International Law, 88*, 477–499. doi:10.2307/2203716

Sumaila, U. R., Lam, V. W. Y., Miller, D. D., Teh, L., Watson, R. A., Zeller, D., … Pauly, D. (2015). Winners and losers in a world where the high seas is closed to fishing. *Scientific Reports, 5*(8481), 1–6. doi:10.1038/srep08481

Teh, L. S., Lam, V. W., Cheung, W. W., Miller, D., Teh, L. C., & Sumaila, U. R. (2016). Impact on high seas closure on food security in low income fish dependent countries. *PloS ONE, 11*(12), e0168529. doi:10.1371/journal.pone.0168529

Teh, L. S., & Sumaila, U. R. (2013). Contribution of marine fisheries to worldwide employment. *Fish and Fisheries, 14*, 77–88. doi:10.1111/j.1467-2979.2011.00450.x

U. N. Economic and Social Council. (2017). *Members*. Retrieved from https://www.un.org/ecosoc/en/content/members

U. N. Office of the High Representative for the Least Developed Countries, Landlocked Developing Countries and Small Island Developing States (UN-OHRLLS). (2017). *Least developed countries*. Retrieved from http://unohrlls.org/about-ldcs/

U. N. Secretary-General. (n.d.). *Former secretaries-general*. Retrieved from https://www.un.org/sg/en/content/former-secretaries-general

U. N. Security Council. (n.d.). *Members*. Retrieved from https://www.un.org/securitycouncil/content/current-members

United Nations. (1945). *Charter of the United Nations and statute of the international court of justice*. Signed at San Francisco, California, 26 June 1945, entered into force 24 October 1945. Retrieved from https://www.un.org/en/charter-united-nations/index.html

United Nations. (1982). *United Nations convention on the law of the sea of 10 December 1982.* Retrieved from https://www.un.org/Depts/los/convention_agreements/texts/unclos/unclos_e.pdf

United Nations. (1995). *Fish stocks agreement.* Retrieved from https://www.un.org/Depts/los/convention_agreements/convention_overview_fish_stocks.htm

United Nations. (2015a). *Eleventh round of informal consultations of States parties to the agreement for the implementation of the provisions of UNCLOS: Report.* Retrieved from https://www.un.org/Depts/los/convention_agreements/fishstocksmeetings/icsp11_final_fsa.pdf

United Nations. (2015b). *United Nations general assembly resolution 69/292.* Development of an internationally legally binding instrument under the United Nations Convention on the Law of the Sea on the conservation and sustainable use of marine biological diversity of areas beyond national jurisdiction. Retrieved from https://undocs.org/en/a/res/72/249

United Nations. (2016). *Main organs.* Retrieved from https://www.un.org/en/sections/about-un/main-organs/

United Nations. (2017a). *Meetings coverage: Adopting two texts on oceans, seas, general assembly also tackles sustainable management, conservation of marine life beyond national jurisdiction.* 63rd & 64th Meetings of the Seventy-Second Plenary Session of the United Nations General Assembly, New York, NY, GA/11985. Retrieved from https://www.un.org/press/en/2017/ga11985.doc.htm

United Nations. (2017b). *Meetings coverage: Concluding main part of seventy-second session, general assembly adopts $5.397 billion budget for 2018-2019, as recommended by fifth committee.* 76th Meeting of the Seventy-Second Plenary Session of the United Nations General Assembly, New York, NY, GA/11997. Retrieved from https://www.un.org/press/en/2017/ga11997.doc.htm

United Nations. (2017c). *Member states.* Retrieved from https://www.un.org/en/member-states/

Visbeck, M., Kronfeld-Goharani, U., Neumann, B., Rickels, W., Schmidt, J., van Doorn, E., ... Proelss, A. (2014). A sustainable development goal for the ocean and coasts: Global ocean challenges benefit from regional initiatives supporting globally coordinated solutions. *Marine Policy, 49,* 87–89. doi:10.1016/j.marpol.2014.02.010

White, C., & Costello, C. (2014). Close the high seas to fishing? *PLoS Biology, 12*(3), e1001826. doi:10.1371/journal.pbio.1001826

World Bank. (2017). *World Bank open data.* Retrieved from https://data.worldbank.org

Part II

Ecological Injustices from the Legacy of Colonialism

Collective survival strategies and anti-colonial practice in ecosocial work

Finn McLafferty Bell, Mary Kate Dennis, and Amy Krings ⓘ

ABSTRACT
Oppressed communities have long used strategies of caring for and protecting each other to ensure their collective survival. We argue for ecosocial workers to critically interrogate how agency, history, and culture structure environmental problems and our responses to them, by developing a resilience-based framework, collective survival strategies (CSS). CSS consider power, culture and history and build upon the strengths of oppressed communities facing global environmental changes. We challenge the dominant narrative of climate change as a "new" problem and connect it to colonization. We discuss implications by examining a social work program explicitly built on Indigenous knowledges and anti-colonial practice.

The only way to survive is by taking care of one another, by recreating our relationships to one another. Grace Lee Boggs (1915-2015)

As social work confronts the severity of the ecological crisis, it becomes increasingly clear that the human- and social-focused logics that dominate the field are not sufficient. Liberal notions of rights and entitlements undergird social work as a discipline, but global environmental changes[1] also necessitate conversations about responsibilities and natural limits. While social work has long used systems theory and ecological perspectives to analyze persons in environment, we rarely acknowledge the natural environment in a meaningful way (Närhi & Matthies, 2016). With the development of ecosocial work as a subfield, scholars and practitioners are developing ways to seriously consider the natural environment (Boetto, 2018). This has included a turn toward resilience (Case, 2017; Peeters, 2012a). Resilience is an essential framework for ecosocial work because by focusing on "the zone of stable functioning" for our ecosystems, resilience insists that we recognize natural limits and our responsibilities for staying within those natural limits (Cretney, 2014). However, resilience is not a normative concept, and incorporating resilience thinking into practice could make conditions more or less just (Walsh-Dilley, Wolford, & McCarthy, 2016). Further, social scientists have rightly criticized resilience scholarship for its disregard for power, culture, and history (Cretney, 2014).

This article builds upon those debates. We develop a new framework, collective survival strategies (CSS), by thinking through a resilience approach that seriously considers power, culture, and history, and squarely focusing on the strengths of oppressed communities. In doing so, we recognize, as North Americans, that we cannot seriously consider power, culture, and history without directly addressing settler colonialism and embracing anti-colonial practice, particularly as ecosocial work incorporates Indigenous[2] knowledges (Gray, Coates, & Hetherington, 2007; Ramsay & Boddy, 2017). By focusing on CSS, we learn from communities that have fought for environmental justice and collective survival for generations. After all, for many on this planet, the threat to collective survival did not begin in this new era of ecological crisis, and failing to recognize and learn from people who have prolonged experience in struggling for their collective survival could diminish the liberatory potential of ecosocial work.

This article focuses on the strategies that oppressed communities have historically used to ensure their collective survival. We argue that ecosocial work has a role in critically interrogating how agency, history, and culture structure environmental problems, as well as responses to those problems. In doing so, ecosocial workers can humbly learn from oppressed communities to uplift and enable their work. Hence, we start by critically examining resilience, including its varied definitions and applications. We then consider Indigenous conceptualizations of climate change that connect it to the colonization of North America. Next, we briefly examine the existing scholarship on ecosocial work and the importance of considering history, culture, and agency. We then present a framework, CSS, by which to understand a historically and culturally relevant approach to resilience that acknowledges both structural forces that have created the climate crisis and the agency that people continue to exercise in organizing for their own collective survival. Finally, we discuss practice implications through an examination of a social work program explicitly built upon Indigenous knowledges and anti-colonial practice.

We are a collective of scholars concerned about the impact of environmental injustice on oppressed communities that social workers are ethically bound to serve (Canadian Association of Social Workers [CASW], 2005; National Association of Social Workers [NASW], 2017), as well as on all other beings. Our diverse social locations, including as settlers and Indigenous, as clinicians and organizers, give us different starting points in considering the sources of environmental degradation and what is yet to be done. This article is the result of us grappling with each other, and with so many significant others, on these existential questions.

Resilience

Ecosocial work takes on the natural environment in a way that social work more broadly has generally neglected (Boetto, 2018). Ecosocial work's use of resilience is an important part of this shift. Resilience emerged from complex systems theory (Chandler, 2014; Vrasti & Michelsen, 2017) and refers to "the capacity of a system to absorb disturbance and reorganize while undergoing change so as to still retain essentially the same function, structure, identity, and feedbacks" (Walker et al., 2004 in Peeters, 2012a, p. 16). Yet, the articulation and application of resilience varies greatly (Cretney, 2014), and the usage of resilience across academic disciplines, policy realms, and popular discourse are contested (Boonstra, 2016; Davoudi, Brooks, & Mehmood, 2013; Hornborg, 2013; Ingalls & Stedman, 2016; Vrasti & Michelsen, 2017).

Resilience emerged in engineering and ecology, but it was soon adopted as a framework to understand the nexus between the social and the ecological (Davoudi et al., 2013). However, with the application of the scientific concept of resilience onto social actors came a number of critiques from social scientists (Boonstra, 2016; Fabinyi, Evans, & Foale, 2014; Ingalls & Stedman, 2016). Social scientists argued that resilience frameworks have not seriously considered power, culture, and agency (Boonstra, 2016; Fabinyi et al., 2014; Ingalls & Stedman, 2016; Ungar, Ghazinour, & Richter, 2013).

Nonetheless, the development in resilience discourse that has provoked the most controversy is the cooptation of resilience by neoliberal forces, wherein individuals and groups are expected to continually build their capacity to "bounce back" from the crises and depredations endemic to neoliberal capitalist society (Cretney, 2014; Hornborg, 2013). The ascent of community resilience – defined as "a process of adaptation in a community following a disruption" (Cretney, 2014, p. 629) – as a dominant goal for disaster response by governmental and foundation actors has proved particularly controversial (Cretney, 2014; Tierney, 2015).

Tierney (2015) incisively critiques community resilience discourse in disaster response as reifying inequality. Although community resilience is framed as a means to empower communities to take control of their circumstances in an uncertain world and build capacity to bounce back from disasters, too often community resilience discourse fails to acknowledge the historical and structural factors that are exposing communities to such risks, and take for granted that the status quo is a desired place to return (Tierney, 2015). Further, the neoliberal discourse on resilience does not take culture into account, both in terms of proposing universalizing interventions, and in terms of failing to draw from cultural traditions that have sustained oppressed communities and enabled their collective survival (Cretney, 2014; Ungar et al., 2013).

Tierney (2015) suggests that the same neoliberal policymakers who advance community resilience also created the climate crisis that they now assert only they can solve. Neoliberal proponents of community resilience see it as the only reasonable reaction to a world defined by disruption caused by rapid urbanization, climate change, and globalization. However, doing so naturalizes disruption and frames it is as inevitable. Contrary to some scientific and transformative articulations of resilience (Cretney, 2014; Hornborg, 2013), neoliberal proponents insist that instead of addressing the root causes of disasters, we must adapt to them. Thus, Tierney (2015) contends that "resilience discourse frames members of at-risk populations as increasingly pressured to adapt to depredations that are the direct result of the historic and contemporary forces of neoliberalization" (p. 1333). In this framework, resilient subjects are not political actors; they must constantly focus on adapting to external conditions, rather than changing those conditions. Again, it should be noted that resilience theorists challenge this neoliberal discourse, noting that all subjects are part of multiple systems, and simultaneously impact those systems and are impacted by them (Chandler, 2014; Davoudi et al., 2013).

Social scientific critiques of how resilience researchers represent the social world and how neoliberal ideologues have co-opted its use have strengthened social-ecological resilience frameworks. These critiques have caused resilience scholars to seriously wrestle with issues of power (Boonstra, 2016), agency (Davoudi et al., 2013), and culture (Cretney, 2014). In doing so, resilience scholars have established a body of evidence supporting the liberatory and transformative potential of a "resilience from below" (Vrasti & Michelsen, 2017).

We locate CSS as one practice of "resilience from below" that is a necessary step in recognizing and increasing marginalized communities' adaptive capacity. While CSS are a necessary component of building resilience, they are by no means sufficient in addressing environmental changes on their own. As local climates may change rapidly, CSS are not enough to ensure collective survival. Yet, they are an important component that draws upon oppressed communities' strengths and histories. We see CSS as part of a larger movement that uses resilience as a basis for climate justice organizing (Movement Generation, 2013). In addition, in the North American context, any resilience framework that seeks to seriously engage history, culture, and power in addressing global environmental change is incomplete without examining settler colonialism as the foundation upon which all of these forces are playing out. Thus, we need to address Indigenous conceptions of global environmental changes, including how they are continuations of colonization.

Settler colonialism and climate change

In his prolific writing on climate change, Indigenous philosopher, Whyte (2016, 2017)), has challenged the dominant narrative propagated by mostly white environmentalists that climate change represents a coming dystopia that has heretofore not existed in the modern world. Rather, Whyte (2017) argues that many of the worst expected outcomes of a changing climate – species extinction, forced migration, hunger, disease, lack of clean water, rapidly shifting environmental changes – are all conditions that European invaders, settlers, and their descendants forced upon North American Indigenous people and continue to do so. Sharpe (2016) makes a parallel argument that we can only understand the current plight of African-Americans in the US "in the wake" of slavery: how being violently ripped from their homelands (another massive change in climate) and enslaved has shaped their experiences.

It is important to understand that Whyte does not make this argument to minimize the dangerous effects of global environmental change, particularly as Indigenous peoples will continue to be impacted first and worst. Instead, Whyte (2016) wants us to take colonialism seriously as both a key cause of climate change and as a factor that prevents Indigenous and other people from effectively "adapting." Waziyatawin (2012) elaborates this paradox when noting that the climate crisis (as part of a series of converging crises) represents a decolonizing opportunity for Indigenous peoples, but also threatens the continuation of life on this planet, including Indigenous communities and all of the lifeways[3] that support them.

Settler colonialism is distinct from other forms of colonialism in that the colonizers do not solely seek to export wealth from their colonies by exploiting its natural resources and native labor; rather, settler colonialism operates under a logic of elimination and domination: destroy to replace (Wolfe, 2006). Alfred (2009) argues this process began with the doctrine of *terra nullius*, or "empty lands" asserting that North America was not populated by humans before the arrival of Christian Europeans and rationalizing the dispossession of Indigenous peoples from their lands. Settler colonialism is fundamentally about land and resources. Settlers seek to destroy the native population, native culture, native ecologies, and native sovereignty in order to replace them with their own population, culture, ecologies, and institutions (Waziyatawin, 2012; Whyte, Caldwell, & Schaefer, 2018). Settler colonialism is not an event that happened in the past; rather it is the structure of settler colonial societies, such as the United States, Canada, Australia, and Israel (Wolfe, 2006). In North America, the arrival and violent settling practices of Europeans brought a literal apocalypse to the Indigenous population. Population estimates are difficult to determine prior to 1492, and the devastating effects vary across tribal groups; however, the Indigenous population was reduced by roughly 80–90% by 1890 (Thornton, 2000).

Whyte (2016) shows that traditional Indigenous governance structures and ways of life are not only in tune with the natural environment, but also are eminently adaptable to fluxes in the natural environment. The continual removal and forced relocation of Indigenous peoples into smaller and smaller tracts of less desirable land caused not just immeasurable loss and grief but also a profound disconnection from an Earth-based way of life (Brewer & Dennis, 2019). Further, the intentional destruction of Indigenous cultures through residential and boarding schools, religious conversion, and other means has disrupted the intergenerational flow of traditional environmental knowledge that teaches Indigenous peoples how to live in right relationship with all their relations in a specific place, thus ensuring collective survival (Hart, 2009; Waziyatawin, 2012).

The forced climate change of colonization is the foundation on which both the US and Canadian industrial societies were built, to the benefit of their settlers and settler descendants, and to the detriment of the planet due to the disproportionate responsibility that North America has in causing the global environmental changes that we see today. We cannot effectively address these changes without simultaneously dismantling one of the foundations on which they were built: colonialism.

We draw particular attention to climate change as a continuation of colonization, because in a rush to place global environmental change on the social work agenda – which is incredibly important and necessary – ecosocial work should not fail to acknowledge how the very real threat to collective survival is historically and culturally situated. Thus, climate change lands very differently on disparate groups, particularly for Indigenous people who have long experienced threats to their futurity. For many of the white environmentalists that Whyte (2017) challenges, threats to their collective survival as a people does indeed feel new, as generally white North Americans are not used to having their futurity threatened. Whyte et al. (2018) describe futurity as:

> the idea that members of a society ought to be able to experience that their own efforts and contributions to their society play a part in making it so that a vibrant future is possible for the coming generations ... Futurity [is] significant for Indigenous peoples, for one way of understanding settler colonialism is as a form of oppression that destroys Indigenous futurity. (p. 163)

In thinking about our futurity as a species, it is vital that ecosocial work attends to the ways that settlers have materially benefitted from the threat to Indigenous futurity.

Ecosocial work: an emerging field

Ecosocial work is a growing field of social work scholarship (Krings, Victor, Mathias, & Perron, 2018; Mason, Shires, Arwood, & Borst, 2017) and a means to promote environmental sustainability at all levels of practice (Norton, 2012). It draws upon a deep ecological awareness of humans' relationship with nature and the built environment and, thus, focuses on protecting and sustaining the natural environment in an equitable way (Gray et al., 2007). Ecosocial work helps to build community resilience, but endeavors to do so in service of social-political change rather than the status quo (Peeters, 2012b; Teixeira & Krings, 2015). In their conceptual analysis, Ramsay and Boddy (2017) found that four key attributes define environmental social work: (1) the application of social work skills to the environment; (2) openness to different values and ways of being or doing, including learning from Indigenous cultures; (3) adopting a change orientation, which includes critiquing hegemony; and (4) working across boundaries and in multiple spaces, which includes working in multidisciplinary teams with communities and individuals. Gray et al. (2007) argue that ecosocial work "articulates and privileges local Indigenous cultures" (p. 56) through its emphasis on the importance of place, alternative worldviews, celebration of diversity, and sharing of knowledge related to humans' interdependence and connectedness to the Earth. As ecosocial work embraces Indigenous knowledges and practices, it is important to acknowledge the work of Indigenous scholars (Billiot et al., 2017), and seriously engage with the ways that colonialism has erased, and continues to erase, Indigenous knowledges and practices in favor of Western ones.

The importance of history, culture, and agency

Ecosocial work prioritizes social change, including in its orientation toward resilience (Case, 2017; Peeters, 2012b). To do so effectively, engaging seriously with the places that resilience frameworks have traditionally struggled – history, culture, and power – is essential. We agree with much of Tierney's (2015) critique of community resilience discourse as overemphasizing agency at the expense of structure, and yet, this critique leaves few options in terms of how marginalized communities can organize to protect and care for themselves. Her critique does not build on the strengths that communities have long held in surviving colonization, enslavement, exploitation and oppression, and it is profoundly demobilizing. Tierney critiques community resilience discourse for putting all of the focus on what marginalized groups need to do to make themselves resilient to disaster without acknowledging the historical and structural factors that put them at risk. Thus, Tierney is constructively demystifying history and structure on one hand, while completely disregarding individual and collective agency on the other. Further, neither community resilience discourse, nor Tierney's critique of it seriously consider culture as an enabler of collective survival. We examine how history, agency, and culture all need to be seriously considered in responding to environmental crises and how a focus on CSS does that.

Historical context

As discussed in Whyte's (2016, 2017) work, understanding the history that has brought us to this moment is essential to effectively addressing climate change. While Tierney (2015) argues that the world's poor, who are simultaneously most at risk from and least responsible for the ecological crisis, should not have to adapt, even if we were to take serious, commensurate global action now, the impacts of global environmental change will continue (Intergovernmental Panel on Climate Change [IPCC], 2018). Thus, understanding the historical roots of the ecological crisis – and how, for many oppressed communities, this is an intensification of already dystopian conditions – is key to understanding how those same communities can approach collective survival now, by building on many of the same practices that have enabled their collective survival thus far. For ecosocial work, the question then is: how can we learn from this history, including our place in it, and support oppressed communities in facilitating CSS? As Anishinaabe Elder, Art Solomon, explains:

> In order to know where we are going, we need to know where we are. In order to know where we are, we need to know who we are. And, in order to know who we are, we need to know where we come from (in Hart et al., 2014, p. 7).

This matters because an ahistorical understanding of resilience to rapid change denies community members their ancestors' experiences of resisting, surviving, and continuing despite horrific conditions being imposed upon them by the same forces that are largely responsible for global environmental change.

Understanding the tension between agency and structure

Similar to the critique of community resilience discourse, Mullaly (1997) has criticized mainstream social work for paying insufficient attention to changing the structural factors that impact clients and communities. However, in bringing attention to structural factors, we must not lose sight of individual and collective agency. Agency is the foundation for self-determination, and collective agency, in the form of collective action for social change, is the only force powerful enough to change structural conditions, as ecosocial work recognizes (Närhi & Matthies, 2016). An over-deterministic focus on structure produces incisive critiques of the world as it is while leaving little room for the political project of building the world that we want. CSS show the power of collective agency not just to directly overthrow oppression, but also to create liberated spaces where people are cared for and safe as a resistance to oppression.

The importance of culture

Ecosocial work has called for engagement with Indigenous cultures and traditional environmental knowledge (Gray et al., 2007; Ramsay & Boddy, 2017), but we must take seriously how those cultures are situated within settler colonial states. Communities have maintained cultural practices despite attempts to violently destroy their traditions. This is true for people who were colonized, as well as people who were enslaved. For example, enslaved African women secretly braided okra and rice seeds into their hair to bring vital pieces of their culture with them through the Middle Passage (Bandele & Myers, 2016). Culture is a strength upon which many communities have built their ability to survive and thrive despite oppressive conditions, which explains why cultural imperialism – convincing the colonized that their culture is inferior and that they must adopt the superior culture of their colonizers – is such a prevalent tool amongst oppressors (Said, 2012). As Nobel Peace Prize winner, Wangari Maathai, stated when discussing the violence of colonialism (Dater & Merton, 2008):

> Culture is coded wisdom. Wisdom that has been accumulated for thousands of years and generations … . All people have their own culture. But when you remove that culture from them, then you kill them in a way. You kill them. You kill a very large part of them.

As ecosocial work scholars recognize, attempts to help a community adapt to environmental change need to fit the unique culture(s) of that community, but they also need to consider what that culture has needed to survive.

Collective survival strategies

CSS are fundamentally about how communities protect and care for each other, and always have. Rather than representing an innovation, CSS are an old technology. There are five key components to CSS, as we define them. They are: (1) communal and cooperative, not individualistic; (2) rooted in place and existing cultural traditions; (3) focus on basic survival needs – food, water, shelter, protection, culture; (4) self-organized and autonomous – not reliant upon outside actors; and (5) address both quotidian and spectacular disasters – making everyday life better and reducing vulnerability to larger crises.

First, the practice must be collective, not individualistic. CSS involve people working cooperatively for the good of the whole. This is a key distinction between CSS and the survivalist practices of predominantly white, male segments of the population who identify as "preppers" (Schneider-Mayerson, 2015). While preppers engage in survival practices that incorporate other components of CSS, the prepper narrative of the rugged individual who must engage in all-against-all warfare to survive is antithetical to CSS (Schneider-Mayerson, 2015).

Second, CSS are rooted in place and existing cultural traditions. There is no single universal approach to CSS because practices are tailored to meet unique needs in a particular place by the people themselves. For instance, Lakota elders living on the Pine Ridge Indian Reservation continue the traditions that they learned as children when their families were self-sufficient on their homesteads: raising animals, growing vegetables, and harvesting wild foods on the land as Lakota people have for millennia (Brewer & Dennis, 2017). These harvesting trips taught children the location and Lakota names for wild foods, thereby helping them to maintain a place-based and spiritual connection to their food system. As older adults, they carry this knowledge and have the skills to achieve food security for younger generations on this reservation (Brewer & Dennis, 2017). A social work approach to CSS recognizes the traditional environmental knowledge that people who are rooted in a specific place carry, and helps to remove the barriers that exist so that those people can exercise that knowledge.

Third, community survival strategies focus on basic human survival needs. These include food, shelter, water, protection, and culture. In the US, where a shifting racialized capitalist economy has left low-income Black communities without access to basic survival needs, struggles are increasingly, explicitly waged over control of food, land, and water (Krings, Kornberg, & Lane, 2019; Krings & Thomas, 2018). In describing Black-led agriculture work in Detroit, Quizar (2018) argues that "growers often characterize farming, accessing food, and having control over one's own food supply as issues of survival – of day-to-day livelihood and also more broadly of Black and poor people's survival" (p. 82). For some Black Detroiters, growing food is an important CSS because it entails reclaiming agricultural labor from its association with enslavement and exploitation as a site to build self-reliance and self-determination (Quizar, 2018; White, 2011, 2017).

Fourth, CSS are self-organized and autonomous; although they could receive assistance from outside actors, they are not created or led by governments or exogenous non-profits. Communities working to meet collective survival needs may form non-profits or apply for government funding to support their work, but they generally do so with a wariness of becoming dependent on such sources or giving them undue influence (Krings, Spencer, & Jimenez, 2014). For example, some climate adaptation planning happening amongst Indigenous people in the US is being financially supported by the federal government, and yet, the initiatives are explicitly and unapologetically by and for Indigenous people (Whyte et al., 2018).

Finally, CSS are not just about preparing for spectacular disasters that may come; they are responses to the disastrousness of everyday life in so many communities. As disaster studies recognize, the destructiveness of what we call disasters are not anomalies, they are magnifications of the injustices and social vulnerabilities of everyday life (Klinenberg, 2015). CSS do make people more resilient to spectacular disasters, but, crucially, they do so by improving their everyday lives. Thus, CSS takes an inverse approach to a neoliberal conception of resilience, rather than focusing on how to "bounce back" to a supposedly stable and socially just point of stasis, CSS address the *instability* and *injustice* that is the lived reality in marginalized communities. In doing so, CSS reduce the community's social vulnerability to both quotidian and spectacular disasters. Going back to Detroit, Black food growers use that practice to reduce their reliance on precarious paid labor and to prevent health problems caused by lack of access to fresh, healthy food: two key factors in the disastrousness of everyday life for many low-income, Black Detroiters (Quizar, 2018; White, 2011). In case of disaster, bouncing back to the unjust and unstable status quo in Detroit is not a worthy goal, rather, farmers in the city are proactively changing the status quo by building food sovereignty in the Black community.

Again, CSS are fundamentally about how communities protect and care for each other. Particularly in communities that have long experienced oppression, exploitation, and colonization, these habits are what have enabled their collective survival thus far and are key to understanding how to continue into the future. These strategies happen at multiple levels and incorporate diverse tactics, which is essential in building resilience (Davoudi et al., 2013).

Protecting and caring for each other happens in both political and seemingly non-political realms. In order to address the root causes of injustice, communities need to address their oppressors directly or build alternative systems, called autonomous zones (Peña, 2005), whereby they can be free of their oppressor. Often both approaches must be undertaken for either to be successful. When oppressed groups manage to free themselves, but do not have already existing alternative systems or institutions, they run the risk of recreating their oppressor's system. When groups successfully build alternative, more just institutions, they often face state violence and repression, which they then need to confront or evade to continue their alternative institutions.

Further, communities need a certain guarantee of rights to access means of survival, such as land and clean water (Walsh-Dilley et al., 2016). Hence, movements may start out with seemingly non-political aims, and yet find themselves engaging in power struggles in order to meet their survival needs. Walsh-Dilley et al. (2016) argue that by embracing food sovereignty's focus on communal rights, resilience scholars can meaningfully incorporate a power analysis into their framework while challenging liberal notions of individual rights.

Anti-colonial practice and collective survival strategies

Anti-colonial practice is a model that provides a way for ecosocial work to support CSS, while challenging colonialism, which is a root cause of the ecological crisis and hinders Indigenous communities' ability to adapt to environmental change. Anti-colonialism is a social, cultural, and political position rooted in the collective and common consciousness that colonialism was imposed and dominating (Hart, 2009). It is also the resistance that Indigenous people have enacted against colonial frameworks since colonialism began (Smith, 1999). One method of anti-colonialism is the recovery and practice of traditional Indigenous knowledge while employing a critical analysis of colonialism.

Indigenism is one stance of anti-colonialism that, like CSS, is tied to a place and a time, as Indigenous people are bounded to a space from which their culture and values are derived. They do not occupy a place but are "children of that place" (Moore et al. in Hart, 2009, p. 33). Indigenous people have "the responsibility to practice kinship roles of their bioregional habitat, manifested through cultural beliefs, rituals and ceremonies that cherish biodiversity" (Hart, 2009, p. 33). Indigenism prioritizes Indigenous rights, and cultural traditions uphold these rights. Without rights, Indigenous people are prevented from exercising their responsibility of kinship roles and meeting their collective survival needs (Waziyatawin, 2012). Further, self-sufficiency is a necessary condition for Indigenous collective action (Tarrow, 1998 in Hart, 2009).

Anti-colonial practice builds social work capacity to support Indigenous communities in collectively surviving global environmental change in a way that is culturally centered, historically relevant, and focused on collective agency. While anti-colonial practice is an emerging framework in social work (Hart, Straka, & Rowe, 2017), there are models we can look to of this framework in action. The Master of Social Work based in Indigenous Knowledges (MSW-IK) program at the University of Manitoba was created in response to the important need for social workers to explore and incorporate Indigenous forms of caring applicable to the unique circumstances of Indigenous people and their communities (Hart et al., 2014). Indigenous forms of caring are rooted in traditional values, social structures, and healing practices. In particular, students are encouraged to practice from an anti-colonial lens in which they learn: the location of Indigenous people in the colonial context and how this context hinders Indigenous self-determination and development; about colonial oppression and its relation to parallel forms of oppression; and to confront issues of oppression in practice by advocating for partnership with Indigenous peoples on matters related to self-determination (Hart et al., 2014).

The MSW-IK program was specifically created by Indigenous social workers, scholars, and elders to train Indigenous social workers for the benefit of Indigenous communities (Hart et al., 2014). We encourage using this program as a model for how to build social work capacity for practitioners who are a part of a community to develop culturally relevant healing and social change practices in partnership with that community. Nonetheless, given the marginalization of Indigenous people, specifically, in social work, partnerships often must be built across settler/Indigenous boundaries in anti-colonial research and practice (Hart et al., 2017). Hart et al. (2017) provide an excellent guide for how researchers can approach these partnerships in a way that maintains the anti-colonial and Indigenist integrity of the practice. Examining this guide, as well as other anti-colonial scholarship by Indigenous people, is an essential first step for ecosocial workers who are starting to include Indigenous knowledges.

Anti-colonial practice enacts ecosocial work principles. Ecosocial work aims to learn from Indigenous knowledges and encourages working with diverse communities while critiquing hegemony (Gray et al., 2007; Ramsay & Boddy, 2017). Anti-colonial social work also requires a critique of colonialism and resistance to its dominance, but demands that research, interventions, and planning for Indigenous communities be led by those communities themselves (Hart et al., 2017). Such self-determination facilitates renewal of Indigenous responsibilities to the sustainable practice of Indigenous livelihoods (Alfred, 2009; Corntassel, 2012; Whyte et al., 2018). The decolonizing praxis must move beyond political awareness or symbolic gestures, and instead engage in daily truth telling and resistance to colonial encroachments, in addition to the struggles to reclaim, restore, and regenerate relationships to the land (Corntassel, 2012).

Adopting anti-colonial practice allows ecosocial work to further support Indigenous communities as they resist climate change and lead environmental movements such as the Dakota Access Pipeline resistance at Standing Rock. As ecosocial work further develops, many practitioners will grapple with not only learning from Indigenous and marginalized communities, but intentionally following the lead of those communities, especially elders and the knowledges they hold. Social workers are trained to serve as bridges between diverse stakeholders and to reduce oppressive power dynamics between professionals and communities (CASW, 2005; NASW, 2017). In order to do so, ecosocial workers must examine their own role in colonialism and resist re-enacting it in their practice. Acknowledging that social workers are part of multiple, intersecting complex systems includes recognizing that we are never acting upon a system as an outside agent; rather, we are always a part of that system (Chandler, 2014). Locating ourselves within systems of power, including colonization, requires critical reflexivity (Hart et al., 2017).

Anti-colonialism and ecosocial work share the outlook that addressing global environmental change necessitates further examination of interlocking oppressions. Addressing the root causes of the climate crisis is essential to building resilience and achieving climate justice (Cretney, 2014; Hornborg, 2013; Movement Generation, 2013). Further, addressing root causes includes marginalized communities being able to provide for their own needs in their own way (Hart, 2009), so that they are not vulnerable to white supremacist economic coercion (Nembhard, 2014; Waziyatawin, 2012; White, 2017). Anti-colonial practice supports CSS, which enables effective collective action and social movements led by frontline communities.

Conclusion

We offer CSS as a framework by which to understand practices that have sustained communities who have experienced colonization, enslavement, exploitation, and oppression. CSS guide us to a way of living in right relationship with the Earth. Doing so is essential to building resilience (Cretney, 2014) and realigns our loyalty to the actual basis of life, the Earth, rather than a fossil fuel-powered industrial society (Waziyatawin, 2012). The de-sanctification of nature is both a key strategy of colonization and a key cause of ecological crises (Waziyatawin, 2012). In restoring communities' abilities to live in right relationship with the Earth, CSS enact climate mitigation and adaptation on a micro-scale. Anti-colonial practice is a framework that encourages CSS and guides us in living in right relationship with each other. As ecosocial work embraces traditional environmental knowledges, considering how mainstream social work and academia more broadly, as settler-imposed institutions (Hart et al., 2017), have constricted Indigenous knowledges and cultures is vital, particularly as settler colonialism already caused a climate change dystopia for Indigenous people. Anti-colonial social work offers a framework for addressing the root causes of environmental crisis and enabling collective survival.

Notes

1. We use global environmental change and environmental (or ecological) crisis to refer to the current large-scale changes that our planet is experiencing due to primarily human causes, including climate change. When authors cite climate change specifically, as does Whyte (2016, 2017), we follow their language.
2. We define and use Indigenous as: The diverse peoples who originally inhabited a particular place (in North America, this includes people referred to as Native American, American Indian/Alaska Native, and Aboriginal), whose culture, way of life, and knowledge systems developed in relationship to that place, and who are the targets of colonial logic to destroy and replace in settler colonial societies (adapted from Brewer & Dennis, 2017).
3. Relationships and daily subsistence practices.

Disclosure statement

No potential conflict of interest was reported by the authors.

ORCID

Amy Krings ⓘ http://orcid.org/0000-0001-5499-5101

References

Alfred, T. (2009). Colonialism and state dependency. *Journal of Aboriginal Health, 5*, 42–60.
Bandele, O., & Myers, G. (2016). Roots of black agrarianism. *Dismantling Racism in the Food System, 4*, 1–7. Oakland, CA: Institute for Food and Development Policy.
Billiot, S., Beltran, R., Teyra, C., Fernandez, A., Black, J. C., Brown, D., … Walters, K. (2017, January). *Strengthening social responses to global environmental changes grand challenge: An indigenous approach.* Roundtable conducted at Society for Social Work and Research Annual Conference, New Orleans.
Boetto, H. (2018). Transformative ecosocial work: Incorporating being, thinking, and doing in practice. In M. Pawar, W. Bowles, & K. Bell (Eds.), *Social work: Innovations and insights* [Google Book Version]. Retrieved from. https://books.google.com/books?hl=en&id= Lh9sDwAA QBAJ&oi=fnd&pg=PT114&ots=eGD6c6cRop&sig= I0IpDGYNkMhYfpHw4D4fd7jJ8fc
Boonstra, W. J. (2016). Conceptualizing power to study social-ecological interactions. *Ecology and Society, 21*(1), 21–32. doi:10.5751/ES-07966-210121
Brewer, J. P., & Dennis, M. K. (2017). An offering: Lakota elders' contributions to the future of food security. *Journal of Indigenous Social Development, 6*(2), 1–22.
Brewer, J. P., & Dennis, M. K. (2019). A land neither here nor there: Voices from the margins & the untenuring of Lakota lands. *GeoJournal, 84*(3),571 - 591.
Canadian Association of Social Workers. (2005). *Code of ethics.* Retrieved from https://www. casw-acts.ca/en/Code-of-Ethics
Case, R. A. (2017). Community resilience and eco-social work practice: Insights from water activism in Guelph, Ontario, Canada. *Journal of Social Work, 17*(4), 391–412. doi:10.1177/ 1468017316644695
Chandler, D. (2014). Beyond neoliberalism: resilience, the new art of governing complexity. *Resilience, 2*(1), 47–63. doi:10.1080/21693293.2013.878544
Corntassel, J. (2012). Re-envisioning resurgence: Indigenous pathways to decolonization and sustainable self-determination. *Decolonization: Indigeneity, Education & Society, 1*(1), 81–101.
Cretney, R. (2014). Resilience for whom? Emerging critical geographies of socio-ecological resilience. *Geography Compass, 8*(9), 627–640. doi:10.1111/gec3.v8.9
Dater, A., & Merton, L. (2008). *Taking root: The vision of Wangari Maathai* [Motion Picture]. United States: Independent Lens.
Davoudi, S., Brooks, E., & Mehmood, A. (2013). Evolutionary resilience and strategies for climate adaptation. *Planning, Practice and Research, 28*(3), 307–322. doi:10.1080/ 02697459.2013.787695
Fabinyi, M., Evans, L., & Foale, S. J. (2014). Social-ecological systems, social diversity, and power: insights from anthropology and political ecology. *Ecology and Society, 19*(4), 28–39. doi:10.5751/ES-07029-190428
Gray, M., Coates, J., & Hetherington, T. (2007). Hearing indigenous voices in mainstream social work. *Families in Society, 88*(1), 55–66. doi:10.1606/1044-3894.3592
Hart, K., Rowe, G., Hart, M. A., Pompana, Y., Halonen, D., Cook, G., … Coggins, K. (2014). A proposed master of social work based in indigenous knowledges program in Manitoba. *Journal of Indigenous Social Development, 3*(2), 1–18.

Hart, M. A. (2009). Anti-colonial Indigenous social work: Reflections on an Aboriginal approach. In G. Bruyere, M. A. Hart, & R. Sinclair (Eds.), *Wicihitowin: Aboriginal social work in Canada* (pp. 25–41). Halifax, Canada: Fernwood Pub.

Hart, M. A., Straka, S., & Rowe, G. (2017). Working across contexts: Practical considerations of doing Indigenist/anti-colonial research. *Qualitative Inquiry, 23*(5), 332–342. doi:10.1177/1077800416659084

Hornborg, A. (2013). Revelations of resilience: From the ideological disarmament of disaster to the revolutionary implications of (p)anarchy. *Resilience, 1*(2), 116–129. doi:10.1080/21693293.2013.797661

Ingalls, M. L., & Stedman, R. C. (2016). The power problematic: exploring the uncertain terrains of political ecology and the resilience framework. *Ecology and Society, 21*(1), 6–16. doi:10.5751/ES-08124-210106

Intergovernmental Panel on Climate Change. (2018, October 8). *Summary for policymakers of IPCC special report on global warming of 1.5°C approved by governments* [Press Release]. Retrieved from https://www.ipcc.ch/pdf/session48/pr_181008_P48_spm_en.pdf

Klinenberg, E. (2015). *Heat wave: A social autopsy of disaster in Chicago.* Chicago, IL: University of Chicago Press.

Krings, A., Kornberg, D., & Lane, E. (2019). Organizing under austerity: How residents' concerns became the Flint Water Crisis. *Critical Sociology, 45*(4–5), 583–597. doi:10.1177/0896920518757053

Krings, A., Spencer, M. S., & Jimenez, K. (2014). Organizing for environmental justice: From bridges to taro patches. In S. Dutta & C. Ramanathan (Eds.), *Governance, development, and social work* (pp. 186–200). New York, NY: Routledge.

Krings, A., & Thomas, H. (2018). Integrating green social work and the U.S. environmental justice movement: An introduction to community benefits agreements. In L. Dominelli (Ed.), *The Routledge handbook of green social work* (pp. 397–406). New York, NY: Routledge.

Krings, A., Victor, B. G., Mathias, J., & Perron, B. E. (2018). Environmental social work in the disciplinary literature, 1991 – 2015. *International Social Work,* 002087281878839. doi:10.1177/0020872818788397

Mason, L. R., Shires, M. K., Arwood, C., & Borst, A. (2017). Social work research and global environmental change. *Journal of the Society for Social Work and Research, 8*(4), 645–672. doi:10.1086/694789

Movement Generation. (2013). *The work of love and the love of work: Resilience-based organizing as a path forward.* Retrieved from https://movementgeneration.org/wp-content/uploads/2014/03/WorkOfLoveAndLoveOfWork.pdf

Mullaly, R. (1997). *Structural social work.* Toronto, Canada: Oxford University Press.

Närhi, K., & Matthies, A.-L. (2016). Conceptual and historical analysis of ecological social work. In J. McKinnon & M. Alston (Eds.), *Ecological social work: Towards sustainability* (pp. 21–38). London, UK: Palgrave MacMillan.

National Association of Social Workers. (2017). *Preamble to the code of ethics.* Retrieved from https://www.socialworkers.org/About/Ethics/Code-of-Ethics/Code-of-Ethics-English

Nembhard, J. G. (2014). *Collective courage: A history of African American cooperative economic thought and practice.* University Park, PA: Penn State University Press.

Norton, C. L. (2012). Social work and the environment: An ecosocial approach. *International Journal of Social Welfare, 21*(3), 299–308. doi:10.1111/j.1468-2397.2011.00853.x

Peeters, J. (2012a). Social work and sustainable development. Towards a social-ecological practice model. *Journal of Social Intervention: Theory and Practice, 21*(3), 5–26.

Peeters, J. (2012b). The place of social work in sustainable development: Towards ecosocial practice. *International Journal of Social Welfare, 21*(3), 287–298. doi:10.1111/j.1468-2397.2011.00856.x

Peña, D. G. (2005). Autonomy, equity, and environmental justice. In D. N. Pellow & R. J. Brulle (Eds.), *Power, justice, and the environment: A critical appraisal of the environmental justice movement* (pp. 131–151). Cambridge, MA: MIT Press.

Quizar, J. (2018). Working to live: Black-led farming in Detroit's racialized economy. In L. Nishime & K. D. Hester Williams (Eds.), *Racial ecologies* (pp. 76–89). Seattle, WA: University of Washington.

Ramsay, S., & Boddy, J. (2017). Environmental social work: A concept analysis. *The British Journal of Social Work*, *47*(1), 68–86.

Said, E. W. (2012). *Culture and Imperialism*. New York, NY: Random House.

Schneider-Mayerson, M. (2015). *Peak oil: Apocalyptic environmentalism and libertarian political culture*. Chicago, IL: University of Chicago Press.

Sharpe, C. (2016). *In the wake: On blackness and being*. Durham, NC: Duke University Press.

Smith, L. (1999). *Decolonizing methodologies: Indigenous peoples and research*. New York, NY: Zed Books.

Teixeira, S., & Krings, A. (2015). Sustainable social work: An environmental justice framework for social work education. *Social Work Education*, *34*(5), 513–527. doi:10.1080/02615479.2015.1063601

Thornton, R. (2000). Population history of native North Americans. In M. R. Haines & R. H. Steckel (Eds.), *A population history of North America* (pp. 12–50). Cambridge, UK: Cambridge University Press.

Tierney, K. (2015). Resilience and the neoliberal project: Discourses, critiques, practices—and Katrina. *American Behavioral Scientist*, *59*(10), 1327–1342. doi:10.1177/0002764215591187

Ungar, M., Ghazinour, M., & Richter, J. (2013). Annual research review: What is resilience within the social ecology of human development? *Journal of Child Psychology and Psychiatry*, *54*(4), 348–366. doi:10.1111/jcpp.12025

Vrasti, W., & Michelsen, N. (2017). Introduction: On resilience and solidarity. *Resilience*, *5* (1), 1–9. doi:10.1080/21693293.2016.1228155

Walsh-Dilley, M., Wolford, W., & McCarthy, J. (2016). Rights for resilience: Food sovereignty, power, and resilience in development practice. *Ecology & Society*, *21*(1), 11–20. doi:10.5751/ES-07981-210111

Waziyatawin. (2012). The paradox of Indigenous resurgence at the end of empire. *Decolonization: Indigeneity, Education & Society*, *1*(1), 68–85.

White, M. M. (2011). D-Town Farm: African American resistance to food insecurity and the transformation of Detroit. *Environmental Practice*, *13*(4), 406–417. doi:10.1017/S1466046611000408

White, M. M. (2017). "A pig and a garden": Fannie lou hamer and the freedom farms cooperative. *Food and Foodways*, *25*(1), 20–39. doi:10.1080/07409710.2017.1270647

Whyte, K., Caldwell, C., & Schaefer, M. (2018). Indigenous lessons about sustainability are not just for "all humanity.". In J. Sze (Ed.), *Sustainability: Approaches to environmental justice and social power* (pp. 149–179). New York, NY: NYU Press.

Whyte, K. P. (2016). Is it colonial déjà vu? Indigenous peoples and climate injustice. In J. Adamson, M. Davis, & H. Huang (Eds.), *Humanities for the environment: Integrating knowledges, forging new constellations of practice* (pp. 88–104). New York, NY: Routledge.

Whyte, K. P. (2017). Indigenous climate change studies: Indigenizing futures, decolonizing the Anthropocene. *English Language Notes*, *55*(1–2), 153–162. doi:10.1215/00138282-55.1-2.153

Wolfe, P. (2006). Settler colonialism and the elimination of the native. *Journal of Genocide Research*, *8*(4), 387–409. doi:10.1080/14623520601056240

Indigenous perspectives for strengthening social responses to global environmental changes: A response to the social work grand challenge on environmental change

Shanondora Billiot, Ramona Beltrán, Danica Brown, Felicia M. Mitchell ⓘ, and Angela Fernandez

ABSTRACT
The "Grand Challenges for Social Work," is a call to action for innovative responses to society's most pressing social problems. In this article, we respond to the "Grand Challenge" of *Creating Social Responses to a Changing Environment* from our perspective as Indigenous scholars. Over the last several decades, diminishing natural resources, pollution, over-consumption, and the exploitation of the natural environment have led to climate change events that disproportionately affect Indigenous peoples. We present how environmental changes impact Indigenous peoples and suggest culturally relevant responses for working with Indigenous communities. We propose a decolonizing cyclical, iterative process grounded in Indigenous Ways of Knowing.

Introduction

Positioned as the "wicked problem" of the 21st-century environmental change is projected to impact all forms of life on earth (Moran, 2010). Global environmental changes include human-induced shifts in the earth's long-term climatic cycle that influence climate change, repeated weather-based disasters, and technological disasters (Moran, 2010). Common anthropogenic causes of environmental change include human population growth, material and resource consumption, energy and land use, and pollution (Ford, 2012; Moran, 2010). While all humans are exposed to the effects of climate, some individuals and communities are disproportionately vulnerable to environmental changes due to their social, economic, and geographic characteristics (Moran, 2010). For instance, Indigenous peoples are particularly susceptible to and affected by climate change due to their close ties to the land and its resources.

Historically, humans were adept at observing, interpreting, and adapting to climate changes in their surrounding environment (McLean, 2010). As societies began to modernize, many cultures experienced a separation from the natural environment and the subsistence lifestyles of generations past. However, many Indigenous peoples remain connected to the land and maintain an understanding of the seasons despite their shared experiences of colonization, forced assimilation, and removal and relocation from their traditional lands; all of which attempted to sever their ties with the land (McLean, 2010; Walters, Beltran, Huh, & Evans-Campbell, 2011; Wildcat, 2009). In recent decades, Indigenous peoples have observed and documented changes in climate through warming temperatures, fluctuations in water quantity and quality, biodiversity loss, coastal erosion, uncharacteristic weather patterns, melting and thinning of snow, ice, and permafrost, as well as pollution (Ford et al., 2014; Furgal & Seguin, 2006; Tam, Gough, Edwards, & Tsuji, 2013). Indigenous peoples manage, use, or occupy nearly 22% of the Earth's land surface(McLean, 2010). In other words, approximately 6% of the world's population maintains about 80% of the world's biodiversity (McLean, 2010), which highlights the importance of acknowledging Indigenous peoples' observations and insights to changes in the environment.

The root causes of environmental issues faced by Indigenous peoples are intimately tied to remarkably similar histories of colonization and ongoing neo-colonial processes. These changes manifest differently among Indigenous peoples but occur consistently across the globe (McLean, 2010).[1] Global environmental change affects Indigenous peoples' livelihood strategies, local knowledge, and their physical and mental health both directly and indirectly (Cunsolo Willox et al., 2012; Snodgrass, 2013). Indigenous peoples' vulnerability to climate change often manifests through food insecurity, changes in traditional knowledge, and the need for climate adaptation and management of environmental resources (Ford, 2012).

In 2015, the American Academy for Social Work and Social Welfare launched the "Grand Challenges for Social Work," which is a call to action for innovative responses to the most pressing contemporary social problems. *Strengthening the Social Response to the Human Impacts of Environmental Change Grand Challenge* identifies four challenges to social justice that social work should have an essential role in addressing, these include: disaster preparedness and response, population dislocation, community-based adaptation, and mitigation (Kemp & Palinkas, 2015). Kemp and Palinkas (2015) suggest that existing social work activities could address these challenges through core activities of social work practice: 1. Intervention development 2. Implementation 3. Coordination, and 4. Education. In this article, we expand the discourse on the grand challenge titled, *Creating Social*

Responses to a Changing Environment Grand Challenge, by presenting an Indigenous perspective of how social work can integrate Indigenous Knowledge into the core activities. Further, we provide case studies of these core activities in social work education, fieldwork, and research.

As Indigenous scholars, we have a unique perspective about traditional knowledge based on sophisticated Indigenous epistemologies that center on place and connection to the land. As such, we provide context to the Grand Challenges on the impact of environmental changes on Indigenous peoples by highlighting anthropogenic causes of environmental disparities and appropriate responses from an Indigenous perspective. We also seek to enhance community practice by illuminating culturally centered solutions that originate from our Indigenous communities and can offer practical strategies for bringing these culture-centered solutions into the social work profession. In this paper, we provide a summary of Indigenous ontology and epistemology as it relates to land and place. Next, we give an overview of the impacts of environmental change and historically traumatic events on Indigenous peoples globally. The last two sections, proposed solutions and case studies, are from a U.S.-based Indigenous perspective as we are all U.S. Indigenous scholars and limit our case studies to communities whose stories we have permission to share. As the social work profession develops a deeper understanding of these ways of being and doing, social workers can illuminate entry points for action toward environmental justice and balance for Indigenous peoples and beyond.

Indigenous peoples connection to land

A profound relationship with the land is fundamental to Indigenous cosmology, epistemology, and lived experience. Many Indigenous communities view the land[2] as a relative and describe it with familial reverence (e.g., mother earth, pacha mama, tonantzin). From creation stories to the concept of the interconnectedness of all things, Indigenous peoples embody socio-cultural earth-based ethics and values that inform daily ceremonial and sustainability practices relating to ecological management as well as social, familial, and intimate relationships. Indigenous scholars and community members developed conceptual frameworks, such as Traditional Ecological Knowledge (TEK) (Pierotti & Wildcat, 2000), Sacred Ecology (Sheridan & Longboat, 2006), and Indigenous Knowledge (IK) (Simpson, 2004), that considers the fundamental care and sophisticated understanding of the relationship between humans and the rest of creation (Pierotti & Wildcat, 2000; Simpson, 2004). For this paper, we will focus on incorporating IK into practices within social work classrooms, field, and research.

Indigenous Knowledge is a community knowledge base of TEK and Sacred Ecology that is informed by places from which the community originates and believes in a spiritual, intimate relationship with the land that is not one of personal ownership but of love and reverence between the land and humankind (Settee, 2008). IK allows communities to survives because of the core virtue that nature and humans are dependent upon each other for existence (Pierotti & Wildcat, 2000). IK was formed through generations of multi-disciplinary, empirical Indigenous observations of the natural world, is grounded in place and provides theory and the praxis of both politics and ethics for many Indigenous communities (Pierotti & Wildcat, 2000). While place-based knowledge is rooted in original lands specific and unique to tribal groups, *IK acknowledges that this knowledge is also embodied and transportable.* Through forced relocation as well as voluntary migration, Indigenous peoples have maintained the ties and knowledge connected to their original lands, which contributes to their survival (Walters et al., 2011). As such, recognizing the importance of Indigenous knowledge through connection to place can help community social workers to address challenges of environmental changes.

The relationship between settler-colonialism and environmental changes

Extensive government reports and emerging empirical literature document Indigenous peoples observations and experiences of environmental changes and strategies used to mitigate or adapt to these changes (see McLean, 2010; United Nations, 2008). As noted earlier, environmental changes are occurring globally but expressed differently and at varying magnitude by region and locality. Indigenous peoples across the Arctic, Africa, Australia, and Latin America observe warming temperatures and deforestation creating changes to their food and water quality, access and availability (Berrang-Ford et al., 2012; Cunsolo Willox et al., 2012; Healey et al., 2011; Hofmeijer et al., 2013). Also, changes in wildlife and vegetation patterns, subsistence agriculture and forest health creates both food insecurity and water insecurity (Brubaker, Berner, Chavan, & Warren, 2011; Hofmeijer et al., 2013). In the United States, anthropogenic activities creating environmental changes are activities related to natural resource extraction (such as daming, drilling, and dredging), population growth and pervasive consumerism culture (Moran, 2010).

In the following section, we transition from a global perspective of Indigenous peoples to an United States (U.S.) Indigenous perspective. We include a review of historical trauma to emphasize the link between settler-colonialism activities and environmental changes from first European contact with U.S. Indigenous peoples. Settler-colonialism is the process of erasing

Indigenous peoples presence, history, and meaning through population control, sovereignty, consciousness, and narrative (Veracini, 2010). In the U.S., erasure continues through exposure to environmental toxins and changes primarily through natural resource extraction.

Natural resource extraction creating environmental changes

Five% of oil, 10% of gas reserves, 30% of low sulfur coal reserves, and 40% of privately held uranium deposits, are located on American Indian reservations (American Indian Resource Center, n.d.). The most prolific and contemporary examples include the Peabody Energy Company (Women's Earth Alliance, 2014); the Fort Berthold Reservation (Tuti & Northern, 2015); and Energy Transfer Partners (Energy Transfer Partners, 2014).

Peabody Energy Company, the world's largest mining company, a strip-mining operation in Black Mesa, has depleted the watershed of the Hopi and Navajo Nations' area, severely impacting the use of water for drinking and sheep farming (Women's Earth Alliance, 2014). This project is an agreement between the Tribes and Peabody Energy, which provided an unusually generous mineral lease. The Peabody Energy company's use and degradation of a potable source of water continue to have a significant impact on tribal people's access to clean water that has also affected their ability to engage in traditional agriculture and herding practices. Additionally, the transport of coal via a pipeline from the mine to a power plant hundreds of miles away has created a public health and environmental impacts of strip mining on tribal lands.

The Fort Berthold Reservation, of the confederated tribes of the Mandan, Hidatsa, and Arikara Nations, has become a center of oil extraction in North Dakota where over 35 corporations extract natural resources from their territory (Tuti & Northern, 2015), commonly known as the Bakken Tar Sands Project. Bakken's shale oil extraction comes at a high environmental price, as it has a substantial impact on water resources, land use, wildlife and habitat, and on the fabric of tribal communities. For every gallon of gasoline made from tar sands, 5.9 gallons of fresh water are used for extraction and processing – that is three times more resources needed than for traditional oil (Wu, Mintz, Wang, & Arora, 2009). Although the oil boom has contributed to financial stability for local tribes, it also created new social and environmental justice issues.

The Dakota Access Pipeline (DAPL) is a $3.8 billion project that transfers shale oil from the Bakken Tar Sands project in Canada to Louisiana and then transferred to other countries for production. The pipeline crosses significant water sources, including the Missouri and Mississippi Rivers, as well as Indigenous lands such as the Standing Rock Sioux Reservation (Partners, 2014). Despite significant protest from tribal communities along the pipeline,

DAPL has been transferring shale oil from the Bakken fields at a rate of over 500,000 barrels per day, with plans for expansion through additional tribal lands. Energy Transfer Partners continues construction of this controversial project, despite knowing they are destroying traditional sacred lands and burial sites (Wells, 2017). In particular, the environmental impact statement for the Enbridge Line 3 project in Minnesota has stressed that damages to tribal natural and cultural resources along that pipeline's pathway are "not quantifiable" and "cannot be mitigated" due to recorded five leaks in 2017 (Minnesota Commerce Department, 2019). April 2019 DAPL leaked 168-gallons in Patoka, Illinois.

Beyond the environmental and economic impacts on Indigenous communities, natural resource extraction, and other anthropogenic activities creating environmental changes are impacting the health and wellbeing of Indigenous peoples. Addressing current removal and land exploitation efforts require developing interventions that understand and disrupt structural and symbolic societal norms that equate Indigenous communities as deserving of removal (Holmes, 2013). Developing effective community-engaged interventions first requires a nuanced look at the impacts of the settler-colonialism on Indigenous peoples. Adverse consequences of colonization on Indigenous health, well-being, and sovereignty, is also understood within the context of historical trauma, which began with the colonial pursuit of Indigenous land and natural resources.

Historical trauma

In contrast to Western biomedical understandings of health as the absence of individual psychological disturbances and disease, Indigenous peoples conceptualize health as a holistic connection between physical, emotional, mental, and spiritual dimensions, as well as connectedness with the natural environment (Vukic, Gregory, Martin-Misener, & Etowa, 2011).

Historical trauma, defined as collective and cumulative trauma across generations is attributable to large-scale events targeted at a specific community (Brave Heart, 2003; Evans-Campbell & Walters, 2006), has played a crucial role in severing cultural connections. Historically traumatic events refer to specific acts that cause extensive destruction to a group or community (Evans-Campbell, 2008). These events, either acute (e.g., targeted massacre) or persistent (e.g., policies that are enacted over time) can be physical, spiritual, and also environmental (Walters, Mohammed et al., 2011). Mass genocide, the introduction of disease, and federal policies aimed at land grabbing Indigenous territories resulted in an estimated loss of millions of lives, long-term rates of population decline, reduced fertility and increased infant mortality (Thornton, 1997). According to one estimate, as many as 90% of the Indigenous population died in the 1700s – from 100 million to

10 million people (Dunbar-Ortiz, 2015). Indigenous people were coerced into migrations that interrupted their relationships with culture, spirituality, and land (Walters, Beltran et al., 2011). Persistent and ongoing traumatic events exacerbate the cumulative impact of historical trauma at multiple levels, through environmental dispossession,[3] disproportionally high rates of violence against Native women, and racial discrimination including microaggressions and cultural appropriation of sacred Indigenous regalia and objects (Evans-Campbell, 2008). Together, the interaction of such historical and contemporary traumas are collectively defined as colonial trauma (Evans-Campbell, 2008).

Stress & trauma embodiment

The multiple forms of colonial trauma previously discussed were designed to disrupt Indigenous peoples' relationship with place through land loss and destruction that limit access to healthy land environments (Walters, Beltran et al., 2011). Such traumatic events can become cumulative stressors, resulting in the embodiment of stress and trauma, contributing to adverse health consequences (Walters, Beltran et al., 2011). Krieger (2005) conceptualizes embodiment as a biological incorporation of social and ecological events – such as colonial traumas like racism or displacement, as well as responses of resilience. For many Indigenous people, the ontology of place claims that humans are part of the land and hold obligations to it, as it does to humans in mutual reciprocity (Coulthard, 2010). Given such intimate, interdependent relationships between health and place for many Indigenous people (Vukic et al., 2011; Walters, Mohammed et al., 2011), disruptions to these relationships are linked to both physical and mental health outcomes that can manifest in poor health outcomes across generations (Krieger & Davey Smith, 2004; Walters et al., 2011).

Poor physical health outcomes can specifically be linked to federal assimilation policies that result in displacement, land loss, restrictions on land usage, and disruption of traditional agricultural practices. Loss of connection with the land is central to dramatic dietary changes, mental health, and sedentary lifestyles (Billiot, Kwon, & Burnette, 2019; Ford, 2012). Food insecurity is linked to several health disparities, such as alarming rates of diabetes, obesity, and heart disease among Indigenous people in the U.S. (First Nations Development Institute, 2013). Similarly, poor mental health outcomes can be linked to boarding school attendance and the prohibition of participation in spiritual and cultural practices (many of which are place-based). Such restrictions also played a significant role in systematically attacking traditional means of stress-coping, reducing opportunities for the intergenerational transmission of Indigenous knowledge and engagement in activities that are perceived as buffers from stress and illness (Billiot, Kwon,

& Burnette, 2019b). Individual and collective responses to such historically traumatic events may include high rates of depression, anxiety, substance abuse, and other forms of somatization (Evans-Campbell, 2008; Evans-Campbell & Walters, 2006). For many Indigenous peoples, preserving relationships with place and adapting to environmental changes through transmitting Indigenous knowledge about place relationships is essential. Thus, for many American Indians, whose identities are rooted in the sense of personal identity within a relational (i.e., human, environment) context, knowledge of and connection with place may be a crucial part of health and well-being. The next section will provide suggestions for working with Indigenous people to address environmental changes in ways that are grounded in Indigenous knowledge–knowledge integral to the health and well-being not only of Indigenous people but also of the planet.

Proposed social work responses to environmental changes with Indigenous communities

In this section, we propose how to utilize IK in social work research and practice to understand the natural world and our relation to it. Addressing the challenges of environmental changes with Indigenous communities begins with a broad societal movement away from western science and toward a holistic and ethical paradigm in order to create opportunities for effective and productive collaboration. It is in this perspective that we propose a cyclical and iterative Indigenous worldview of social work solutions to addressing environmental changes based on Linda Tuhiwai Smith's Indigenous Research Agenda and the medicine wheel conceptualized in many American Indian and Alaska Native communities (Smith, 2012) (Figure 1). Incorporating IK into mainstream education, healing through

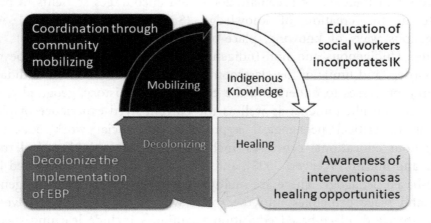

Figure 1. Indigenous worldview of social work activities to address environmental changes.

intervention development, decolonizing implementation activities, and mobilizing communities for coordination activities promotes holistic approaches to addressing environmental changes and reiterates tribal communities' self-determination (Lucero, 2011).

Education utilizing indigenous knowledge

Establishing environmental education programs based on Indigenous knowledge is essential to fortify culture, build up environmental protection practices, and promote sustainability in local and tribal economies (Simpson, 2004). Developing these programs with and for Indigenous communities also empowers Indigenous students to decolonize[4] and heal from legacies of western education and colonial processes related to land exploitation. It also allows non-Indigenous students to learn about the damage of these legacies and assists them in identifying ways to disrupt ongoing colonial land occupation and exploitation. Understood through the fundamental Indigenous ecological concept of interconnectedness, the benefits of Indigenous knowledge in education are inclusive and expansive. The necessary components of Indigenous environmental education programs include involving Elders in all processes of program development and implementation as well as a commitment to a consistent process and evaluation of decolonizing for students and teachers (Simpson, 2004). Based on land and place principles, Indigenous environmental education offers concrete and practical approaches to education that appreciates the role of Elders and community knowledge systems, the importance of developing a relationship to the land, and the process of decolonizing from Western education practices.

Place-based education principles emphasize experiential, hands-on engagement with local and regional places, communities, and the natural environment (Semken & Freeman, 2008) and encourages students to participate in the creation of knowledge (Smith, 2002). Consistent with Indigenous ways of knowing, place-based education allows students and teachers (Indigenous and non-Indigenous) the freedom to explore beyond the borders and limits of the classroom, prescriptive textbooks, and didactic learning processes to understand the complexity of history, geography, and socio-cultural phenomena, as well as the current lived-experience of place. Similar to critical pedagogical approaches for social work education, Indigenous educational processes, including collective thinking, oral traditions, and holism (Weaver, 2008), and are valued and easily integrated into place-based pedagogy. There are multiple strategies for bringing Indigenous land and place principles into the social work classroom. Innovative yet straightforward, place-based education techniques include learning specific local geographic history (e.g. learning the original peoples of a region), group field trips, engagement with community members, stakeholders, and Indigenous experts, consideration of the group and self as related to place for greater ecological consciousness and corresponding practice skills (Beltrán, Hacker, & Begun, 2016). Such efforts, as described, build critical thinking skills needed to understand sociocultural influences on maintaining traditional ecological knowledge and motivates community members to begin to create social networks (Sullivan & Syvertsen, 2018). They also disrupt many of the historical colonial narratives that have omitted Indigenous history from educational spaces.

Coordination through mobilizing communities

In response to environmental changes, Indigenous communities are taking collective action through mobilization. Decolonizing community mobilizing efforts challenges the silo mentality by calling attention to the interconnectedness of the physical, social, spiritual, and emotional ways of knowing and relating to the environment to address the causes of suffering (Smith, 2012). Indigenous community mobilizing efforts are activities *within* Indigenous communities rather than *for* them.

Indigenous groups are documenting long-term changes in their local climates, such as noticeable changes in the timing of the seasons and changes in snowfall and precipitation (Doyle, Redsteer, & Eggers, 2013). In response, Indigenous communities are continually utilizing adaptive strategies to respond to environmental change in their communities (Cozzetto et al., 2013; Tam et al., 2013). Without national climate change policies in the United States, U.S. tribal governments are developing climate change policies and adaption strategic plans to address natural resource management (Billiot & Parfait, 2019). Social workers can participate in these activities through mobilizing communities for planning and advocacy. To do this, researchers, governments, and organizations who wish to partner with tribal and marginalized communities should develop an awareness of traditional ecological knowledge, acknowledgment that environmental injustices today are re-traumatization of historical colonization efforts, and honor tribal sovereignty & and community individuality.

Interventions begin with healing

Intervention development that recognizes Indigenous conceptions of resilience begin with healing. Mainstream literature regards resilience as sustained and healthy functioning when faced with adversity (Southwick, Bonanno, Masten, Panter-Brick, & Yehuda, 2014). For Indigenous people, however, resilience is defined contextually and holistically, as "a dynamic process of social and psychological adaptation and transformation … characteristic of individuals, families, communities or larger social groups and is manifested as positive outcomes in the face of historical and current stresses" (Kirmayer, Dandeneau, Marshall, Phillips, & Williamson, 2011). Resilience is also an ongoing resistance to social and structural barriers of the dominant society (Kirmayer et al., 2011), a form of "survivance" characterized by Indigenous individual and collective capacities to persist in the face of colonially imposed adversities (Vizenor, 2008). Resistance for Indigenous people is a coping mechanism for persisting in the face of colonial oppression through maintaining Indigenous identity, ontology, and lifeways (Caxaj, Berman, Ray, Restoule, & Varcoe, 2014). Foundations of Indigenous resistance are identified as healthy families, grounding in community, connection to land, language, storytelling, and spirituality, and their interrelationships (Cunsolo Willox, Harper, & Edge, 2013). Social work can build upon specific examples of resistance to develop therapies or interventions that assist in changing personal narratives of health, the continuation of Indigenous cultural and spiritual lifeways, opposition to racial discrimination and the racialization of place, and embracing and protecting Indigenous ontology and identity (Caxaj et al., 2014; Vizenor, 2008). Understanding and honoring Indigenous definitions of historical trauma and healing is crucial in each step of community-engaged development and implementation of culturally congruent environmental change adaptation and mitigation interventions and policies.

Decolonizing implementation activities

Leading Indigenous scholars point out that there is a lack of consensus regarding the process of cultural adaptation of evidence-based practices with Indigenous communities (Weaver, 2008; Wilson, 2004). Some scholars argue that in order to decolonize science, evidence should begin within the Indigenous community through the communities' cultural ways of knowing and expression. Others counter that cultural adaptation is possible and advocate for a mixed methods approach of Indigenous knowledge expression and western science. Regardless of one's stance on the appropriateness of evidence-based practices, it is crucial to recognize the notion of evidence-based practice is a western concept developed through a specific set of values regarding the theoretical development, measurement, and other forms of acquiring knowledge that is considered "evidence." Social worker techniques (e.g., reflexivity), which recognize power and privilege, acknowledge Indigenous rights and knowledge are key to decolonizing implementation activities (Briskman, 2008).

Proposed solutions summary

Incorporating Indigenous knowledge can enhance social work's efforts to develop social responses to global environmental changes. The framework presented above provides a decolonized perspective of core social work activities that are iterative and nonlinear approaches to working with Indigenous and marginalized communities who are impacted by environmental changes. In the following section, we present case studies of applying these practices in social work education, field, and research.

Case studies

Indigenous knowledge in the classroom: place-based education, University of Denver and the sand creek massacre

Arguably, all land in North America is occupied Indigenous territory. From all of the historical and current examples described above, there has been a multitude of ways that Indigenous peoples have been stripped of their inherent rights to their original lands and territories. If we merely dig into the historical record of the places where our classrooms stand, we can often make connections to these histories. Accordingly, we illuminate the historically anchored and ongoing institutional occupation of Indigenous land and implicate ourselves and our students in need to demand institutional accountability, shift the mythological narratives of American exceptionalism, and co-create new (old) knowledge in solidarity Indigenous communities toward environmental justice and sustainability. One of the key concepts embedded in historical trauma theory is the idea that narrative can buffer the impacts of historically traumatic events on health, mental health, and social outcomes (Beltrán, Hacker, & Begun, 2016; Evans-Campbell, 2008). As we collaborate in communities, our institutions, as well as our social work classrooms, have the opportunity to engage in historical truth-telling that will re-cast deliberately obscured narratives and, optimally, point us toward disciplinary leadership in creating policies and practices that leverage Indigenous knowledge rather than marginalize it. Utilizing the place-based education techniques described above, social work educators can combine narrative and experiential learning to engage students in critical learning about the inextricably linked experiences of colonial violence, settler occupation, and environmental injustice.

The University of Denver is located in Denver, Colorado, the traditional homelands of Cheyenne, Arapaho, and Ute tribes. In 2014, the University of Denver John Evans Committee released a report on the role of the university's founder, John Evans, in the events leading up to the Sand Creek Massacre[5]. In response, a faculty-led committee, led by Nancy Wadsworth, worked with descendant members of Cheyenne and Arapaho tribes, Sand Creek historians, and Native community members to bring this previously hidden history into the classroom to educate students on the ways our educational institutions are deeply implicated in historical colonial violence as well as current settler occupation (see Clemmer-Smith et al., 2014). Combining this historical truth-telling with place-based experiential activities that encourage students to consider the deep connections of land and place to historical and ongoing colonial trauma facilitates a deep and embodied learning that, ultimately (hopefully), promotes action toward social and environmental justice.

Graduate social work students at the University of Denver explore these connections through field trips that focus on engaging with the places these events occurred. Although colonial violence is written on this land, students are encouraged to consider the ways that Native and marginalized peoples also write their own narratives on the land as evidenced by the memorials of Silas Soule and the corrected historical plaques. Often, students who engage in these activities express a multitude of emotions including rage and betrayal for not having learned the history before graduate education as well as responsibility for educating themselves and others on the complex colonial history of this country.

As described in this brief case example, engaging with history and place allows students, across positional identities, to participate in critical truth-telling toward identifying openings for place-based educational interventions. While uncovering this history can be shocking, it is also necessary. Some place-based and Indigenous focused strategies that educators can use are: 1) Begin all classes with a land acknowledgment. Educators can do this by researching the original Indigenous people of the land occupied by the respective academic institutions. The U.S. Department of Arts and Culture has a useful guide (see https://usdac.us/nativeland); 2) Expand beyond the classroom and explore land and place as it connects to both academic institutional and Native peoples' history and current context.; and 3) Encourage students to learn the history and to make land acknowledgment a practice everywhere they may go.

Indigenous knowledge in the field: Yappalli, the Choctaw road to health

Choctaw scholars have theorized that the Trail of Tears is a historically anchored event that continues to impact health issues in the lives of tribal members whose ancestors were displaced through the Indian Removal Act of the 1830s (Schultz, Walters, Beltran, Stroud, & Johnson-Jennings, 2016; Walters et al., 2018). *Yappallí Choctaw Road to Health* is a culturally focused, strengths-based outdoor experiential obesity-substance use risk prevention and health leadership program for Choctaw Nation of Oklahoma (CNO) women that utilize Indigenous knowledge of the Choctaw worldview. The 3-month intervention (i.e., individual meetings; group sessions, culture camp, and Choctaw Trail of Tears walk) is grounded in the Indigenist Stress Coping model (Walters & Simoni, 2002).

Yappallí, translated in the Choctaw language means "to walk slowly and softly," seen as walking "with reverence" and "blessing the grounds" (Schultz et al., 2016). The Yappallí project recognizes Indigenous conceptions of resilience and healing in place and community. This health promotion intervention empowers women to address and change their personal narratives of health and wellness, supports them to learn about their ancestral, cultural and spiritual lifeways, connects them to the place where their ancestors walked, to the sacrifices their ancestors made for them to be Choctaw and embracing and protecting Indigenous ontology and identity by revisiting the vision of health for future generations. The Yappallí project contributes to the empirical literature on stress and trauma embodiment by suggesting that reconnecting with ancestral land can evoke ancestral memories of resilience and health (Schultz et al., 2016).

Specifically, Yappallí is a place-based healing project that focuses on IK in education and healing by returning to the place where their historical trauma occurred. It provides a concrete and practical approach to environmental education that centers the role of the Choctaw worldview, elders, and community knowledge systems. This project utilizes place-based education principles, which emphasize experiential, hands-on engagement with the Trail of Tears, CNO community members, and the natural environment. The project reiterates the IK concept of healing community is synonymous with healing the environment around them.

Indigenous knowledge in research: research to build community-based adaptation strategies

After every natural or human-made disaster, the media and researchers often barrage marginalized and vulnerable communities with requests for interviews regarding how their community is responding. One Indigenous community aptly recognized that disasters are acute-onset, time-delineated events, and following the 3 to 36-month recovery time frame (Sheikhbardsiri, Yarmohammadian, Rezaei, & Maracy, 2017), the media and researchers disappear until the next disaster. What was not studied are the chronic and ongoing environmental changes within their community. Empirical science has not fully explored how such environmental changes are experienced and how they affect human systems. Also, future disasters will become more frequent and more impactful, especially in marginalized populations. Therefore, when approached by an Indigenous scholar of their community, they asked her to study how these environmental changes are affecting tribal members.

In a concurrent mixed methods community-engaged research project, the results highlighted the importance of connection to land among participants and the interconnectedness between sociocultural events, physical environmental changes, and impacts on culture and health. Participants were dependent on the land for their basic subsistence and thus observed changes to their environment daily. The environmental changes led to a loss of medicines and harvest, which led to impacts on health and livelihoods and then to loss of cultural knowledge transmitted and reiterated between generations (Billiot, Kwon, & Burnette, 2019).

After reporting the extent of exposure to environmental changes among tribal members and willingness among participants to be involved in adaptation activities, the Indigenous scholar worked with her community to utilize the findings to develop an adaptation behavioral health intervention that incorporates traditional ecological knowledge and culture through youth education and fieldwork. When researchers use principals of community-based participatory research, the process respects Indigenous knowledge and incorporates traditional ecological knowledge as an integral component to social responses of education, healing, mobilizing and implementation needed for addressing environmental changes.

Conclusion

As environmental change events are predicted to increase in frequency in the future, culturally appropriate responses to environmental change will likely become a higher priority for Indigenous peoples and their allies. Additionally, as the health impacts of environmental change are not entirely understood, addressing environmental change will require participatory approaches and partnerships to understand better and improve our responses to environmental change and its impact on tribal health and well-being. Ultimately, it is through strengthening tribal capacity that Indigenous communities will be able to effectively respond to and mitigate from the effects of environmental change in their communities.

In this article, we contribute to the social work "Grand Challenges" discussion by proposing how community social work practice can benefit from understanding Indigenous Knowledge for future and ongoing social responses to addressing detrimental environmental changes. We provide a summary of Indigenous ontology and epistemology as it relates to place. Next, we presented historical and current trauma through examples of environmental change impacts on Indigenous communities and the embodiment of traumatic race and class-based experiences. We further the social work grand challenges discussion on environmental changes by proposing Indigenous inspired social responses in addressing a changing environment. Indigenous peoples are resisting settler-colonialism, reclaiming traditional knowledge, and translating it into practices of renewed connection to the land and environmental sustainability. Finally, we suggested social work community practices of social responses to environmental change through education, community mobilization, healing, and implementation that are both culturally relevant to Indigenous communities and responsive to environmental change for all. We propose that these recommendations are cyclical and iterative processes based on Indigenous ways of knowing.

Notes

1. Specific examples include: 1) the forced removal of the American Indian Choctaw (1831–1833) approximately 500 miles from their original homelands (Akers, 2004), 2) the forcible removal of over 100,000 Australian Aboriginal children (1910–1970) to residential schools and orphanages as well as through adoption (Human Rights and Equal Opportunities Commission, 1997), and 3) ongoing exploitation and contamination of Indigenous lands through gold mining operations leading to adverse health outcomes in a Guatemalan Mayan community (Caxaj, Berman, Ray, Restoule, & Varcoe, 2014).
2. In this paper we use "land" to refer to all landscapes and seascapes from which Indigenous peoples belong.
3. Defined as "the processes through which Aboriginal people's access to the resources of their traditional environments is reduced," (Richmond & Ross, 2009, p. 403). Examples include "widespread displacement, environmental contamination, forced assimilation, unprecedented resource extraction, and land rights disputes," (Tobias & Richmond, 2014, p. 26).
4. Yellow Bird defines decolonization as actions taken to "weaken the effects of colonialism and create opportunities to promote traditional health practices in present-day settings" (Yellow Bird 2016, p. 65).
5. On November 29, 1864, a U.S. militia attacked a peaceful village of Cheyenne and Arapaho tribal members, killing an estimated 160 women, children, and elders near what is present day Eads, Colorado. John Evans was governor of Colorado territory and territorial superintendent of Indian affairs (Clemmer-Smith et al., 2014).

Summary of Declarations

Competing interests: None declared

Ethical approval: Not required (the development of this conceptual model did not involve human subject research).

Declarations of interest: none declared

Acknowledgment

We would like to thank our senior mentors who encouraged this publication, Karina Walters and Susan Kemp.

Disclosure statement

No potential conflict of interest was reported by the authors.

Funding

Research reported in this publication was supported by the National Institute on Drug Abuse of the National Institutes of Health under award number HHSN271201200663P and award number R01DA037176 and the National Institute on Minority Health and Health Disparities of the National Institutes of Health under award number P60MD006909.

ORCID

Felicia M. Mitchell ⓘ http://orcid.org/0000-0002-8156-9818

References

Akers, D. (2004). *Living in the Land of Death: The Choctaw Nation, 1830–1860* Michigan State University Press. Retrieved from http://www.jstor.org/stable/10.14321/j.ctt7zt650

American Indian Resource Center. (n.d.). *Law reform.* Retrieved from http://indianlaw.org/lawreform

Beltrán, R., Hacker, A., & Begun, S. (2016). Environmental justice is a social justice issue: Incorporating environmental justice into social work practice curricula. *Journal of Social Work Education, 52*(4), 493–502. doi:10.1080/10437797.2016.1215277

Berrang-Ford, L., Dingle, K., Ford, J. D., Lee, C., Lwasa, S., Namanya, D. B., … Edge, V. (2012). Vulnerability of Indigenous health to climate change: A case study of Uganda's Batwa Pygmies. *Social Science & Medicine, 75*(6), 1067–1077. doi:10.1016/j.socscimed.2012.04.016

Billiot, S., & Parfait, J. (2019). Reclaiming land: Adaptation activities and global environmental change challenges within Indigenous communities. In L. Mason & J. Rigg (Eds.), *People and climate change: Vulnerability, adaptation, and social justice* (pp. 108–121). New York, NY: Oxford University Press.

Billiot, S., Kwon, S., & Burnette, C. (2019). Repeated disasters and chronic environmental changes impede generational transfer of Indigenous knowledge. *Journal of Family Strengths.* [in press].

Brave Heart, M. Y. H. (2003). The historical trauma response among Natives and its relationship with substance abuse: A Lakota illustration. *Journal of Psychoactive Drugs, 35*(1), 7–13. doi:10.1080/02791072.2003.10399988

Briskman, L. (2008). Decolonizing social work in Australia: Prospect or illusion. In M. Gray, J. Coates, & M. Yellow Bird (Eds.), *Indigenous social work around the world: Towards culturally relevant education and practice* (pp. 83–93). Hampshire, England: Ashgate Publishing.

Brubaker, M., Berner, J., Chavan, R., & Warren, J. (2011). Climate change and health effects in Northwest Alaska. *Global Health Action, 4,* 1–5. doi:10.3402/gha.v4i0.8445

Caxaj, C. S., Berman, H., Ray, S. L., Restoule, J. P., & Varcoe, C. (2014). Strengths amidst vulnerabilities: The paradox of resistance in a mining-affected community in Guatemala. *Issues in Mental Health Nursing, 35*(11), 824–834. doi:10.3109/01612840.2014.919620

Clemmer-Smith, R., Gilbert, A., Halaas, D. L., Stratton, B. J., Tinker, G. E., Wadsworth, N. D., & Fisher, S. (2014). *Report of the John Evans study committee.* Denver, CO. Retrieved from https://portfolio.du.edu/evcomm/page/52699

Coulthard, G. (2010). Place against empire: Understanding Indigenous anti-colonialism. *Affinities: A Journal of Radical Theory, Culture, and Action, 4*(2), 79–83.

Cozzetto, K., Chief, K., Dittmer, K., Brubaker, M., Gough, R., Souza, K., ... Chavan, P. (2013). Climate change impacts on the water resources of American Indians and Alaska Natives in the U.S. *Climatic Change, 120*(3), 569–584. doi:10.1007/s10584-013-0852-y

Cunsolo Willox, A., Harper, S. L., & Edge, V. L. (2013). Storytelling in a digital age: Digital storytelling as an emerging narrative method for preserving and promoting Indigenous oral wisdom. *Qualitative Research, 13*(2), 127–147. doi:10.1177/1468794112446105

Cunsolo Willox, A., Harper, S. L., Ford, J. D., Landman, K., Houle, K., & Edge, V. L. (2012). "From this place and of this place:" Climate change, sense of place, and health in Nunatsiavut, Canada. *Social Science & Medicine, 75*(3), 538–547. doi:10.1016/j.socscimed.2012.03.043

Doyle, J., Redsteer, M., & Eggers, M. (2013). Exploring effects of climate change on Northern Plains American Indian health. *Climatic Change, 120*(3), 643–655. doi:10.1007/s10584-013-0799-z

Dunbar-Ortiz, R. (2015). *An Indigenous Peoples' history of the United States*. Boston, MA: Beacon Press.

Energy Transfer Partners. (2014). *Dakota access pipeline facts*. Retrieved from http://daplpipelinefacts.com

Evans-Campbell, T., & Walters, K. L. (2006). Indigenist practice competencies in child welfare practice: A decolonization framework to address family violence and substance abuse among First Nations Peoples. In R. Fong, R. McRoy, & C. Ortiz Hendricks (Eds.), *Intersecting child welfare, substance abuse, and family violence: Culturally competent approaches* (pp. 266–290). Washington, DC: CSWE Press.

Evans-Campbell, T. (2008). Historical trauma in American Indian/Native Alaska communities: A multilevel framework for exploring impacts on individuals, families, and communities. *Journal of Interpersonal Violence, 23*(3), 316–338. doi:10.1177/0886260507312290

First Nations Development Institute. (2013). *Reclaiming Native food systems: Part I*. Longmont, CO: Author.

Ford, J. D. (2012). Indigenous health and climate change. *American Journal of Public Health, 102*(7), 1260–1266. doi:10.2105/ajph.2012.300752

Ford, J. D., Cunsolo Willox, A., Chatwood, S., Furgal, C., Harper, S., Mauro, I., & Pearce, T. (2014). Adapting to the effects of climate change on Inuit health. *American Journal of Public Health, 104*(S3), e9–e17. doi:10.2105/ajph.2013.301724

Furgal, C., & Seguin, J. (2006). Climate change, health, and vulnerability in Canadian Northern Aboriginal communities. *Environmental Health Perspectives, 114*(12), 1964–1970. doi:10.1289/ehp.8433

Healey, G. K., Magner, K. M., Ritter, R., Kamookak, R., Aningmiuq, A., Issaluk, B., ... Moffit, P. (2011). Community perspectives on the impact of climate change on health in Nunavut, Canada. *Arctic, 64*(1), 89–97. doi:10.14430/arctic4082

Hofmeijer, I., Ford, J. D., Berrang-Ford, L., Zavaleta, C., Carcamo, C., Llanos, E., ... Namanya, D. (2013). Community vulnerability to the health effects of climate change among Indigenous populations in the Peruvian Amazon: A case study from Panaillo and Nuevo Progreso. *Mitigation and Adaptation Strategies for Global Change, 18*(7), 957–978. doi:10.1007/s11027-012-9402-6

Holmes, S. M. (2013). *Fresh fruit, broken bodies: Migrant farmworkers in the United States* (1st ed.). Berkeley: University of California Press.

Kemp, S. P., & Palinkas, L. A., (with Wong, M., Wagner, K., Mason, L. R., Chi, I., Nurius, P., Floersch, J., & Rechkemmer, A.). (2015). *Strengthening the social response to the human impacts of environmental change* (Grand Challenges for Social Work Initiative Working

Paper No. 5). Cleveland, OH: American Academy of Social Work and Social Welfare. Retrieved from http://grandchallengesforsocialwork.org/wp-content/uploads/2015/12/

Kirmayer, L., Dandeneau, S., Marshall, E., Phillips, M., & Williamson, K. (2011). Rethinking resilience from Indigenous perspectives. *Canadian Journal of Psychiatry, 56*(2), 84–91. doi:10.1177/070674371105600203

Krieger, N. (2005). Embodiment: A conceptual glossary for epidemiology. *Journal of Epidemiology & Community Health, 59*(5), 350–355. doi:10.1136/jech.2004.024562

Krieger, N., & Davey Smith, G. (2004). "Bodies count, " and body counts: Social epidemiology and embodying inequality. *Epidemiological Review, 26,* 92–103. doi:10.1093/epirev/mxh009

Lucero, E. (2011). From tradition to evidence: Decolonization of the evidence-based practice system. *Journal of Psychoactive Drugs, 43*(4), 319–324. doi:10.1080/02791072.2011.628925

McLean, K. (2010). *Advance guard: Climate change impacts, adaptation, mitigation, and Indigenous Peoples.* Darwin, Australia: United Nations University – Traditional Knowledge Initiative. Retrieved from https://i.unu.edu/media/ourworld.unu.edu-en/article/1148/Advance_Copy-Advance_Guard_Compendium.pdf

Minnesota Commerce Department. (2019). *Line 3 pipeline replacement.* Retrieved from https://mn.gov/commerce/energyfacilities/line3/

Moran, E. (2010). *Environmental social science: Human-environmental interactions and sustainability.* West Sussex, UK: Wiley-Blackwell Publishing.

Pierotti, R., & Wildcat, D. (2000). Traditional ecological knowledge: The third alternative. *Ecological Applications, 10*(5), 1333–1340. doi:10.1890/1051-0761

Rights, Human, &. (1997). Annual Report (ISSN 1031–5098), Sydney, NSW

Richmond, C. A. M., & Ross, N.A. (2009). The determinants of First Nation and Inuit health: a critical population health approach. *Health Place, 15*(2), 403–411. doi:10.1016/j.healthplace.2008.07.004

Schultz, K., Walters, K. L., Beltran, R., Stroud, S., & Johnson-Jennings, M. (2016). "I'm stronger than I thought": Native women reconnecting to body, health, and place. *Health Place, 40,* 21–28. doi:10.1016/j.healthplace.2016.05.001

Semken, S., & Freeman, C. B. (2008). Sense of place in the practice and assessment of place-based science teaching. *Science Education, 92*(6), 1042–1057. doi:10.1002/sce.20279

Settee, P. (2008). Indigenous knowledge as the basis for our future. Rochester, VT: Bear and Company. (p. 42-47.

Sheikhbardsiri, H., Yarmohammadian, M. H., Rezaei, F., & Maracy, M. R. (2017). Rehabilitation of vulnerable groups in emergencies and disasters: A systematic review. *World Journal of Emergency Medicine, 8*(4), 253–263. doi:10.5847/wjem.j.1920-8642.2017.04.002

Sheridan, J., & Longboat, R. H. C. T. S. D. (2006). The Haudenosaunee imagination and the ecology of the sacred. *Space and Culture, 9*(4), 365–381. doi:10.1177/1206331206292503

Simpson, L. R. (2004). Anticolonial strategies for the recovery and maintenance of Indigenous knowledge. *The American Indian Quarterly, 28*(3), 373–384. Retrieved from http://www.jstor.org/stable/4138923

Smith, G. A. (2002). Place-based education: Learning to be where we are. *Phi Delta Kappan, 83*(8), 584–594. doi:10.1177/003172170208300806

Smith, L. T. (2012). *Decolonizing methodologies* (2nd ed.). New York, NY: Zed Books.

Snodgrass, J. (2013). Health of Indigenous circumpolar populations. *Annual Review of Anthropology, 42,* 69–87. doi:10.1146/annurev-anthro-092412-155517

Southwick, S. M., Bonanno, G. A., Masten, A. S., Panter-Brick, C., & Yehuda, R. (2014). Resilience definitions, theory, and challenges: interdisciplinary perspectives. *European Journal of Psychotraumatology, 5.* doi:10.3402/ejpt.v5.25338

Sullivan, T. K., & Syvertsen, A. K. (2018). Conservation leadership: A developmental model. *Journal of Adolescent Research, 34*(2), 140–166. doi:10.1177/0743558417752638

Tam, B. Y., Gough, W. A., Edwards, V., & Tsuji, L. J. S. (2013). The impact of climate change on the well-being and lifestyle of a First Nation community in the western James Bay region. *Canadian Geographer, 57*(4), 441–456. doi:10.1111/j.1541-0064.2013.12033.x

Tobias, J. K., & Richmond, C. A. M. (2014). "That Land Means Everything to Us as Anishinaabe..": Environmental Dispossession and Resilience on the North Shore of Lake Superior. *Health & Place, 29*, 26–33

Thornton, R. (1997). Aboriginal North American population and rates of decline, ca. A.D. 1500-1900. *Current Anthropology, 38*(2), 310–315. doi:10.1086/204615

Tuti, Y., (Writer), & Northern, C., (Director). (2015). American by the numbers with Maria Hinojosa: Episode 4. In C. Readdean (Producer) (Ed.), *Native American Boomtown*. Boston, MA: The Futuro Media Group in Association with WGBH for the Public Broadcasting Service.

United Nations. (2008). *Inter-agency support group on Indigenous Peoples' issues collated paper on Indigenous Peoples and climate change*. New York, NY: Author. Retrieved from https://www.un.org/esa/socdev/unpfii/documents/2016/egm/IASG-Collated-Paper-on-Indigenous-Peoples-and-Climate-Change.pdf

Veracini, L. (2010). *Settler colonialism: A theoretical overview*. Hampshire, UK: Palgrave Macmillian.

Vizenor, G. R. (2008). *Survivance: Narratives of Native presence*. Lincoln: University of Nebraska Press.

Vukic, A., Gregory, D., Martin-Misener, R., & Etowa, J. (2011). Aboriginal and Western conceptions of mental health and illness. *Pimatisiwin: A Journal of Aboriginal & Indigenous Community Health, 9*(1), 65–86. Retrieved from https://journalindigenouswellbeing.com/aboriginal-and-western-conceptions-of-mental-health-and-illness/

Walters, K. L., Beltran, R., Huh, D., & Evans-Campbell, T. (2011). Dis-placement and disease: Land, place, and health among American Indian and Alaska Natives. In L. M. Burton, S. P. Kemp, M. C. Leung, S. A. Matthews, & D. T. Takeuchi (Eds.), *Communities, neighborhood, and health: Expanding the boundaries of place* (pp. 163–199). Philadelphia, PA: Springer Science+ Business Media, LLC.

Walters, K. L., Johnson-Jennings, M., Stroud, S., Rasmus, S., Charles, B., John, S., … Boulafentis, J. (2018). Growing from our roots: Strategies for developing culturally grounded health promotion interventions in American Indian, Alaska Native, and Native Hawaiian communities. *Prevention Science*. doi:10.1007/s11121-018-0952-z

Walters, K. L., Mohammed, S. A., Evans-Campbell, T., Beltran, R., Chae, D. H., & Duran, B. (2011). Bodies don't just tell stories, they tell histories: Embodiment of historical trauma among American Indian and Alaska Natives. *Du Bois Review, 8*(1), 179–189. doi:10.1017/S1742058X1100018X

Walters, K. L., & Simoni, J. M. (2002). Reconceptualizing Native women's health: An 'Indigenist' stress-coping model. (Cover story). *American Journal of Public Health, 92*(4), 520–524. doi:10.2105/ajph.92.4.520

Weaver, H. (2008). Indigenous social work in the United States: Reflections on Indian tacos, Trojan horses and canoes filled with Indigenous revolutionaries. In M. Gray, J. Coates, & M. Yellow Bird (Eds.), *Indigenous social work around the world: Towards culturally relevant education and practice* (pp. 71–82). Hampshire, UK: Ashgate Publishing.

Wells, M. (2017). In defense of our relatives. *Studies in Arts and Humanities, 3*(2), 142–160. doi:10.18193/sah.v3i2.111

Wildcat, D. (2009). *Red alert! Indigenous call for action*. Golden, CO: Fulcrom Publishing.

Wilson, A. (2004). Reclaiming our humanity: Decolonizing and the recovery of Indigenous knowledge. In D. A. W. Mihesuah (Ed.), *Indigenizing the academy* (pp. 70–87). Lincoln: Univeristy of Nebraska.

Women's Earth Alliance. (2014). *Violence on the land, violence on our bodies: Building an Indigenous response to environmental violence.* Retrieved from http://landbodydefense.org

Wu, M., Mintz, M., Wang, M., & Arora, S. (2009). Water consumption in the production of ethanol and petroleum gasoline. *Environmental Management, 44*(5), 981–997. doi:10.1007/s00267-009-9370-0

Yellow Bird, M. (2016). Neurodecolonization: Applying Mindfulness Research to Decolonize Social Work. In M. Gray, J. Coates, M. Yellow Bird, & T. Hetherington (Eds.). *Decolonizing Social Work.* London, UK: Taylor and Francis.

"Let's talk about the real issue": Localized perceptions of environment and implications for ecosocial work practice

Joonmo Kang, Vanessa D. Fabbre, and Christine C. Ekenga

ABSTRACT
This interpretive study investigated how residents from socio-economically challenged communities in North St. Louis understand and make meaning of environmental change and its impact on their well-being. Based on these localized data, we argue that racial minorities facing socioeconomic challenges may experience some environmental issues as less of an immediate concern than violence and racism. However, race and racism shape both the realities of environmental threats as well as residents' perceptions about environmental injustice in their communities. This study informs ecosocial work practices such as educating communities on local environmental issues and mobilizing community members toward environmental decision-making.

Unprecedented environmental changes have become an existential challenge for all living beings. While environmental change affects everyone, it disproportionately impacts people with few social and economic resources, which points to a fundamental relationship between existing social problems and environmental crisis, what Peeters (2012) referred to as a *social-ecological crisis*. The deleterious impact of environmental changes has also been conceptualized as *slow violence* (Nixon, 2011) that "occurs gradually and out of sight, a violence of delayed destruction that is dispersed across time and space, an attritional violence that is typically not viewed as violence at all" (p. 2). Slow violence affects the poor more than other groups because it compounds existing injustices. These environmental, social, and political forces are deeply troubling for those concerned about the health and well-being of vulnerable populations and form the landscape for social work practice that aims to promote environmental justice.

Coates and Gray (2012) argued that in response to the social-ecological crisis, the field of social work needs to transform to *ecosocial work* by broadening its scope of person-in-environment to better attend to the natural world in our views of social welfare. Ecosocial work, which Dominelli (2015) calls green social work, "respects and values the physical or 'natural' environment as an entity in its own right, albeit a socially constructed one, while simultaneously recognizing that people use its bounty to meet their needs" (p. 25). Many scholars have argued that social workers are uniquely suited to deal with emerging social problems caused by environmental changes and could serve as agents in transitioning to an ecosocial society (Coates, 2004; Dominelli, 2015; Närhi & Matthies, 2018) and increasing social work research is focused on these topics (Krings, Victor, Mathias, & Perron, 2018; Mason, Shires, Arwood, & Borst, 2017). However, despite these theoretical contributions to ecosocial work, practical approaches to achieving these ideals have not yet been fully articulated in the literature (Bexell, Sparks, Tejada, & Rechkemmer, 2018; Molyneux, 2010; Ramsay & Boddy, 2017). Thus, the aims of this study were to learn how residents of socioeconomically challenged communities – who are often hit first and worst by the impacts of environmental change – experience their local environments and to derive implications from these experiences for the practice of ecosocial work.

Localized perceptions of environment

Exploring localized perceptions of environmental change at the community level can shed light on the ways that global environmental changes manifest and impact human beings in context-specific and proximal ways (Pyhälä et al., 2016). In this vein, Närhi and Matthies (2018) suggested that the practical implementation of ecosocial transition must occur at the local level, which is echoed by Kemp's (2011) emphasis on eliciting local knowledge (through engagement with clients, communities, practitioners, and local programs or initiatives) to enhance environmentally oriented practice in social work.

Studying localized experiences, perspectives, and insights is also important for promoting social justice. First, it allows the voices of many individuals and communities that have been historically marginalized from mainstream conversations about the environment to be heard. Poor communities and communities of color have been easier targets of industry and government with respect to environmental issues (Mohai, Pellow, & Roberts, 2009), and even in organizations working on environmental issues, people of color have not been equally represented by membership and leadership (Taylor, 2014). Second, reflecting localized perceptions of environmental risks is essential because a community's perception of environmental issues can influence the mental and physical well-being of its residents (Wen, Hawkley, & Cacioppo, 2006). This potential impact on people's health and well-being point to the importance of studying people's perceptions of their environment and its relationship to their own well-being. Finally, local knowledge and experience are important because people's perceptions not only influence the ways in which they mitigate or adapt to environmental changes (Pyhälä et al., 2016) but also inform the decision-making of community development practitioners and policymakers (Mason, Ellis, & Hathaway, 2017). For example, Petts and Brooks (2006) promote paying attention to the "lay expert"

(p. 1048) in addressing responses to environmental change because they have insight and knowledge that facilitates collaboration and trust building, which in turn facilitates social and environmental justice.

Method

Stemming from these calls to attend to localized perceptions of environmental issues, this study investigated how residents living in socioeconomically challenged communities in St. Louis, Missouri, perceive and make meaning of their local environmental conditions (e.g., air, water, climate and built environment) and risks, especially with respect to their health and well-being. We used abductive reasoning as the epistemological underpinning of this study, which meant first seeking out relevant literature and reflecting on the nature of our prior knowledge about this topic and then engaging in an iterative and recursive process of generating data through semi-structured interviews and making sense of these data with respect to our analytical aims (Schwartz-Shea & Yanow, 2012).

Study participants

Geography was central to our recruitment strategy in this interview-based study. We used purposive sampling (Padgett, 2017) to recruit individuals who resided in the northern part of the St. Louis, Missouri, metropolitan area, which includes a contiguous group of 25 zip codes in North St. Louis City and North St. Louis County. For background, the St. Louis metropolitan area – which includes the City of St. Louis, St. Louis County, and East St. Louis, Illinois – needs to be understood in the context of its long history of residential segregation by both race and social class. In general, socio-economically challenged neighborhoods located in North St. Louis County, North St. Louis City, and parts of Central and South St. Louis City, have high concentrations of African American residents and high poverty rates (Cambria, Fehler, Purnell, & Schmidt, 2018). Disparities in health outcomes and other quality of life measures are also associated with living in these neighborhoods. These local disparities and inequities are likely to exacerbate the impact of environmental change, which motivated our focus on understanding residents' first-hand perceptions of these issues.

We used facility-based and chain-referral techniques to recruit participants from North St. Louis City (sometimes referred to by study participants as "the City") and North St. Louis County (sometimes referred to as "the County"). The research team first recruited through a local community development nonprofit organization that advocates for low-income families in metropolitan St. Louis. We put up flyers in the organization's building, which is located in the northern part of the City, emailed recruitment information to its members, and passed out fliers at their events. We also reached out to the Urban League of St. Louis, whose leadership sent recruiting emails to their members. Furthermore, we utilized the Washington University School of Medicine's Research Engagement to Advance Community Health Initiative, which includes outreach sites such as libraries, food pantries, and employment agencies in North St. Louis City and North St. Louis County. Last, we recruited through chain referral from participants' social networks by asking participants to share information about this study with their friends, families and neighbors. Washington University's Institutional Review Board approved this study for the ethical conduct of research with human subjects (# 201,707,138).

We were able to recruit 15 study participants. Twelve participants identified as female and three as male. Eleven participants identified as African American, two as White, one as Moor, and one as mixed-race. Four participants were 30–40 years old, two were 41–50 years old, four were 51–60 years old, four were 61–70 years old, and one participant was 83 years old. In regard to annual household income, two identified as $70,000 or more, one as $60,000–69,999, one as $50,000–59,000, two as $40,000–49,000, five as $20,000–29,999, three as less than $20,000 and one did not reveal the information. In terms of education, four participants had a graduate degree, four were college graduates, five had experienced some college or had a degree from a technical school, and two had a high school diploma or equivalent.

Interviews

We conducted semi-structured interviews with participants that focused on their perceptions of environmental issues at varying scales (neighborhood, city, national) and health. The term "environmental issues" can mean "different things to different people" (Harvey, 1993, p. 1); for the purposes of this study we used this term to refer to environmental pollution and climate change. We developed interview questions to address the following elements: (a) participants' perceptions of and response to environmental issues at the neighborhood and city level; (b) participants' perceptions of the health issues at the neighborhood and city level as well as their connection to environmental issues; (c) participants' perception of climate change; and (d) source of information on environmental issues, method of obtaining information, and communication with others.

Developing the interview protocol was an iterative process. The first author conducted a pilot interview, after which we revised the questions slightly in order to more effectively elicit perceptions about environmental issues. Then, two more pilot interviews were conducted and reviewed with a faculty member in the Department of Anthropology at Washington University who is knowledgeable in environmental issues in St. Louis. Many of our final questions sought to elicit perceptions of locally relevant issues. For example, according to the

Asthma and Allergy Foundation of America (2018), St. Louis was 30th on its list of the most challenging places to live with asthma, so we asked participants if they knew anyone with asthma and whether they connected this condition to air pollution in St. Louis. Another local topic we raised was the media coverage of the 2016 water fountain contamination at 12 St. Louis Public Schools, which elicited participants' perceptions of this issue and associations with other environmental issues.

The first interviews were conducted at Washington University's main campus due to some delays on the part of the research team in planning adequately for field work, but then several interviews were conducted off-campus near participants' homes (see Limitations for a more in-depth discussion of this issue). Most interviews lasted about one hour, with the exception of two interviews that lasted for about 30 minutes. All interviews were audio recorded and transcribed verbatim by a professional transcription company. Participants received a $25 gift card for their participation in the project.

Data analysis

We analyzed the interviews in three stages to develop the most salient themes in participants' perceptions of environmental and health issues in their community and develop implications for ecosocial work practice. In the first stage, we developed a priori structural codes (Saldaña, 2016) to capture and organize data that fell into the four main elements of the interviews (see above, research questions A, B, C, and D). For example, some of our structural codes captured *neighborhood environmental issues, city level environmental issues,* and *climate change.* We applied these codes throughout the interview transcripts to draw our attention to the data most directly relevant to our research focus and interview questions. In the second stage of analysis, we conducted open/inductive coding to immerse ourselves in the data free from a priori categories (Padgett, 2017; Saldaña, 2016); this stage of analysis sensitized us even more to participants' various forms of meaning-making and contextual knowledge, the hallmark of an interpretive approach (Schwartz-Shea & Yanow, 2012). This open/inductive coding also facilitated a more nuanced look at the variation of responses within each category and formed the foundation for our thematic development. Examples of open codes that we developed and applied in this phase were *violence is the real issue, a sense of vagueness, environmental justice* and *people's perception of the impact of climate change.*

After we completed the open/inductive coding, we generated themes that we felt best illuminated the main perceptions and concerns that participants shared in the interviews. The most salient themes from this stage of the analysis focused on (a) participants' desire to discuss pressing problems in their communities, such as violence and racism; and (b) the impact of race and racism in shaping their perception of environmental issues. As we developed these themes, we relied on our abductive reasoning process by continually going back to the raw interview data to check and refine our thematic development. We present some of these raw data in our findings section to foster trustworthiness about our analytical process. After these first stages of a priori structural coding, open/inductive coding, and thematic development, the first author carried out an interpretive reading of the coded data and themes in order to develop implications for ecosocial work practice. By interpretive reading, we mean that the first author read and reviewed the coded text and themes closely, while applying an ecosocial work lens and writing analytical memos about implications for practice. This close reading served as an analytical bridge between the thematic analysis and the practice implications we drew from it.

Findings

Our interpretive analyses suggest that residents of these socioeconomically challenged communities, particularly African Americans, perceived and identified violence and racism as far more immediate concerns than environmental issues. However, residents' awareness of racial injustice also extended to environmental issues through their own application of an environmental justice perspective to make sense of their lived experiences.

"Let's talk about the real issue": violence and racism in St. Louis

Our interviews illuminated the ongoing challenges of living with threats of violence and the effects of racism on a daily basis, which constitute real vulnerabilities for residents of North St. Louis and North St. Louis County. Residents recounted multiple experiences with violence and racism, and particularly police racism, as shaping their immediate sense of well-being. Throughout the interviews, even though the interview questions specifically asked about environmental conditions and risks, many participants often redirected the conversation to crime and violence. For example, when asked to share his experience about living close to a factory growing up, Chris (all names in this paper are pseudonyms), an African American man in his 50s who grew up in a neighborhood with many factories and who suffered asthma since he was a child, replied:

> Well, a lot of times, when you live in neighborhoods like that you are not worried about factories [*laughs*] or pollution killing you. You're worried about crime mostly killing you ... [you know] that pollution is hurting my health – but yeah – but let's talk about the real issue that's hurting my health – the drugs, the alcohol, you know? Those are things that hurt more than anything, you know? ... the environment is never a priority living in what I quote unquote call the hood.

Like Chris, almost all participants conveyed concerns about violent crime, reflecting the reality of St. Louis which continues to be one of the most dangerous cities in the United States, even reaching the highest urban murder rate for the country in 2017 (Beyond Ferguson, 2017). Even when questions regarding health and environmental issues in St. Louis were asked, many participants pointed out crime and violence as the most important issue impacting their well-being and at times leading to feelings of powerlessness. For example, Denise, an African American woman in her 50s from North St. Louis County, reflected on a recent shooting in her neighborhood:

> I think even in my neighborhood, there was a young man that was shot. He got shot 25 times … [He was a] 17-year-old child. You didn't see anything about it on the news and then, maybe, about a week later, you seen it on the news where he got shot because, in 2015, he accidentally shot a 3-year-old. The people that were related to the 3-year-old, who were also 17 [years old], they came and shot him in Bellefontaine, where I live at … It was a concern. If you are gonna get killed in the broad daylight – that happened in broad daylight!

Denise's telling of her experience illustrates that violent crime has a palpable impact on her sense of well-being where she lives, and residents like her are often left feeling helpless in the face of these types of crimes. Stories like Denise's were common among interview participants in this study. For example, Adeline, an African American woman in her 60s, also emphasized "the guns and violence" as the most serious health issue in St. Louis. She said, "I mean, every weekend, in a week, at least you have two or three gunshots, people shot to death and all that." Concerned about their personal safety, David and Marcus, male participants living in North St. Louis County, revealed that they possess a weapon for protection. David, an African American man in his 60s, purchased a gun after his house was robbed. Marcus, an African American man in his 50s, after sharing three incidents of robbery and gun violence he recently witnessed, revealed he has been carrying a boxcutter knife for the past five years. He shared:

> … the three incidents I just described to you, that's just a microcosm of things that's been happening, just being out and about. Like I said, I take public transportation. I have to walk to, I have to walk from … work … I'm mostly by myself, so I have to have some kind of means to protect myself in case something comes my way, that I can deal with it.

Along with fear of violence, many expressed their concerns about and distrust towards ongoing police racism and brutality in St. Louis. When asked about their dislikes about the neighborhood the first thing Whitney, a 31-year-old African American woman, mentioned was that "the police officers are all White." She continued, "They stereotype the community in a way … they don't understand people or just don't even know." When asked, "Who is 'they'?", she answered, "The government, the mayor, the police department." Sophia, an African American woman in her 80s, pointed to the disproportionate force used by the police on African Americans as one of the main issues that needs to be addressed in St. Louis after sharing that her daughter, who "wears her hair short," got pulled over by the police. Whitney and Sophia's concerns reflect the reality of police racism in St. Louis, where African American drivers are stopped at a rate 85% higher than White drivers (Missouri Attorney General, 2017). Participants' concerns reflected the widespread distrust of police on the part of African Americans in St. Louis, particularly for residents of neighborhoods similar to Ferguson in St. Louis County where Michael Brown was shot and killed by a White police officer in 2014 (Kochel, 2015). Taken together, these concerns suggest that the necessity of attending to the threats posed by violence and racism renders environmental pollution as a secondary concern, or as Chris put it, hardly a "real issue."

"I'm concerned because the area that they've chosen happens to be the area that's dominated by minorities": environmental injustice in St. Louis

Although issues of violence and racism were often prioritized over environmental issues in these interviews, the theme of racial injustice was also extended to environmental issues with many participants applying an environmental justice perspective to their lived experiences.

For example, Ronda, an African American woman in her 40s, was faced with an environmental condition that was directly affecting her life. She was dealing with a constant flood from the river, which had already caused $20,000 in damage, and shared:

> Me, personally, I've lost thousands of dollars in furniture [and] irreplaceable things … because of my basement having two-foot flooded water in it. It's difficult to get the insurance companies to pay me for it. Prior to getting my home, it wasn't disclosed to me that there was any type of flood plain or anything. Being a first-time homebuyer, being African American, not knowing a lot, I just feel bamboozled.

In addition to her sense of frustration for not being informed about these environmental conditions when she purchased her home, she was deeply concerned about the Metropolitan St. Louis Sewer District's (MSD) recent plan to build a sewage storage tank in a residential area of her neighborhood as part of Project Clear (MSD's long-term initiative to improve water quality and alleviate waste water concerns). She believed this was clearly an example of environmental racism and said, "I'm concerned because the area that they've chosen happens to be the area that's dominated by minorities – African Americans."

Many participants also underscored the unhealthy surroundings of their neighborhood, which echoes the long history of urban decline in St. Louis, which is marked by deep racial and economic segregation. Darlene, an African American woman in her 50s and long-time city resident said, "Everywhere you look, there's a liquor store … that's what stuck out to me when I first moved. I've been here for over 25 years. That's the first thing that stuck out to me." She continued, "Liquor store everywhere. Everywhere you turn, there's a – you could walk to the liquor store. It's just sad because you have substance abuse – it's right there! It's right there!"

Participants also shared concerns about the lack of grocery stores and presence of fast food chains in their neighborhoods. Julia, an African American woman in her 30s shared, "I mean it's not any secret that this is one of the poorer communities, as you drive through all you see is [fast food chains]. Where's Trader Joe's? Where's Whole Foods … you know?" Sophia wished she "had quality stores, where we could buy lots of fruits and vegetables" in her neighborhood rather than fast food chains. David, who lives in Spanish Lake in North County where almost 80% of residents are African American, shops at a supermarket chain in Florissant – an adjacent neighborhood that is majority White – rather than using the same chain in his neighborhood because "the quality is better, as far as expiration dates … [It] just seems like more quality food goes into certain neighborhoods." Chris also described how, compared to the higher income suburbs which he recently moved to that have "retail stores, restaurants, things of that nature," the neighborhood in North County that he used to live in had "no money coming into the community 'cause everything – well, the only money that's being made in the community is the liquor store … cigarette ads and stuff like that."

On top of the inequity in healthy food sources, many participants appeared to be impacted by environmental issues like air pollution and climate change. In discussing air pollution, almost all participants had or knew someone who had asthma. This result aligns with previous case studies of environmental injustice in St. Louis showing that minorities and low-income residents live disproportionately closer to industrial pollution sources (Abel, 2008) and that socioeconomically challenged neighborhoods have higher rates of childhood asthma (Harris, 2019). Interestingly, despite observed environmental health risks, many participants did not perceive air pollution as making a direct impact in their lives. For example, when asked "Where did [your] asthma come from?" Sophia, who not only has asthma herself but also had a nephew who died of asthma, replied "I can't understand it. I can't, but it's very annoying." When we asked the same question to Amber, an African American woman in her 40s whose friend had asthma since she was a little girl, she replied, "It could be the air. It could be her environment, the way she was raised, how she was – I don't know. They say asthma comes from a lot of stuff. It could be a whole bunch of stuff."

In discussing climate change, all participants were aware of climate change and believed it was real. Most participants, with an exception of a few who thought it had gotten cooler, believed the weather was warmer or more unpredictable than in years past. Roxy, a St. Louis native, shared:

> Even here in St. Louis, I'm noticing differences. Because as a kid, like I told you, you know, we could get through the summer with our windows [open], because we couldn't afford [air conditioning]. We didn't even have fans and stuff when I was growing up. You know, I just can't remember it being so intense, the heat, and lasting so long.

Increasingly hot weather may be particularly concerning for low-income residents who cannot afford air conditioning, since many homes in St. Louis were built between 1900 and 1940, using locally sourced brick that retains heat. In fact, this construction makes many homes unsuitable for hot summers, according to a case study of heat-related mortality in St. Louis (Smoyer, 1998). This study showed that mortality rates during heat waves tend to be higher in economically stressed areas, compared to affluent parts of the city.

During our interviews, the first author often followed these types of comments by inquiring whether participants had seen a change in utility bills or knew anyone who has struggled to pay their utility bills – since climate change is thought to increase power costs (Auffhammer, Baylis, & Hausman, 2017). Most participants either struggled themselves or knew someone who struggled to pay their utility bills, which suggests that climate change has already had an impact on their lives. Amber said, "[Utility bills] go up and down. Sometimes, some years it's really, really low, and then the next year it's super high … the bill just seems to fluctuate up and down." For example, Susan, whose electricity company recently threatened to cut off her electricity, said, "I pay what I can and beg for mercy … I had to pay it off with my credit card. It makes it very tough." She explained, "I'm on a fixed income. I'm on disability and able to work only about 15 or 18 hours a week just to buy groceries. That makes less groceries if I have to pay more for utility bills."

Similar to air pollution, while many participants felt changes in weather patterns through the changes in their utility bills, most participants did not perceive climate change as having a direct impact on their daily lives. When asked what kind of impact climate change has on their lives, Amber, who also knew many people who had trouble paying utility bills, said: "Not directly. Probably indirectly, some kind of way. Probably with the universe, probably with stuff that's goin' on that's gonna eventually probably affect the utility bills in some kind of way." To many, the idea of climate change having a direct impact seemed difficult to understand and its impact felt somewhat remote. For example, when we asked Sophia whether she has seen a change in her utility bills, she answered, "I think it's about two weeks of the year that I just really get stressed, 'cause my bills get so high during summer." However, when we asked if she ever felt the impact of climate change, she answered, "I don't think it reaches all the way here, but … it's gotta be affecting somebody."

Although participants did not readily perceive air pollution or climate change as having a direct impact on their lives, environmental injustice still loomed large in their minds. Almost all participants were not only aware of and influenced by the Flint Water Crisis but also believed in the possibility of a similar crisis happening in St. Louis because of its history of systemic racism. Flint made Ronda "extremely paranoid" and believed MSD's plan to build sewage tanks in her neighborhood was similar. When asked about the likelihood of a similar event taking place in St. Louis she said, "No doubt.

No doubt. Yes ... I really do feel like it would take place in the areas where there's not affluent people." Moreover, when the recent report on lead contamination of water fountains in 12 St. Louis Public Schools that exceeded the levels in Flint (Crouch & Bernhard, 2016, August, p. 25) was brought up during the interview, many were initially shocked but not surprised that it happened in St. Louis. For example, Roxy responded, "I wouldn't doubt that. I'm gonna tell you why. I'm a product of the St. Louis Public Schools." She then shared that her school also had "old lead paint in the building" and talked about the history of lead poisoning in St. Louis (see Lewis, Collins, & Wilson, 1955) which still continues to today. More than 6% of African American children under the age of 6 have blood lead levels above the Centers for Disease Control and Prevention's (CDC) safe threshold, which is more than twice the percentage of White children in St. Louis City and County (Hudson, 2016).

On the whole, participants' perspectives reverberated the long history of racial inequality in St. Louis and demonstrated an awareness of environmental injustice and disproportionate health risks for African Americans. Although they did not immediately see environmental issues like air pollution or climate change as having a direct impacts on their lives, they were sensitive to race-based environmental injustices, as Ronda demonstrated, "I just feel like a lot of times, African Americans, particularly descendants of slaves, I feel like we get bamboozled." This somewhat contradictory finding may reflect the perception that air pollution and climate change do not stem from overtly racist actions, while water contamination and cover-ups like those in Flint and the St. Louis Public Schools are more readily perceived as being driven by racism.

Discussion

While our analytical focus in this study was the perceptions of environmental issues from people living in socioeconomically challenged communities, our findings show that race and racism are central aspects of their lived experiences and influence the ways in which environmental change impacts their well-being. We found that those living in socioeconomically challenged communities, particularly African Americans, have been enduring, as one participant said – "real problems" that are perceived as more immediate. The impact of violence and racism was the issue that participants viewed as most salient to their well-being. This finding highlights the specific role that perceptions of violence and racism play in creating a barrier to attending to environmental change and suggests imminent threats must be addressed alongside efforts to draw attention to environmental issues.

Despite this prioritization of violence and racism on the part of community residents, our findings also show that racial injustice is perceived to extend to environmental issues as well. Participants were concerned about their neighborhood environments, noting too many liquor stores and unequal access to healthy food, which Hilmers, Hilmers, and Dave (2012) have described as the subtle inequities that promote unhealthy eating. The high prevalence of asthma and struggles to pay utility bills also point toward the disproportionate impact of air pollution and climate change on poor communities, or what Shonkoff, Morello-Frosch, Pastor, and Sadd (2009) called the *climate gap* – the disproportionate burden of urban heat and air pollution on people of color and the poor.

Although many of our study participants did not see themselves as directly affected by air pollution or climate change, this finding is not surprising given the theory that the non-immediacy, gradual impact, and complexity of environmental issues create cognitive barriers to developing environmental awareness (Kollmuss & Agyeman, 2002). This finding also echoes results of a study about how low-income residents and people of color experience climate change in Seattle, Washington, which found that only 24% of this group thought they would be most impacted by climate change in their area (Got Green & Puget Sound Sage, 2016). Taken together, we conclude that threats like violence and racism play a significant role in shaping people's awareness of and engagement with environmental issues; this conclusion also adds to knowledge that perceived racism is associated with psychological distress (Pieterse, Todd, Neville, & Carter, 2012) and that poverty-related concerns are known to reduce cognitive capacity, leaving less mental space for other tasks (Mani, Mullainathan, Shafir, & Zhao, 2013).

Finally, our findings show that despite some disconnection from pollution and climate change, many study participants actually applied an environmental justice lens to their experiences. As Marcus explained, "If you aren't of a certain group, you don't have the power to decide where the things go … it's called environmental racism. Certain types of factories, certain types of businesses tend to be located in lower-income areas." Moreover, given the history of racism and localized environmental injustices like lead poisoning in the St. Louis Public Schools, they viewed environmental crises like Flint as something that could happen to them at anytime. While this finding echoes the dark side of history in St. Louis, this degree of alertness could serve as an opportunity in mobilizing in the face of these types of threats. This finding also supports the model of pro-environmental behavior by Kollumus and Agyeman (2002) which hypothesizes that fear, sadness, pain and anger trigger pro-environmental behavior because emotional activation increases environmental awareness. In addition, while our research highlights the experiences of those impacted by violence and racism, this does not necessarily mean they perceive their communities as defined by these issues, as one participant emphasized, "People don't know it's nice over there 'cause … when Mike Brown got killed, they just focused on the negative part of Ferguson, but they got a lotta nice stuff over there in Ferguson too."

Limitation

A limitation of our study is that we fell short in prioritizing participants' comfort, as initial interviews were conducted on the campus of Washington University, an elite private institution in St. Louis. Although interviews were conducted in a private setting and after work hours, one potential impact of this choice is that being in an unfamiliar place could have diminished participants' ease in sharing their thoughts and feelings. After one of our participants pointed out that some might be "intimidated by coming out here to Washington University," we conducted later interviews off-campus in a location closer to people's residences.

Implications for ecosocial work practice

These findings reiterate that social justice and environmental issues are intrinsically connected and reaffirm that social workers are well positioned to facilitate awareness and action to address environmental injustice. Particularly in places like St. Louis, where racism informs the realities of people's daily lives and the meanings people generate with respect to environmental issues, social workers who are knowledgeable about racism and environmental justice are well-positioned to carry out ecosocial work practice.

Two ways social workers can put this knowledge into practice is by serving as educators on environmental issues and securing resources to help vulnerable people respond to environmental challenges. Along these lines, one recommendation by Got Green and Puget Sound Sage (2016) is to educate and organize around communities of color because the reason that community members may not see themselves as the most impacted by climate change is due to the climate movement's failure to adequately acknowledge this impact and convey that information. As informed understanding of environmental issues can inspire environmental action (Macias, 2015), social workers can promote environmental knowledge as a means of facilitating action. For example, in our study a person like Sophia, who suffers from asthma and has trouble paying her utility bills a few times a year, might feel more empowered by connecting her struggles with larger environmental forces. Similarly, Ronda's experience as a first-time homeowner dealing with constant flooding coupled with her concern about the proposed sewage tank in her neighborhood serves as an illustration of this potential role for social workers. Ronda sharing that one of her struggles was "understanding what my responsibilities are, versus what's the City's and the County's and the environment," provides a helpful example of an opportunity for social workers to intervene as educators or advocates.

Furthermore, while serving as educators and advocates, social workers can also enhance clients' exposure to environmental issues by strategically finding ways to increase experiences with the natural world. In this regard, Heinsch (2012) argued that all types of interaction with the natural environment hold the potential to have therapeutic effects and Boetto (2016) proposed that subtle awareness-raising techniques can be used by clinical social workers to increase clients' psychological connection to their environment. Specifically, Boetto suggested increasing clients' interactions with nature, such as engaging with clients in a green space, providing information on local environmental groups, including environment-related questions during assessments, and incorporating eco-therapy methods into psychotherapeutic work.

Another role for ecosocial workers is to help mobilize communities in response to environmental threats, particularly by building upon community members' awareness of environmental racism and how it impacts their decision-making. This work would specifically respond to Got Green and Puget Sound Sage's (2016) recommendation to "put racial equity at the center of climate adaptation decision-making" (p. 40). Organizing to increase representation of communities of color in decision-making processes that impact the natural environment may also empower people to develop a *locus of control* – the individual-level perception that one can bring about actual change – which may then promote environmental responsibility, values, and attitudes (Kollmuss & Agyeman, 2002). With respect to our study, the City of St. Louis's recent resolution to pursue 100% renewable energy by 2035 (i.e., its commitment to the Paris Climate Agreement), provides one opportunity to put these ideas into practice. This long-term transformation will entail partnerships between governments, the private sector, and other civil society groups, which challenges local social workers to get involved and push for environmental justice in urban climate adaptation discourse (see Shi et al., 2016). Specifically, social workers can intervene by supporting communities of color to influence these types of civic plans and to assert environmental justice perspectives in the decision-making process.

St. Louis's own local history provides inspiration for this work: in 1970, Freddie Mae Brown, an African American social worker in St. Louis, wrote and staged the play Black Survival: A Collage of Skits for that year's Earth Day celebration. The play specifically emphasized the problems of urban pollution for African Americans, but also challenged the assumption that environmentalism was a White movement, which Brown was known to speak up about frequently and forcefully as a community organizer (Gioielli, 2019). In many ways, Freddie Mae Brown's pioneering work laid the groundwork for contemporary developments in ecosocial work practice, which our findings suggest must incorporate localized perceptions of environment and attention to environmental racism in any education or community mobilization for environmental decision-making.

Disclosure statement

No potential conflict of interest was reported by the authors.

References

Abel, T. D. (2008). Skewed riskscapes and environmental injustice: A case study of metropolitan St. Louis. *Environmental Management, 42*(2), 232–248. doi:10.1007/s00267-008-9126-2

Asthma and Allergy Foundation of America (2018). *Asthma capitals 2018: The most challenging places to live with asthma.* Retrieved from http://www.aafa.org/media/AAFA-2018-Asthma-Capitals-Report.pdf

Auffhammer, M., Baylis, P., & Hausman, C. (2017). Climate change impacts on US electricity demand. *Proceedings of the National Academy of Sciences, 114*(8), 1886–1891. doi:10.1073/pnas.1613193114

Bexell, S. M., Sparks, J. L., Tejada, J., & Rechkemmer, A. (2018). An analysis of inclusion gaps in sustainable development themes: Findings from a review of recent social work literature. *International Social Work., 62*(2), 864–876. doi:10.1177/0020872818755860

Beyond Ferguson: Millennials really like St. Louis. (2017, April 12). *The Economist.* Retrieved from https://www.economist.com/united-states/2017/04/12/millennials-really-like-st-louis

Boetto, H. (2016). Developing ecological social work for micro-level practice. In J. McKinnson & M. Alston (Eds.), *Ecological social work* (pp. 59–77). New York, NY: Palgrave.

Cambria, N., Fehler, P., Purnell, J. Q., & Schmidt, B. (2018). *Segregation in St. Louis: Dismantling the Divide.* St Louis, MO: Washington University in St. Louis.

Coates, J. (2004). *Ecology and social work: Toward a new paradigm.* Black Point, Canada: Fernwood Publishing Co.

Coates, J., & Gray, M. (2012). Guest editorial: The environmental and social work: An overview and introduction. *International Journal of Social Welfare, 21*(3), 230–238. doi:10.1111/j.1468-2397.2011.00851.x

Crouch, E., & Bernhard, B. (2016, August 25). Report details lead contamination in water at St. Louis schools. *St. Louis Post-Dispatch.* Retrieved from https://www.stltoday.com/news/local/education/report-details-lead-contamination-in-water-at-st-louis-schools/article_6e0bbeae-b273-58e7-8662-95281e175a3d.html

Dominelli, L. (2015). *Green social work: From environmental crises to environmental justice.* Malden, MA: Polity.

Gioielli, R. (2019). *Black survival: Mainstream environmentalism's missed opportunities.* Retrieved from http://enviro-history.com/black-survival

Got Green & Puget Sound Sage. (2016). *Our people, our planet, our power.* Retrieved from http://gotgreenseattle.org/wp-content/uploads/2016/03/OurPeopleOurPlanetOurPower_GotGreen_Sage_Final1.pdf

Harris, K. M. (2019). Mapping inequality: Childhood asthma and environmental injustice, a case study of St. Louis, Missouri. *Social Science and Medicine, 230*, 91–110. doi:10.1016/j.socscimed.2019.03.040

Harvey, D. (1993). The nature of environment: Dialectics of social and environmental change. *Socialist Registar, 29.* Retrieved from https://socialistregister.com/index.php/srv/article/view/5621

Heinsch, M. (2012). Getting down to earth: Finding a place for nature in social work practice. *International Journal of Social Welfare, 21*(3), 309–318. doi:10.1111/j.1468-2397.2011.00860.x

Hilmers, A., Hilmers, D. C., & Dave, J. (2012). Neighborhood disparities in access to healthy foods and their effects on environmental justice. *American Journal of Public Health, 102*(9), 1644–1654. doi:10.2105/AJPH.2012.300865

Hudson, N. (2016, November 29). Seeing inequity: A St. Louis lead crisis. *Medium.* Retrieved from https://medium.com/forward-through-ferguson/seeing-inequity-a-st-louis-lead-crisis-1c55dd24d1e1

Kemp, S. (2011). Recentring environment in social work practice: Necessity, opportunity, challenge. *British Journal of Social Work, 41*, 1198–1210. doi:10.1093/bjsw/bcr119

Kochel, T. R. (2015). *Assessing the initial impact of the Michael Brown shooting and police and public responses to it on St Louis County residents' views about police.* Retrieved from https://opensiuc.lib.siu.edu/cgi/viewcontent.cgi?article=1001&context=ccj_reports

Kollmuss, A., & Agyeman, J. (2002). Mind the gap: Why do people act environmentally and what are the barriers to pro-environmental behavior? *Environmental Education Research, 8* (3), 239–260. doi:10.1080/13504620220145401

Krings, A., Victor, B. G., Mathias, J., & Perron, B. E. (2018). Environmental social work in the disciplinary literature, 1991–2015. *International Social Work.* doi:10.1177/0020872818788397

Lewis, B. W., Collins, R. J., & Wilson, H. S. (1955). Seasonal incidence of lead poisoning in children in St. Louis. *Southern Medical Journal, 48*, 298–301. doi:10.1097/00007611-195503000-00013

Macias, T. (2015). Risks, trust, and sacrifice: Social structural motivators for environmental change. *Social Science Quarterly, 96*(5), 1264–1276. doi:10.1111/ssqu.12201

Mani, A., Mullainathan, S., Shafir, E., & Zhao, J. (2013). Poverty impedes cognitive function. *Science, 341*(6149), 976–980. doi:10.1126/science.1238041

Mason, L. R., Ellis, K. N., & Hathaway, J. M. (2017). Experiences of urban environmental conditions in socially and economically diverse neighborhoods. *Journal of Community Practice, 25*(1), 48–67. doi:10.1080/10705422.2016.1269250

Mason, L. R., Shires, M. K., Arwood, C., & Borst, A. (2017). Social work research and global environmental change. *Journal of the Society for Social Work and Research, 8*(4), 645–672. doi:10.1086/694789

Missouri Attorney General. (2017). *Annual report Missouri vehicle stops.* Retrieved from https://www.ago.mo.gov/home/vehicle-stops-report/2017-executive-summary

Mohai, P., Pellow, D., & Roberts, J. T. (2009). Environmental justice. *Annual Review of Environment and Resources, 34*(1), 405–430. doi:10.1146/annurev-environ-082508-094348

Molyneux, R. (2010). The practical realities of ecosocial work: A review of the literature. *Critical Social Work, 11*(2), 61–69.

Närhi, K., & Matthies, A. (2018). The ecosocial approach in social work as a framework for structural social work. *International Social Work, 61*(4), 490–502. doi:10.1177/0020872816644663

Nixon, R. (2011). *Slow violence and the environmentalism of the poor.* Cambridge, MA: Harvard University Press.

Padgett, D. (2017). *Qualitative methods in social work research.* Los Angeles, CA: Sage.

Peeters, J. (2012). Sustainable development: a mission for social work? A normative approach. *Journal of Social Intervention: Theory and Practice, 21*(2), 5–22. doi:10.18352/jsi.306

Petts, J., & Brooks, C. (2006). Expert conceptualisations of the role of lay knowledge in environmental decisionmaking: Challenges for deliberative democracy. *Environment and Planning A, 38*(6), 1045–1059. doi:10.1068/a37373

Pieterse, A. L., Todd, N. R., Neville, H. A., & Carter, R. T. (2012). Perceived racism and mental health among Black American adults: A meta-analytic review. *Journal of Counseling Psychology, 59*(1), 1–9. doi:10.1037/a0026208

Pyhälä, A., Fernández-Llamazares, Á., Lehvävirta, H., Byg, A., Ruiz-Mallén, I., Salpeteur, M., & Thornton, T. F. (2016). Global environmental change: local perceptions, understandings, and explanations. *Ecology and Society, 21*(3), Retrieved from https://www.ecologyandsoci ety.org/vol21/iss3/art25/.

Ramsay, S., & Boddy, J. (2017). Environmental social work: A concept analysis. *British Journal of Social Work, 47*, 68–86. doi:10.1093/bjsw/bcw078

Saldaña, J. (2016). *The coding manual for qualitative researchers.* Los Angeles, CA: Sage.

Schwartz-Shea, P., & Yanow, D. (2012). *Interpretive research design: Concepts and processes.* New York, NY: Routledge.

Shi, L., Chu, E., Anguelovski, I., Aylett, A., Debats, J., Goh, K., ... VanDeveer, S. D. (2016). Roadmap towards justice in urban climate adaptation research. *Nature Climate Change, 6* (2), 131–137. doi:10.1038/nclimate2841

Shonkoff, S. B., Morello-Frosch, R., Pastor, M., & Sadd, J. (2009). Minding the climate gap: Environmental health and equity implications of climate change mitigation policies in California. *Environmental Justice, 2*(4), 173–177. doi:10.1089/env.2009.0030

Smoyer, K. E. (1998). Putting risk in its place: methodological considerations for investigating extreme event health risk. *Social Science and Medicine, 47*(11), 1809–1824. doi:10.1016/s0277-9536(98)00237-8

Taylor, D. (2014). *The state of diversity in environmental organizations.* Retrieved from http://vaipl.org/wp-content/uploads/2014/10/ExecutiveSummary-Diverse-Green.pdf

Wen, M., Hawkley, L., & Cacioppo, J. (2006). Objective and perceived neighborhood environment, individual SES and psychosocial factors, and self-rated health: An analysis of older adults in Cook County, Illinois. *Social Science and Medicine, 63*(10), 2575–2590. doi:10.1016/j.socscimed.2006.06.025

Urban flooding, social equity, and "backyard" green infrastructure: An area for multidisciplinary practice

Lisa Reyes Mason ⓘ, Kelsey N. Ellis ⓘ, and Jon M. Hathaway

ABSTRACT
"Backyard" green infrastructure programs are an innovative way to manage urban stormwater, with many social and ecologic benefits. In many programs, however, residents with lower incomes are not reached, though they could benefit from participation, and though their participation could benefit the socioecological system. We examined awareness of and interest in backyard green infrastructure among lower- and moderate-income residents (N = 234). Awareness among our study population is low to moderate, but interest is moderate to high, with variability by some demographic and other characteristics. A spouse/partner, city agency, and/or neighbor may have influential roles in increasing participation in backyard green infrastructure.

Introduction

Urban flooding is a social, environmental, and engineering concern in many cities. As populations surge in urban areas, impervious surfaces increase. When open lands and green space are replaced with pavement and new buildings, the rainfall absorption capacity of watersheds decreases, creating more runoff that can overwhelm aging stormwater infrastructure. Increased imperviousness can cause hydrologic imbalance, stream bank erosion, and urban flooding, with consequent impacts on human and ecosystem health (Hammond, Chen, Djordjević, Butler, & Mark, 2015; Klein, 1979). With climate change comes a greater chance of more frequent and severe flood events in the future (Gao, Fu, Drake, Liu, & Lamarque, 2012; Schreider, Smith, & Jakeman, 2000), and with more flooding comes greater threat to human well-being and, in some cases, survival (National Weather Service, 2019). The sustainable management of urban stormwater is thus critical for a healthy and sustainable urban environment.

Despite this understanding, there are limitations to what can be achieved by traditional municipal interventions. Improvements in urban infrastructure, such as installing larger stormwater conveyances, can lessen the effects of urban flooding, but these efforts are more effective when paired with initiatives to store rainwater throughout the watershed, thereby reducing the amount quickly conveyed to local waterways (Pennino, McDonald, & Jaffe, 2016). Storing rainwater in innovative ways requires engagement with a diversity of stakeholders, leading to new challenges for municipalities interested in working with individuals to achieve societal benefits (Heckert & Rosan, 2016).

Green infrastructure (GI) is an innovative way to manage urban stormwater with many social and ecologic benefits (U.S. Environmental Protection Agency, 2018). Under the core principles of GI-based stormwater management, runoff is stored and treated in a highly localized manner, as close to its origin as possible. Common types of GI include bioretention ponds, bioswales, rain gardens, and rain barrels. A substantial amount of the impervious area in an urban watershed where GI could be beneficial, however, is on private property, where traditional stormwater abatement programs (e.g., large bioretention areas) cannot be implemented. At the same time, this creates potential for rich community engagement around urban flooding and stormwater management through programs that connect people with "backyard" GI (e.g., Shuster & Rhea, 2013). These programs work directly with residents to install and maintain small-scale GI on their property (e.g., rain gardens). These programs have the potential to generate positive, collective impacts at both community and watershed scales. Reduced urban flooding and improved water quality help utilities and stormwater managers achieve their goals of environmental stewardship and provision of clean water to the public. Meanwhile, residents can benefit from improved quality of life due to more green space exposure and less damage and stress from property flooding (U.S. Environmental Protection Agency, 2018).

Research on backyard GI programs, however, is only recently emerging. Further, and of importance to social work, there is an overlooked dimension of social equity in many programs. Lower- and moderate-income residents are often not reached by these programs, even though people in these groups often live in areas of cities that are more vulnerable to flooding or have fewer resources to cope with heavy rains (e.g., Few, 2003; Fothergill & Peek, 2004; Wickes, Zahnow, Taylor, & Piquero, 2015).

Grounded in a social work perspective that values equity and opportunity – and also conducted with a multidisciplinary team of the kind needed for collaborative research and practice moving forward – this exploratory study aims to better understand awareness of and interest in backyard GI among a sample of lower- and moderate-income residents in an urban watershed, using survey research methods and descriptive and bivariate analyses. With new knowledge about the potential of backyard GI from a social work lens, results can be used toward multidisciplinary efforts in which community organizers, urban planners, county extension agents, and stormwater personnel work together to identify how to reach groups not traditionally served by backyard GI. If these groups are effectively reached and GI adoption rates increase, both participating individuals and the broader socio-ecological system can benefit from lower flood risk, less property damage, more green space, and improved watershed health.

Background

Backyard green infrastructure

GI is a sociotechnical (Chini, Canning, Schreiber, Peschel, & Stillwell, 2017) or socioecological (Flynn & Davidson, 2016) system, requiring adoption from many stakeholders including municipalities, schools, businesses, and private citizens to successfully improve water issues (Heckert & Rosan, 2016). This provides an opportunity for communities to be involved and to advance inclusive and equitable decisions regarding infrastructure improvements, but also provides the challenge of gaining support and adoption of individuals (Heckert & Rosan, 2016).

The first step to understanding the potential for public support of backyard GI for stormwater management is assessing people's understanding of stormwater related topics and GI capabilities. In previous studies, public understanding of stormwater was site and situation specific. For instance, understanding of stormwater issues may be related to firsthand flood experience (Baptiste, 2014), just as flood protection benefits of GI are likely better understood by those living in an area where GI is already being practiced (Derkzen, van Teeffelen, & Verburg, 2017). Conversely, in Australia where water scarcity is a concern, many residents considered stormwater runoff a benefit to waterways and not a flood risk, for example, by providing flow when water demands are high (Brown, Bos, Walsh, Fletcher, & RossRakesh, 2016). More specific to GI literacy, people with prior knowledge of these practices are more likely to adopt the practices (Gao et al., 2016). As an example, after the "Save the Rain" campaign, residents of two Syracuse, New York, neighborhoods demonstrated a strong understanding of stormwater issues, regardless of demographics (Baptiste, Foley, & Smardon, 2015). This is critical to community buy-in, as practitioners interviewed in one study identified "weak community understanding" of stormwater problems as a barrier to integrating GI (Keeley et al., 2013).

Willingness of an individual to participate in backyard GI for stormwater management depends on a variety of factors, the primary of which is often cost (Brown et al., 2016). Success of financial incentives and potential financial gains are an important topic in prior literature (Baptiste et al., 2015; Tayouga & Gagné, 2016). Newburn and Alberini (2016), for example, found that expected adoption rate of rain gardens tripled when people were offered a one-third government rebate; however, lack of knowledge kept some participants from adopting rain gardens even when the rebate was offered.

While funding is among the most frequently cited barriers to GI adoption by stormwater managers (Flynn & Davidson, 2016) and municipalities (Rowe, Rector, & Bakacs, 2016), other factors have also been shown to matter in the emerging literature. At the individual level––the level of backyard GI implementation––studies have found that social capital and social characteristics of a neighborhood may have a strong influence on adoption (Green, Shuster, Rhea, Garmestani, & Thurston, 2012; Montalto et al., 2013). Stronger relationships with and/or concern for the environment (Ando & Freitas, 2011; Gao et al., 2016; Newburn & Alberini, 2016), a higher income (Ando & Freitas, 2011; Newburn & Alberini, 2016), and being a non-senior citizen (Newburn & Alberini, 2016) may also increase the likelihood of being willing to pay when adopting GI or of having already adopted it. Meanwhile, government distrust led to negative feelings toward some GI stormwater management programs, including fear over formally registering a rain barrel and distrust of pro-environmental causes (Brown et al., 2016). Because some residents may distrust programs encouraging GI, interpersonal approaches to recruitment have been recommended (Bos & Brown, 2015). Finally, and especially relevant for our focus on lower income groups who may be less likely to own their home, landlord-tenant relationships have also been shown to matter in GI adoption (Ando & Freitas, 2011).

Multidisciplinary approaches and the current study

Recent studies such as Gilbert, Held, Ellzey, Bailey, and Young (2015) have suggested the benefits of multidisciplinary approaches to sustainability challenges, particularly those at the interface of social and engineering challenges. Such approaches are critical when attempting to manage stormwater via backyard GI. As noted above, the goal of GI strategies is to treat rainfall in a highly localized manner, which requires engagement of diverse stakeholders to encourage participation across the extent of an urban watershed. Yet, in studies such as Shuster and Rhea (2013) and Jarden, Jefferson, and Grieser (2016), participation in backyard GI programs ranged between just 14 and 32%. Rates of participation must be increased (and maintained long-term) if such programs are to successfully mitigate the impacts of urbanization on local waterways. As noted in Roy et al. (2008), knowledge of innovative stormwater controls is historically limited in communities, contributing to one major barrier to achieving sustainable stormwater management: "resistance to change." However, increased public engagement and awareness has started to prove valuable in gaining more acceptance of GI in some cities in the United States.

Given the salience of financial barriers to backyard GI adoption, the need to diversify and expand program participation for both individual and socio-ecologic benefits, and a social work focus on equity and opportunity, this study examines awareness of and interest in backyard GI among lower- and moderate-income residents of an urban watershed. Our focus on a group of people who are often not participating in backyard GI, but who could potentially benefit from it, reflects social work values of social justice and inclusion. Pursuing this work in an empirically grounded and multidisciplinary way reflects recent calls in the social work profession for new and collaborative research on social aspects of environmental issues that can lead directly to implications for practice and social change (e.g., Kemp & Palinkas, 2015; Krings, Victor, Mathias, & Perron, 2018; Mason, Shires, Arwood, & Borst, 2017).

Methods

Sample and data collection

We surveyed residents of the First Creek Watershed in Knoxville, Tennessee, between November 2017 and March 2018. The First Creek Watershed has an area of approximately 5,320 hectares and is nearly entirely within the Knoxville city limits. The watershed is just over 18% impervious and has a variety of land use/land cover including a small amount of forest, single family residential, and more densely developed commercial and multi-family residential areas (Figure 1). At its terminus, First Creek flows to the west of downtown Knoxville before spilling into the Tennessee River.

First Creek has been one focal point of the City of Knoxville's Stormwater Engineering Division due to historical flooding in the watershed. The city's efforts have included developing hydrologic models to better understand the system and improvement of drainage infrastructure on the main stem, which has the highest risk for flooding. Due to the historical flood risks in this watershed, recent studies have aimed to understand how additional stormwater interventions may benefit the watershed (Epps & Hathaway, 2019). As noted above, efforts to reduce flooding will benefit from providing stormwater storage around the watershed, necessitating engagement with the local community to better understand how individual needs and preferences may affect GI installations in public and private spaces. Further, although catastrophic flooding is most likely along the main stem of First Creek, localized flooding occurs in other locations within the watershed to a degree that concerns residents.

Due to the scope and available budget for the project, we initially recruited randomly-sampled participants by landline and cell phone using a standard, purchased list from a third-party sampling company (in lieu of, for example,

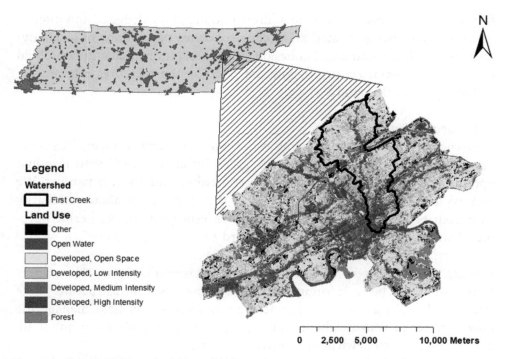

Figure 1. First Creek Watershed, Knoxville, Tennessee

cost-prohibitive, door-to-door surveying across the watershed). However, many of those contacted by cell phone were ineligible because they lived outside of the study's geographic scope. To supplement the sample, we added a non-randomly sampled online recruitment method. We purchased targeted Facebook advertisements, chosen for their affordability with our project budget and due to the wide reach of this social media platform; interested and eligible participants completed a survey instrument online that was identical to the one administered by phone. Participants who completed the survey by cell phone or online received a $5 incentive. A total of 511 participants completed the survey, 396 of whom provided a cross-street that could be mapped as within the watershed boundaries. For the purposes of this study, with its focus on lower- and moderate-income residents, we examine data for the 234 of 396 participants who reported an annual household income up to $50,000.

Measures and analyses

The survey instrument, part of a larger project on social vulnerability to urban flooding, asked 57 questions in the following general order: prior experience with neighborhood flooding and water in the home, individual and household impacts of those experiences (e.g., social, emotional, health, financial), awareness of efforts to address flooding, knowledge of and interest in GI, climate change related knowledge/concerns, perceptions of local governance, neighborhood social cohesion, and several individual and household demographic characteristics. Below, we describe the measures relevant for and analyzed in this study.

Dependent variables

Awareness. We measured general awareness of GI with a Likert-like item, "How familiar are you with the term 'green infrastructure'?" with response options of 1 = not at all, 2 = slightly, 3 = somewhat, and 4 = very familiar. We also asked three dichotomous (1 = yes, 0 = no) questions about familiarity with each of three types of GI (rain barrels, rain gardens, permeable pavement) with the questions: "Have you heard of _____ before?"

Interest. We measured interest in GI with a Likert-like item, "How interested would you be in learning more about how green infrastructure – like rain barrels, rain gardens, or permeable pavement – can help manage the flow of water in your neighborhood?" Response options were 1 = not at all, 2 = slightly, 3 = somewhat, or 4 = very interested.

We also asked about several potential influencers on interest: whether (1 = yes, 0 = no) talking with each of the following people would increase the participant's interest in GI, if the former was to try and encourage the participant to use GI: spouse or partner (if applicable), child (if applicable), someone else in the participant's family, a close friend, a neighbor, someone from the participant's neighborhood association, someone from a City of Knoxville agency or department.

Independent variables

We measured demographic characteristics including gender (1 = female); age (years); race or ethnicity (1 = white or Caucasian, 2 = black or African American, 3 = other which includes American Indian or Alaska Native, Asian, Hispanic or Latino, other (specified by the participant), biracial, and multiracial); marital status (1 = married or living with a long-term partner); education level (1 = high school diploma or less, 2 = some college or technical/associate's degree, 3 = college degree or more); annual household income (1 = $20,000 or less, 2 = $20,000 to less than $35,000; 3 = $35,000 to less than $50,000); and homeownership (1 = yes).

We also measured several non-demographic characteristics: prior experience with flooding/water, perceptions of local government, knowledge and concerns about climate change, and social cohesion. For prior experience with flooding in the neighborhood, we asked, "When there is heavy rain, how often are there pools of standing water in your neighborhood" and "When there is heavy rain, how often do creeks and streams overflow in your neighborhood?" Response options for each item were never, sometimes, often, and always. If a participant responded sometimes, other, or always to either item, the participant was recorded as having prior experience with flooding in the neighborhood (1 = yes). For prior experience with water in the home, we asked, "When there is heavy rain, how often does water get inside your home?" Response options were never, sometimes, often, and always. If a participant responded sometimes, often, or always, the participant was recorded as having prior experience with water in the home (1 = yes).

We measured perceived helpfulness of and trust in the local government. Participants responded to a Likert-like statement, "The City of Knoxville does a good job helping people address concerns they have about their neighborhood," with response options ranging from 1 = strongly disagree to 5 = strongly agree; responses of "do not know" were coded with 3 = neither agree nor disagree. Participants also responded with similar options to the statement, "In general, I trust the city of Knoxville government."

For knowledge and concerns about climate change, we used three Likert-like statements with response options identical to those for perceptions of local government. The statements were: 1) Human activity is the cause of climate change; 2) In the future, rainfall amounts in Knoxville will be affected by climate change; and 3) I feel concerned about climate change.

We measured perceived neighborhood social cohesion with the Social Cohesion and Trust scale (Sampson, Raudenbush, & Earls, 1997). This scale consists of five items that ask the extent of participant agreement (1 = strongly disagree, 5 = strongly agree) with each of the following statements: "People around here are willing to help their neighbors," "This is a close knit neighborhood," "People in this neighborhood can be trusted," "People in this neighborhood generally don't get along with each other," and "People in this neighborhood do not share the same values." We reverse coded the last two items for analysis, replaced any "don't know" responses with a value of 3 = neither agree nor disagree, and averaged the five responses to create a social cohesion score.

Analyses

We conducted descriptive statistics and bivariate analyses in SPSS 25. In some cases, variables were collapsed into fewer categories for analysis, based on the distribution of the data. Select ordinal variables (helpfulness, trust, and social cohesion) were treated as continuous for analysis, also based on data distribution.

Results

Sample characteristics are summarized in Table 1. The typical participant was female, in her mid-60s, white or Caucasian, and with a high school education or less. About one-third of participants (37.2%) were married or living with a long-term partner, and about three-quarters (77.7%) were homeowners.

Table 1. Sample characteristics (N = 234).

Variable	% or Mean (SD)
Demographic characteristics	
Gender, female	71.2
Age, years	65.9 (18.5)[b]
Race or ethnicity	
White or Caucasian	86.7
Black or African American	10.3
Other[a]	3.0
Married or living with a long-term partner	37.2
Education level	
High school diploma or less	51.5
Some college, or technical/associate's degree	26.6
College degree or more	21.9
Income	
Less than $20,000	32.5
$20,000 to less than $35,000	36.3
$35,000 to less than $50,000	31.2
Homeownership	77.7
Non-demographic characteristics	
Prior experience with flooding/water	
In the neighborhood	64.5
In the home	28.3
Perceptions of local government	
Helpfulness	3.2 (1.1)[b]
Trust	3.4 (1.2)[b]
Climate change beliefs or concerns, agree/strongly agree	
Human activity is cause	61.1
Rainfall amounts will increase	62.0
Feel concerned	65.0
Social cohesion, score	3.5 (1.0)[b]

[a] Other includes American Indian or Alaska Native, Asian, Hispanic or Latino, other (specified by the participant), biracial, and multiracial. [b] Mean (SD) is reported.

Despite our efforts to broaden recruitment with a supplemental online component, our sample was not necessarily representative of the First Creek watershed population, a limitation discussed further below.

Awareness of green infrastructure

Most participants (62.9%) had no familiarity with the term "green infrastructure", while 22.4% were slightly familiar, 10.8% were somewhat familiar, and 3.9% were familiar. When specific types of GI were asked about, awareness was higher for one type, and lower for two others. About two-thirds of participants (67.5%) had heard of a rain barrel, whereas only 13.2% had heard of a rain garden, and 13.4% had heard of permeable pavement.

Having any degree of familiarity with the term "green infrastructure", compared to none at all, was associated in bivariate analyses with being younger, having more education, not being a homeowner, having prior experience with neighborhood flooding, and agreement with the climate change knowledge/concern statements in this study (Table 2). No associations were found with gender, race, marital status, income, prior experience with water in the home, perceptions of local government, or social cohesion.

Interest in green infrastructure

Almost 60% of participants reported some degree of interest in learning more about GI (17.5% slightly, 22.2% somewhat, and 18.4% very interested), while 41.9% were not at all interested. Having any degree of interest in GI, compared to none at all, was associated in bivariate analyses with being younger, being married or living with a long-term partner, having more education, not being a homeowner, prior experience with neighborhood flooding or water in the home, and agreement with the climate change knowledge/concern statements in this study (Table 3). No associations were found with gender, race, income, perceptions of local government, or social cohesion.

Table 2. Sample characteristics, by familiarity with green infrastructure (N = 234).

Variable	Not at all; % or Mean (SD)	Slightly, Somewhat, or Very; % or Mean (SD)	p^a
Demographic characteristics			
Gender, female	71.2	70.6	0.917
Age, years	69.3 (16.5)[b]	60.1 (20.2)[b]	**<0.001**
Race or ethnicity, white or Caucasian	88.4	83.5	0.299
Married or living with a long-term partner	38.4	34.9	0.597
Education level			**<0.001[c]**
High school diploma or less	62.1	32.6	
Some college, or technical/associate's degree	24.1	31.4	
College degree or more	13.8	36.0	
Income			0.167[c]
Less than $20,000	35.6	26.7	
$20,000 to less than $35,000	35.6	38.4	
$35,000 to less than $50,000	28.8	34.9	
Homeownership	82.1	70.9	**0.048**
Non-demographic characteristics			
Prior experience with flooding/water			
In the neighborhood	59.6	73.3	**0.035**
In the home	29.7	26.7	0.636
Perceptions of local government			
Helpfulness	3.3 (1.2)[b]	3.2 (1.1)[b]	0.451
Trust	3.4 (1.2)[b]	3.4 (1.2)[b]	0.713
Climate change beliefs or concerns, agree/strongly agree			
Human activity is cause	55.5	70.9	**0.020**
Rainfall amounts will increase	55.5	73.3	**0.007**
Feel concerned	59.6	73.3	**0.035**
Social cohesion, score	3.5 (1.0)[b]	3.6 (1.0)[b]	0.452

[a] All *p* values are from chi-square analyses, except for age, helpfulness, trust, and social cohesion, whose *p* values are from an independent samples t-test; bold indicates statistical significance. [b] Mean (SD) is reported. [c] The *p* value for the linear-by-linear association is reported.

Table 3. Sample characteristics, by interest in green infrastructure (N = 234).

Variable	Not at all; % or Mean (SD)	Slightly, Somewhat, or Very; % or Mean (SD)	p^a
Demographic characteristics			
Gender, female	71.4	71.1	0.958
Age, years	74.3 (14.0)[b]	59.9 (19.0)[b]	**<0.001**
Race or ethnicity, white or Caucasian	86.7	86.7	0.988
Married or living with a long-term partner	29.6	42.6	**0.041**
Education level			**0.001**[c]
High school diploma or less	64.3	42.2	
Some college, or technical/associate's degree	22.4	29.6	
College degree or more	13.3	28.1	
Income			0.902[c]
Less than $20,000	32.7	32.4	
$20,000 to less than $35,000	36.7	36.0	
$35,000 to less than $50,000	30.6	31.6	
Homeownership	85.7	71.9	**0.012**
Non-demographic characteristics			
Prior experience with flooding/water			
In the neighborhood	48.0	76.5	**<0.001**
In the home	20.6	33.8	**0.027**
Perceptions of local government			
Helpfulness	3.4 (1.1)[b]	3.1 (1.1)[b]	0.119
Trust	3.5 (1.2)[b]	3.3 (1.2)[b]	0.112
Climate change beliefs or concerns, agree/strongly agree			
Human activity is cause	50.0	69.1	**0.003**
Rainfall amounts will increase	46.9	72.8	**<0.001**
Feel concerned	50.0	75.7	**<0.001**
Social cohesion, score	3.6 (1.0)[b]	3.4 (1.0)[b]	0.134

[a] All p values are from chi-square analyses, except for age, helpfulness, trust, and social cohesion, whose p values are from an independent samples t-test; bold indicates statistical significance. [b] Mean (SD) is reported. [c] The p value for the linear-by-linear association is reported.

Among those with a spouse or partner, 32.1% said this person could influence them to have increased interest in GI; while 18.1% of those with a child said the same. For other potential influencers on interest, the percentage of positive (yes) responses were as follows: 17.5% if someone else in the participant's family, 22.6% if a close friend, 23.1% if a neighbor, 19.7% if someone from the participant's neighborhood association, 28.6% if someone from a City of Knoxville agency or department.

When potential influence on interest is compared with baseline interest in GI (Table 4), a small percentage of participants (4.2% to 7.9%) whose interest was "none at all" said that talking with the indicated person could increase the participant's own interest; the top three types of possible influencers were spouse or partner (7.9%), city agency (7.2%), and neighborhood association (6.2%). For those whose interest was "slightly", the top three types were spouse or partner (52.9%), city agency (39.4%), and neighborhood association (30.3%). Finally, for those whose interest was "somewhat", the top three types were spouse or partner (52.8%), city agency (47.9%), and neighbor (45.8%).

Table 4. Interest in green infrastructure and the potential influence of encouragement from other people[a.]

Baseline Interest	Spouse or Partner (n = 190)	Child (n = 199)	Other Family Member (n = 210)	Close Friend (n = 214)	Neighbor (n = 211)	Neighborhood Association (n = 217)	City Agency (n = 217)
None at all	7.9	5.4	4.2	5.2	5.2	6.2	7.2
Slightly	52.9	19.4	27.3	26.5	24.2	30.3	39.4
Somewhat	52.8	34.1	21.7	38.3	45.8	22.0	47.9
Very Much	54.8	32.3	51.4	58.3	55.9	51.4	61.5

[a] Values in the table are the percentage of participants, by category of baseline interest in green infrastructure (GI), who said their interest in GI would increase if they were encouraged by the other person to use GI (e.g., spouse or partner, child, other family member, etc.).

Study limitations

Due to the geographic scope of the study (one watershed's boundary), conventional methods of purchasing landline and cell phone samples, and particularly the latter, were a challenge. Though we added an online recruitment and survey method, the final sample is skewed to older adults and females. Thus, results should not be taken as necessarily representative of First Creek Watershed residents. Since similar challenges will likely be present for other studies in individual urban watersheds, which tend to be more limited in size and thus require targeted recruitment efforts, future studies could potentially address these challenges through more intensive, door-to-door recruitment efforts if sufficient funding is secured in advance.

In addition, our measure of prior flooding hinged on the participant's conception of "heavy rain", which may vary among participants. Future studies could consider more detailed explanations of what is meant by "heavy rain" or could gather and analyze open-ended responses from participants to address this.

Discussion and conclusions

Site-specific, community-engaged research on backyard GI is essential for effective program planning and implementation to reach groups not traditionally served by these programs. In this study, we examined awareness of and interest in backyard GI among a sample of lower- and moderate-income residents in an urban watershed. Awareness of GI was low to moderate (about 37% had some familiarity with the general term), with higher awareness of rain barrels, but low awareness of rain gardens or permeable pavement. Meanwhile, interest in GI was moderate to high, at about 60% of the study sample expressing interest. These results suggest that there is substantial room to increase awareness of GI among lower- and moderate-income residents, and that programs intentionally designed to reach this population could be well received.

That younger and more highly educated residents, and ones with prior experience with flooding and/or concerns about the environment (here, measured through climate change statements), had both greater awareness of and interest in GI is not surprising and is consistent with prior research (e.g., Ando & Freitas, 2011; Gao et al., 2016; Newburn & Alberini, 2016). This finding has two possible implications for addressing social equity and expanding opportunities to participate in backyard GI. First, it helps identify which groups have less familiarity and/or interest, and thus who might be targeted through outreach and engagement efforts (e.g., older residents, ones with less education.). Second, if there are positive feedback cycles of how GI can spread in communities as early adopters take a role in informing and influencing others (e.g., Bos & Brown, 2015; Green et al., 2012), then efforts that specifically focus on increasing adoption among these groups could help spread GI to other lower- and moderate-income residents in urban communities.

To create, promote, and expand such efforts, social workers can bring needed skills and perspectives to multidisciplinary teams, drawing on the profession's expertise in program development, participatory approaches, cultural competence, and systems thinking that considers how flood risk and GI may fit in an individual's overall risk milieu or priority of needs. Social workers practicing in community-based organizations can seek new partnerships with city or county offices that manage stormwater or GI programs, as well as university extension programs that already have active GI efforts in wealthier parts of a city or county. These partnerships could take multiple forms. Social workers might engage in door-to-door efforts to raise awareness about GI and available programs, work with children in schools to increase knowledge that they in turn bring home to their parents, or train other professionals in effective communication and engagement strategies for working with lower- and moderate-income residents. Working with existing agencies such as Habitat for Humanity or environmentally-focused AmeriCorps or VISTA programs is another route social workers could explore to address GI awareness and interest.

The finding that homeownership was associated with less familiarity and interest in GI is an interesting finding from this study. Since homeowners have more control over private property investments than non-homeowners (i.e., renters), the opposite relationship is expected, like the one found by Ando and Freitas (2011) for rain barrel adoption. Finding ways to build from non-homeowners' interest in GI to landlord willingness to install GI and meet their tenants' preferences is an interesting avenue for future community-engaged research and practice on this topic, and one little explored in the literature to date. Adding an ecosocial or sustainability element about flood risk and GI to social work practice on tenant rights or neighborhood organizing, for example, would expand existing social work practice in new and innovative ways. Social workers already practicing in these areas might benefit from new post-BSW or post-MSW training (e.g., continuing education units, certificate programs) on environmental justice and sustainability issues, which speaks to the profession's broader effort to infuse environment-related competencies and skills across the profession (e.g., Council on Social Work Education, 2018). To further support such infusion, social work schools and departments can also actively create more field placements to support ecosocial work practice, such as with municipal sustainability offices or local environmental organizations.

Given this study's primary focus on social equity and inclusion in backyard GI among residents with lower incomes, it is interesting that no statistically significant associations were found between income and either awareness of or interest in GI. In fact, the proportion of participants who had at least some interest in GI was nearly equally spread among the three income categories in this study. Since so much prior literature has emphasized the role of financial barriers in GI adoption, this study provides further support for identifying ways – through future research that delves into participant preferences and perspectives in more depth – to overcome these barriers for lower- and moderate-income residents, in particular. Sliding fee scales, rebates, and utility bill reductions are just some of the financial incentives that could be further explored with these specific communities in mind. Social workers engaged in community practice can pursue advocacy with utility companies, stormwater programs, and city or county sustainability offices to create and promote programs that offer such incentives, and help evaluate their uptake and impact.

Finally, prior studies have found that individuals can positively influence GI adoption of other individuals, and that formal social networks such as community meetings (Afzalan & Muller, 2014) and informal social networks (Bos & Brown, 2015) can play important roles. This study provides similar support for efforts to increase awareness and adoption among lower- and moderate-income residents, who have infrequently been the focus of prior research in this area. That city agencies and neighborhood associations (or neighbors) were among the top three potential influencers on someone's self-report likelihood of having greater interest in GI makes community practice that connects these influencers with residents a relevant way forward. In line with the Tayouga and Gagné (2016) recommendation that professional educators, governmental agencies, and non-profits incorporate material on GI into their curricula and outreach efforts, this study suggests that this outreach should include ways of reaching lower- and moderate-income residents in particular, as many people in these groups do indeed have interest in learning more about and potentially participating in backyard GI programs despite the possibility of financial barriers still being a concern. In addition, social workers engaged in policy practice or who work in government can strive to influence trust and rapport from the top-down, by working to influence government agency views of lower- and moderate-income residents and the importance of valuing their perspective and participation, when social workers assess that such views need challenging.

The sustainable management of urban stormwater through backyard GI is an emerging area for multidisciplinary research and practice. Prior studies have identified financial barriers as an important factor, and have also highlighted the need for a site-specific, community engaged understanding of how to best move forward. When social workers, in particular, collaborate with other disciplines and sectors on this work, priorities of social equity and opportunity for all to participate in GI may be more likely to become a priority, or at least remain on the agenda. Through future research and practice at the nexus of urban flooding, stormwater, and the potential role of backyard GI, new efforts can advance the well-being of both social and ecological systems.

Disclosure statement

No potential conflict of interest was reported by the authors.

Funding

This work was funded by the Institute for a Secure and Sustainable Environment at the University of Tennessee.

ORCID

Lisa Reyes Mason http://orcid.org/0000-0001-5386-4425
Kelsey N. Ellis http://orcid.org/0000-0003-1699-6132

References

Afzalan, N., & Muller, B. (2014). The role of social media in green infrastructure planning: A case study of neighborhood participation in park siting. *Journal of Urban Technology, 21* (3), 67–83. doi:10.1080/10630732.2014.940701

Ando, A. W., & Freitas, L. P. (2011). Consumer demand for green stormwater management technology in an urban setting: The case of Chicago rain barrels. *Water Resources Research, 47*(12), W12501. doi:10.1029/2011WR011070

Baptiste, A. K. (2014). "Experience is a great teacher": Citizens' reception of a proposal for the implementation of green infrastructure as stormwater management technology. *Community Development, 45*(4), 337–352. doi:10.1080/15575330.2014.934255

Baptiste, A. K., Foley, C., & Smardon, R. (2015). Understanding urban neighborhood differences in willingness to implement green infrastructure measures: A case study of Syracuse, NY. *Landscape and Urban Planning, 136*, 1–12. doi:10.1016/j.landurbplan.2014.11.012

Bos, D. G., & Brown, H. L. (2015). Overcoming barriers to community participation in a catchment-scale experiment: Building trust and changing behavior. *Freshwater Science, 34* (3), 1169–1175. doi:10.1086/682421

Brown, H. L., Bos, D. G., Walsh, C. J., Fletcher, T. D., & RossRakesh, S. (2016). More than money: How multiple factors influence householder participation in at-source stormwater management. *Journal of Environmental Planning and Management, 59*(1), 79–97. doi:10.1080/09640568.2014.984017

Chini, C. M., Canning, J. F., Schreiber, K. L., Peschel, J. M., & Stillwell, A. S. (2017). The green experiment: Cities, green stormwater infrastructure, and sustainability. *Sustainability, 9*(1), 105. doi:10.3390/su9010105

Council on Social Work Education. (2018). *Committee on environmental justice.* Retrieved from https://www.cswe.org/Centers-Initiatives/Center-for-Diversity/About/Stakeholders/Commission-for-Diversity-and-Social-and-Economic-J/Committee-on-Environmental-Justice.aspx

Derkzen, M. L., van Teeffelen, A. J., & Verburg, P. H. (2017). Green infrastructure for urban climate adaptation: How do residents' views on climate impacts and green infrastructure shape adaptation preferences? *Landscape and Urban Planning, 157*, 106–130. doi:10.1016/j.landurbplan.2016.05.027

Epps, T. H., & Hathaway, J. M. (2019). Using spatially-identified effective impervious area to target green infrastructure retrofits: A modeling study in Knoxville, TN. *Journal of Hydrology, 575*, 442–453. doi:10.1016/j.jhydrol.2019.05.062

Few, R. (2003). Flooding, vulnerability and coping strategies: Local responses to a global threat. *Progress in Development Studies, 3*(1), 43–58. doi:10.1191/1464993403ps049ra

Flynn, C. D., & Davidson, C. I. (2016). Adapting the social-ecological system framework for urban stormwater management: The case of green infrastructure adoption. *Ecology and Society, 21*(4), 19. doi:10.5751/ES-08756-210419

Fothergill, A., & Peek, L. A. (2004). Poverty and disasters in the United States: A review of recent sociological findings. *Natural Hazards, 32*(1), 89–110. doi:10.1023/B:NHAZ.0000026792.76181.d9

Gao, Y., Babin, N., Turner, A. J., Hoffa, C. R., Peel, S., & Prokopy, L. S. (2016). Understanding urban-suburban adoption and maintenance of rain barrels. *Landscape and Urban Planning, 153*, 99–110. doi:10.1016/j.landurbplan.2016.04.005

Gao, Y., Fu, J. S., Drake, J. B., Liu, Y., & Lamarque, J. F. (2012). Projected changes of extreme weather events in the eastern United States based on high resolution climate modelling system. *Environmental Research Letters, 7*(4), 1–12. doi:10.1088/1748-9326/7/4/044025

Gilbert, D. J., Held, M. L., Ellzey, J. L., Bailey, W. T., & Young, L. B. (2015). Teaching 'community engagement' in engineering education for international development: Integration of an interdisciplinary social work curriculum. *European Journal of Engineering Education, 40*(3), 256–266. doi:10.1080/03043797.2014.944103

Green, O. O., Shuster, W. D., Rhea, L. K., Garmestani, A. S., & Thurston, H. W. (2012). Identification and induction of human, social, and cultural capitals through an experimental approach to stormwater management. *Sustainability, 4*(8), 1669–1682. doi:10.3390/su4081669

Hammond, M. J., Chen, A. S., Djordjević, S., Butler, D., & Mark, O. (2015). Urban flood impact assessment: A state-of-the-art review. *Urban Water Journal, 12*(1), 14–29. doi:10.1080/1573062X.2013.857421

Heckert, M., & Rosan, C. D. (2016). Developing a green infrastructure equity index to promote equity planning. *Urban Forestry & Urban Greening, 19*, 263–270. doi:10.1016/j.ufug.2015.12.011

Jarden, K. M., Jefferson, A. J., & Grieser, J. M. (2016). Assessing the effects of catchment-scale urban green infrastructure retrofits on hydrograph characteristics. *Hydrological Processes, 30*, 1536–1550. doi:10.1002/hyp.10736

Keeley, M., Koburger, A., Dolowitz, D. P., Medearis, D., Nickel, D., & Shuster, W. (2013). Perspectives on the use of green infrastructure for stormwater management in Cleveland

and Milwaukee. *Environmental Management*, *51*(6), 1093–1108. doi:10.1007/s00267-013-0032-x

Kemp, S. P., & Palinkas, L. A. (with Wong, M., Wagner, K., Mason, L. R., Chi, I., Nurius, P., Floersch, J., & Rechkemmer, A.). (2015). *Strengthening the social response to the human impacts of environmental change* (Grand Challenges for Social Work Initiative Working Paper No. 5). Cleveland, OH: American Academy of Social Work and Social Welfare.

Klein, R. D. (1979). Urbanization and stream quality impairment. *Water Resources Bulletin*, *15*(4), 948–963. doi:10.1111/j.1752-1688.1979.tb01074.x

Krings, A., Victor, B. G., Mathias, J., & Perron, B. E. (2018). Environmental social work in the disciplinary literature, 1991–2015. *International Social Work*, 0020872818788397. doi:10.1177/0020872818788397

Mason, L. R., Shires, M. K., Arwood, C., & Borst, A. (2017). Social work research and global environmental change. *Journal of the Society for Social Work and Research*, *8*(4), 645–672. doi:10.1086/694789

Montalto, F. A., Bartrand, T. A., Waldman, A. M., Travaline, K. A., Loomis, C. H., McAfee, C., … Boles, L. M. (2013). Decentralised green infrastructure: The importance of stakeholder behaviour in determining spatial and temporal outcomes. *Structure and Infrastructure Engineering*, *9*(12), 1187–1205. doi:10.1080/15732479.2012.671834

National Weather Service. (2019). *Weather related fatality and injury statistics*. Retrieved from https://www.weather.gov/hazstat/

Newburn, D. A., & Alberini, A. (2016). Household response to environmental incentives for rain garden adoption. *Water Resources Research*, *52*(2), 1345–1357. doi:10.1002/2015WR018063

Pennino, M. J., McDonald, R. I., & Jaffe, P. R. (2016). Watershed-scale impacts of stormwater green infrastructure on hydrology, nutrient fluxes, and combined sewer overflows in the mid-Atlantic region. *Science of the Total Environment*, *565*, 1044–1053. doi:10.1016/j.scitotenv.2016.05.101

Rowe, A., Rector, P., & Bakacs, M. (2016). Survey results of green infrastructure implementation in New Jersey. *Journal of Sustainable Water in the Built Environment*, *2*(3), 04016001. doi:10.1061/JSWBAY.0000810

Roy, A. H., Wenger, S. J., Fletcher, T. D., Walsh, C. J., Ladson, A. R., Shuster, W. D., & Brown, R. R. (2008). Impediments and solutions to sustainable, watershed-scale stormwater management: Lessons from Australia and the United States. *Environmental Management*, *42*, 344–359. doi:10.1007/s00267-008-9119-1

Sampson, R. J., Raudenbush, S. W., & Earls, F. (1997). Neighborhoods and violent crime: A multilevel study of collective efficacy. *Science*, *277*, 918–924. doi:10.1126/science.277.5328.918

Schreider, S. Y., Smith, D. I., & Jakeman, A. J. (2000). Climate change impacts on urban flooding. *Climatic Change*, *47*, 91–115. doi:10.1023/A:1005621523177

Shuster, W., & Rhea, L. (2013). Catchment-scale hydrologic implications of parcel-level stormwater management (Ohio USA). *Journal of Hydrology*, *485*, 177–187. doi:10.1016/j.jhydrol.2012.10.043

Tayouga, S. J., & Gagné, S. A. (2016). The socio-ecological factors that influence the adoption of green infrastructure. *Sustainability*, *8*(12), 1277. doi:10.3390/su8121277

U.S. Environmental Protection Agency. (2018). *What is green infrastructure*. Retrieved from https://www.epa.gov/green-infrastructure/what-green-infrastructure

Wickes, R., Zahnow, R., Taylor, M., & Piquero, A. R. (2015). Neighborhood structure, social capital, and community resilience: Longitudinal evidence from the 2011 Brisbane flood disaster. *Social Science Quarterly*, *96*(2), 330–353. doi:10.1111/ssqu.12144

Clean and green organizing in urban neighborhoods: Measuring perceived and objective outcomes

Nicole Mattocks ⓘ, Megan Meyer, Karen M. Hopkins, and Amy Cohen-Callow

ABSTRACT
One way in which urban community organizations attempt to improve neighborhood health is through cleaning and greening efforts. Few studies have evaluated how such efforts are related to changes in both residents' perceptions of neighborhoods and objective community-wide cleaning and greening indicators over time. Drawing upon quantitative and qualitative data collected during an evaluation of a community-building initiative in two communities, results show how neighborhood changes in cleaning and greening were reflected in perceived and objective measures and how these measures compare across different time periods and subgroups of residents within the two target communities. We provide suggestions for additional ways that future evaluations of urban cleaning and greening efforts can examine the impact.

Introduction

Community organizers and foundations supporting their work in low-income urban neighborhoods have long recognized the benefits of community cleaning and greening efforts. "Clean and green" campaigns have been a staple in both large-scale community revitalization initiatives, and smaller community-building efforts led by community-based organizations (CBOs). Indeed, scholars and practitioners recognize that clean and green communities are associated with numerous social and health outcomes, including improved mental health (Gatersleben & Andrews, 2013), reductions in all-cause mortality rates (van Den Berg et al., 2015), reductions in crime and violence (Donovan & Prestemon, 2012), and greater social cohesion among neighbors (Fone et al., 2014).

Greening efforts, in particular, have garnered significant attention in the past few decades as climate change and rapid urbanization have resulted in extraordinary environmental changes, disproportionally affecting marginalized communities and exacerbating existing social and economic inequities. These changes have led government agencies, non-profit organizations, and numerous commissions to establish bold goals for protecting the environment. Examples in the U.S. include large-scale greening initiatives, such as the Atlanta BeltLine and New York City's famous High Line, both of which repurposed abandoned railways as integrated mixed-use park systems (Parkman, 2016).

These environmental and policy changes coincide with the emergence of ecosocial work within the social work profession, illustrated in part with "the changing environment" identified as one of the American Academy of Social Work and Social Welfare's 12 Grand Challenges for Social Work. In their lead paper, Kemp and Palinkas identify core areas requiring an ecosocial work response, including " ... collaborative capacity building to mobilize and strengthen place-based, community-level resilience, assets, and action" (2015, p. 3). An intention of this article is to share lessons learned from our study, which addressed this goal of strengthening community-level resilience through community cleaning and greening initiatives.

We examine the evaluation results of one community-building initiative in Baltimore, Maryland. Baltimore City, like other formerly industrial cities in the U.S., faces significant environmental challenges, such as high rates of toxin exposure (Boone, Fragkias, Buckley, & Grove, 2014), large numbers of vacant lots and homes (American Forests, 2012), and inadequate green spaces (Baltimore Office of Sustainability, 2013). Baltimore City officials began implementing a Climate Action Plan in 2012 to reduce the city's greenhouse gas emissions by 15% by 2020 through a range of greening initiatives. This plan entails numerous greening efforts, including tree plantings to increase the tree canopy, replacing concrete and pavement with vegetation, and providing safe and maintained green spaces within a quarter mile of all residents' homes (Baltimore Office of Sustainability, 2013). Similar efforts have been taking place throughout the city since the early 2000s, such as a citywide schoolyard asphalt removal project, which increases the city's tree canopy coverage around schools (Buckley, Boone, & Grove, 2017).

Within the broader context of these state and city climate initiatives, a community foundation in Baltimore invested in two neighborhoods with three intended outcomes: 1) become safe, vibrant, clean and green, 2) increase involvement and social capital among neighborhood residents, and 3) foster greater equity and inclusion in neighborhood decision-making. An evaluation plan was collaboratively developed and implemented by the University of Maryland School of Social Work (UMSSW); the community foundation; the Baltimore Neighborhood Indicators Alliance – Jacob France Institute (BNIA-JFI); and lead partner agencies in each neighborhood: Hilltop Improvement Association (HIA) and Middlebay Development

Organization (MDO) (names have been changed to ensure confidentiality). The overall evaluation aimed to do the following: (1) gather two waves of data (2013 and 2016) on community members' perceptions of safety, greening, cleanliness, vibrancy, social capital, and equity and inclusion in neighborhood decision-making; (2) examine changes in these conditions over the study period, and (3) assess the initiative's implementation process.

The purposes of this article are to: (1) Discuss the congruence of findings from qualitative and quantitative data collected from two urban neighborhoods on cleaning and greening indicators; (2) Demonstrate the complex relationship between green space and community benefits; and (3) Share lessons learned from using a CBPR approach to measure the effectiveness of a community-level intervention. Drawing primarily upon quantitative survey data, we also integrate qualitative findings to demonstrate how neighborhood changes in cleaning and greening were reflected in both perceived and objective measures and how these measures compare across different time points within the two communities.

Literature review

The person-in-environment perspective established within the field of social work has consistently recognized that an individual's surrounding environment has the potential to both protect and harm their health and well-being. Similarly, the now widely recognized Social Determinants of Health (SDOH) framework, established by the World Health Organization, articulates the ways in which the physical and social environments influence health and other quality-of-life outcomes for individuals (Office of Disease Prevention and Health Promotion, 2018) and largely explain disparities in health across individuals and groups.

Through the lens of the SDOH framework, recent reviews have examined the relationship between the natural environment and a range of public health outcomes, including mental health and well-being, perceived general health, and all-cause mortality (Kabisch, Qureshi, & Haase, 2015; Tzoulas et al., 2007; van Den Berg et al., 2015). Empirical evidence consistently demonstrates a positive relationship between the availability of neighborhood green spaces, such as parks, tree canopies, and community gardens, and mental health outcomes (van Den Berg et al., 2015). Other studies suggest that exposure to signs of social and physical disorder, such as crime and physical hazards (common in high poverty neighborhoods), generates stress, anxiety, and fear (Kuo & Sullivan, 2001; Sampson & Groves, 1989), ultimately leading to poor mental health.

Interestingly, an emerging area in the greening literature indicates a complex relationship between urban green spaces and positive outcomes, particularly in regard to safety concerns. For instance, a qualitative study of Baltimore residents living in high crime neighborhoods (Battaglia, Buckley, Galvin, & Grove, 2014) found that some respondents were concerned about the link between trees and increased opportunities for drug trade. Similarly, an experimental study (Martens, Gutscher, & Bauer, 2011) revealed that exposure to maintained forests resulted in a stronger increase in positive affect than did exposure to less maintained forests, which may be due to safety concerns when visibility is reduced. These studies indicate that the broader context of the neighborhood environment may influence residents' interactions with green spaces, suggesting the importance of assessing residents' perceptions of green spaces.

Individuals residing in low-income urban communities are considered most vulnerable to deleterious health impacts because environmental stressors are especially prevalent in urban settings (Leventhal & Brooks-Gunn, 2003). Given the latest figures from the World Health Organization, which indicate that over 50% of the global population and over 80% of the U.S. population resides in urban areas, both of which are projected to increase every year (World Health Organization, 2016), issues of pollution, overcrowding, and poor sanitation will likely increase the prevalence of poor physical and mental health and well-being for urban populations.

While urbanization is increasing globally, many U.S. cities, like Baltimore, have experienced significant population loss and declining tax bases, threatening the ability of city government to manage basic city services. These trends have collided with neoliberal policies that have driven both a devolution of responsibility for addressing urban problems to cities and nongovernmental actors and a decrease in federal funding to cities. Therefore, CBOs have increasingly filled the gap and have become major players in a bricolage of public, private and nonprofit partnerships to address problematic neighborhood conditions, such as preventing illegal dumping and cleaning up brownfields, planting trees, and converting vacant asphalt lots to community gardens. Few studies, however, have examined how such efforts are related to changes in both residents' perceptions of their neighborhood and objective community-wide indicators. Indeed, most funders and CBOs count their outputs (number of programs, number of people attending an event, etc.), yet few assess their outcomes, because measuring these impacts is time-consuming and fraught with methodological challenges including a dearth of well-developed community measures and inherent difficulties in establishing the counterfactual.

Method

Data for this study are from the evaluation of a 5-year community-building initiative in two Baltimore communities: Hilltop and Middlebay, both funded by a local community foundation. The evaluation process took place from October 2012 through December 2016; this process included (1) qualitative and quantitative data collection for wave 1, (2) analysis of wave 1 data, (3) dissemination of findings to stakeholders through meetings and technical reports, (4) meetings with community stakeholders to revise the wave 2 survey based on wave 1 experiences and findings, and (5) wave 2 data collection, analysis and dissemination to stakeholders.

The initiative supported community partners to engage residents of all ages, build connections between residents and CBOs, and foster equitable and collaborative partnerships among diverse groups. However, the community foundation gave lead CBOs significant leeway to design their community-building efforts. CBOs and their partner organizations worked to implement a range of activities: targeted block clean-ups and garden projects, porch lighting campaigns, public art projects, block parties, parades, and community-wide festivals. While the activities in each neighborhood varied, each included clear goals to increase the number of trees planted and decrease visible litter, particularly on major thoroughfares and entrances to their communities. One significant difference between the efforts in each community was that the Hilltop neighborhood focused much of its effort on the development of an urban farm, engaging youth in farm maintenance and produce sales. Middlebay engaged more effort to organize festivals and art projects, as the community is host to one of the largest parks in the city where annual festivals and parades are held.

Data collection and sample

The data for the cleaning and greening components to this research included surveys with both closed and open-ended questions, and corroboration with existing secondary neighborhood indicator data. The authors developed the surveys in partnership with lead CBOs in each neighborhood, and the surveys used in wave 1 of data collection (2013) were slightly modified in wave 2 (2016) to reflect the prominent interests of the CBOs from each neighborhood. In the Hilltop community, 132 useable surveys were completed in 2013, and 215 useable surveys were completed in 2016. In Middlebay, 283 useable surveys were completed in 2013, and 215 useable surveys were completed in 2016. Tables 1 and 2 note key demographic information on the 2013 respondents, the 2016 respondents, and actual census data for each of the neighborhoods.

The evaluation team used a variety of methods to collect surveys. Community members and graduate students went door-to-door, interviewed residents at community meetings and events, and the survey was available on-line for completion through an anonymous link. A more representative sample was achieved in 2016 in comparison to 2013. In both neighborhoods, the 2016 samples more closely represented the census data based on race, sex, and income. Additionally, surveys were available in Spanish and an incentive of five-hundred dollars in each neighborhood was raffled off to respondents in denominations of $25.00. Quantitative survey data were entered into

Table 1. Hilltop: Demographic and descriptive information for survey respondents.

Variables	Hilltop 2013 Total (N = 132)		Hilltop 2016 Total (N = 215)		2011 – 2015 Census Data Total (N = 6,125)	
	n	(%)	n	(%)	n	(%)
Age	*Mean = 48*		*Mean = 42*		—	
	min = 20 – max = 92		min = 16 – max = 84		—	
Age						
% Under 30	12	(13.0)	45	(20.9)	2,457	(40.1)
% 30 – 59	52	(56.5)	119	(55.3)	2,686	(43.9)
% 60 and Above	28	(30.4)	51	(23.7)	982	(16.0)
Gender						
Male	36	(35)	110	(54.7)	2,853	(46.6)
Female	67	(65)	91	(45.3)	3,272	(53.4)
Missing	29		14			
Race						
White/Caucasian	38	(38)	31	(14.4)	979	(16.0)
Black/African American	59	(59)	147	(68.4)	4,749	(77.5)
Other Races	3	(3)	37	(17.2)	379	(6.5)
Missing	32		0			
Households with children under 18	*(N/A)*		(25.6)		(24.1)	
Homeownership						
Owner	62	(63.3)	55	(29.3)	577	(21.5)
Renter	36	(36.7)	133	(70.7)	2,484	(78.5)
Missing	34		27			
Household Income						
Less than $24,999	23	(24.7)	62	(30.8)	1,073	(40.0)
$25,000 - $74,999	36	(38.7)	102	(50.7)	1.063	(39.7)
$75,000 or Greater	34	(36.6)	33	(16.4)	544	(20.3)
Missing	39		14			

Table 2. Middlebay: Demographic and descriptive information for survey respondents.

Variables	Middlebay 2013 Total (N = 283)		Middlebay 2016 Total (N = 215)		2011-2015 Census Data Total (N = 11,849))	
	n	(%)	n	(%)	n	(%)
Age	*Mean = 38*		*Mean = 36*		—	
	min = 9 – max = 83		*min = 14 – max = 79*		—	
Age						
Under 30 (%)	58	(28.7)	46	(21.4)	5,239 (44.2)	
60 – 59 (%)	122	(60.4)	135	(62.8)	5,278 (44.5)	
60 and Above (%)	22	(10.9)	34	(15.8)	1,332 (11.2)	
Gender						
Male	80	(38.5)	66	(34.9)	6,056	(51.1)
Female	128	(61.5)	123	(65.1)	5,793	(48.9)
Missing	75		26			
Race						
White/Caucasian	146	(74.1)	100	(59.5)	5,775	(48.7)
Black/African American	27	(13.7)	22	(13.1)	3,027	(25.5)
Hispanic/Latino	24	(12.2)	46	(27.4)	2,608	(22.0)
Missing	86		47			
Households with children under 18	*N/A*	*N/A*	(27.3)		(29.8)	
Homeownership						
Owner	130	(67)	79	(42.5)	2,484 (56.9)	
Renter	64	(33)	107	(57.5)	1,883 (43.1)	
Missing	89		29			
Household Income						
Less than $24,999	30	(16)	46	(29.3)	1,154 (26.4)	
$25,000 - $74,999	76	(40.6)	54	(34.4)	1,535 (35.1)	
$75,000 or Greater	81	(43.3)	57	(36.3)	1,678 (38.4)	
Missing	96		58			

158   ECOSOCIAL WORK IN COMMUNITY PRACTICE

a database and analyzed with IBM SPSS version 24. Qualitative data from open-ended questions on the survey were transcribed and compiled in MS Word documents for hand-coding and analysis.

Quantitative measures

Green

In order to assess respondents' attitudes towards neighborhood green spaces, we asked five questions adapted from Balram and Dragićević's (2005) study designed to improve measurement issues related to perceptions of green spaces. Table 3 presents abbreviated versions of each question; for example, "I use the green spaces in my neighborhood to relax". Respondents were asked to what extent they agreed with each statement, and response options ranged from "strongly disagree" to "strongly agree". For the present study, we dichotomized all responses, where "strongly disagree", "disagree" and "neither agree nor disagree" were combined into a "disagree" category (0), and "agree" and "strongly agree" were combined as "agree" (1). We dichotomized responses rather than interpreting mean scores, as we were particularly interested in comparing those in agreement versus everyone else (neutral and/or disagree). Scale reliability was tested for both neighborhoods, and found to be moderate for Hilltop (Cronbach's α = .79) and high for Middlebay (Cronbach's α = .85). Additionally, we examined each item individually, rather than as a complete scale because this approach provided a more detailed account of residents' perceptions on each aspect of cleaning and greening.

To assess residents' perceptions of changes in levels of greening by the end of the initiative, we examined responses to the following question: "Have you seen improvement in greening of the neighborhood over the last few years?" Response options included "no" (0), "yes" (1), and "I have been in the neighborhood less than a year", which we treated as missing.

Using neighborhood-level data obtained from the BNIA-JFI, we measured the number of trees planted each year from 2013 through 2015 for each

Table 3. Greening questions and percent agreeing with statements for both neighborhoods at wave 1 and 2.

Survey Questions	Hilltop		Middlebay	
	2013	2016	2013	2016
Keep the existing green spaces in the neighborhood	81.9	83	87.6	81.8
Green spaces contribute to my quality of life	83.3	81.6	86.8	83.5
I use green spaces to relax	60.4	79.5***	81.5	82.1
I use green spaces for recreation	55.1	78***	80.5	83
This neighborhood needs more trees	73.4	60.7*	80.9	68.9**

Note: Asterisks indicate a statistically significant difference from wave 1 to wave 2, within the same neighborhood.
*p < .05, **p < .01, ***p < .001.

neighborhood. These data were originally derived from TreeBaltimore, a local umbrella organization that coordinates all tree planting efforts citywide.

Clean

We measured residents' perceptions of neighborhood cleanliness and order with eight questions derived from the "Keep America Beautiful" campaign's Community Improvement Checklist. A number of these questions also correspond to commonly used neighborhood disorder measures (Elo, Mykyta, Margolis, & Culhane, 2009; Sampson & Raudenbush, 1999). Examples of questions include "The general appearance of the neighborhood is neat and clean", and "Homes and businesses are painted and in good repair." Abbreviated versions of each item can be found in Table 4. As with the greening questions, all responses were dichotomized to either "agree" (1) or "disagree" (0). Each question was examined individually to assess the percentage of respondents who agreed with each statement. Scale reliability was high for both neighborhood samples: Hilltop (Cronbach's α = .88), Middlebay (Cronbach's α = .84). As with changes in greening, we examined perceptions of changes in neighborhood cleanliness by examining responses to the following question: "Have you seen improvements in the cleanliness of the neighborhood over the last few years?" Responses were dichotomized to "no" (0) and "yes" (1).

Qualitative measures

In order to gain deeper insight into residents' beliefs about greening and cleaning changes in the neighborhood over the prior few years, a number of clarifying questions were included in the survey. For instance, following the question "Have you seen improvement in greening of the neighborhood over

Table 4. Percent of respondents agreeing with clean statements about their community for both neighborhoods at wave 1 and 2.

Survey Questions	Hilltop		Middlebay	
	2013	2016	2013	2016
Parks are maintained and in neat condition	57.3	63.3	73.9	67.9
Playground equipment is painted	72.5	51.6***	60.4	57.1
A visitor would be attracted to become a resident	50.5	77.3***	43.8	48.4
Entrances to neighborhood create favorable impression	35.5	53.8**	42	45.7
Public spaces free from broken structures	45.3	62.2**	46.4	45.4
Trees are in healthy condition	39.4	64***	41.9	44
Homes and businesses are painted	31.5	44.2*	40.8	41.6
General appearance of neighborhood is neat and clean	42.3	72.4***	37.8	40.7

Note: Asterisks indicate a statistically significant difference from wave 1 to wave 2, within the same neighborhood.
$*p < .05$, $**p < .01$, $***p < .001$.

the last few years?", respondents were then asked, "If you answered yes or no to the previous question, please explain." These qualitative data were captured verbatim by interviewers or, in the case of surveys completed on-line, were written by participants.

Representatives from the lead CBO in Middlebay were particularly interested in learning about residents' attitudes regarding tree plantings in 2016, which led to inclusion of questions that asked residents to indicate why they would either support more tree-plantings or not.

Data analysis

We conducted univariate and bivariate analyses to examine respondents' perceptions of cleanliness and greening in both neighborhoods. Independent sample t-tests were used to assess potential differences in cleaning and greening perceptions between our wave 1 and wave 2 samples within each neighborhood. For the purposes of this study, we analyzed our data for each neighborhood separately. Listwise deletion was used to remove those from each dataset that were missing on more than half of the survey questions, yielding a final sample size of $N = 347$ for Hilltop, and $N = 498$ for Middlebay. All data cleaning, coding, and analyses were conducted in IBM SPSS version 24.

Although both quantitative and qualitative data were gathered concurrently for this mixed methods study, the qualitative data for this paper were comprised solely of short answers to open-ended questions on the surveys. These data were analyzed sequentially following the quantitative analysis to supplement, contextualize, and add nuance to the quantitative findings.

As a first step in the qualitative analysis, the comments across all surveys for each neighborhood were transcribed and compiled into separate Word documents for each community. Because of the short-answer nature of the qualitative survey data, no qualitative analysis software was used for data analysis. Data were first categorized into the dominant areas of interest in the study: clean, green, safety, vibrancy, equity, and social capital; only those data relating to greening and cleaning were extracted for analysis. Two members of the study team used a grounded theory approach to independently open code each transcript, capturing those areas of cleaning and greening that drew the most attention. Memos and themes were then used to record discussions among team members to identify points of convergence and divergence (Charmaz, 2006). Overall, the findings presented are a result of triangulation, where the authors wove together respondents' qualitative and quantitative responses, and corroborated these data with ongoing discussions with staff of the lead CBO partners (Padgett, 2008).

Results

Green

Table 3 presents results from bivariate analyses comparing responses of greening questions between wave 1 and wave 2 samples, within each neighborhood. The data represent the percentage of respondents who agreed with each statement (e.g., "Green spaces contribute to my quality of life"). Overall, findings indicate that the majority of respondents agreed with most statements in both waves, suggesting that residents generally support the presence of neighborhood green spaces. However, a comparison of responses from wave 1 to wave 2 indicates some significant differences worth noting. In the Hilltop community, significantly more respondents in wave 2 reported the use of green spaces for recreation ($t_{(189)} = -3.3$, $p = .001$) and relaxation ($t_{(183)} = -2.5$, $p < .05$) when compared to the wave 1 sample.

In the Hilltop neighborhood, 68.4% of the residents surveyed in 2016 perceived an improvement in greening over the last few years. Residents' perceptions of improvements in greening dovetail with the objective neighborhood greening indicator of tree plantings, which shows a significant increase from 2013 to 2015 (see Figure 1). Qualitative data suggest that the top reasons given by respondents for improvement in greening include more trees, presence, and expansion of a local community farm in the community, and more gardens and parks throughout the neighborhood. As one resident said: *"I have seen a big improvement. Gardens are growing all over the neighborhood and there are more trees and the new community space."* Additionally, a vast majority of respondents agreed that they use green spaces for recreation, with a significant increase in agreement from 2013 to 2016.

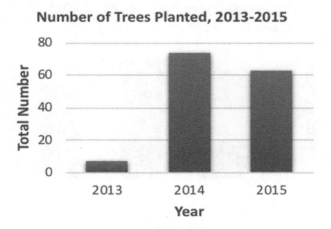

Figure 1. Trees planted in Hilltop neighborhood during the study period.

In the Middlebay neighborhood, 58.4% of the residents surveyed in 2016 perceived an improvement in greening over the last few years. As in the Hilltop community, the qualitative data reveal numerous positive comments by the residents in this community, with the top improvement mentioned being *"more trees"*. Comments like the following from one resident were common: *"Since we bought our house in 2014, there's a new community garden across the street from our house, and our block has 7-8 trees!"* Middlebay residents' perceptions of improvement in greening are also consistent with actual increases in tree plantings from 2013 to 2015 (see Figure 2). Given the increase in tree plantings in both communities, it is not surprising that a significantly lower percentage of respondents in 2016 believed their neighborhoods needed more trees.

Despite the reports that various greening efforts seem to have a positive impact on resident perceptions in both neighborhoods, some also voiced negative perceptions of trees. For instance, in Middlebay's 2016 survey, when asked why they would not support more tree plantings, respondents conveyed multiple concerns related to maintenance, sanitation, and racial disparities. One resident commented, *"People don't take care of them and they become eye sores,"* *"All the leaves blow to my side of the street!,"* Some residents expressed their frustrations about the behaviors they believe the presence of trees invite, pertaining to cleanliness and safety. One resident said, *"Dog poop always ends up where there are trees."* Yet another remarked, *"[I] have found used needles in trees in neighborhood."* This reflects a concern that trees and bushes provide spaces for drugs to be stashed.

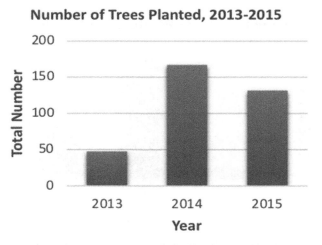

Figure 2. Trees planted in Middlebay neighborhood during the study period.

Clean

Table 4 displays responses to eight survey questions regarding neighborhood cleanliness, as well as bivariate comparisons of responses from wave 1 to wave 2 samples for each neighborhood. As with the previous table, these data represent the percentage of respondents who agreed with each statement (e.g., "Playground equipment is painted"). In the Hilltop community, all but one question yielded significantly more positive responses in wave 2 compared to wave 1. For example, in 2013 only 42% of the respondents felt that the general appearance of the neighborhood was neat and clean, whereas in 2016, 72% of the respondents agreed with this statement ($t_{(207)} = -5.3$, $p < .001$). When asked about changes in cleanliness, 62.4% of the residents surveyed in 2016 perceived an improvement.

In the Middlebay neighborhood, 44.5% of the respondents perceived an improvement in cleanliness over the last few years; however, unlike with Hilltop, there were no statistically significant differences in perceptions of cleanliness between the 2013 and 2016 samples. Qualitative comments from Middlebay residents dovetail with these quantitative findings, where some residents recognized the existence of community cleanups and felt the streets were cleaner, but other residents still perceive trash to be a big problem: *"My street is still swamped with trash on a weekly basis. There is a huge dumpster in the alley next to my house and there is constant dumping trash and rats there. The trash migrates up the alley and onto my street."*

Discussion

As climate change and increasing urbanization harm the environmental and physical health of communities, CBOs and foundations are striving to generate community resilience through cleaning and greening efforts. The rationale for these efforts aligns with research on "neighborhood disorder," which implies that addressing visual indicators of physical deterioration (e.g., vacant buildings, litter, and poorly maintained parks) can influence the perceptions of a neighborhood and subsequent levels of social control and fear (Franklin, Franklin, & Fearn, 2008). Therefore, when prioritizing where to dedicate limited resources, it makes sense for initiatives like the one described here to choose those activities that result in the greatest and most immediate visible changes. Among the changes that positively influence resident perceptions, greening efforts are relatively cost-effective compared to other physical improvements in the urban environment (Jim, 2013).

While measuring the impact of these community initiatives is difficult, this evaluation shows how the lead CBOs in two urban neighborhoods were able to capture changes in resident perceptions which reflected the objective indicator of tree plantings. In both neighborhoods, the majority of respondents perceived a significant increase in greening; additionally, significantly fewer respondents reported a perceived need for more trees in 2016 relative to 2013, which is consistent with the increased number of trees planted during this period.

This paper also adds to the developing body of literature that indicates a complex relationship between green spaces and resident attitudes. Our findings revealed numerous reasons why residents both supported and did not support more tree plantings. Although qualitative and quantitative findings indicated many perceived benefits of greening efforts, residents also expressed concerns. Issues such as maintenance of trees, parks and playgrounds, as well as concerns about cleanliness and safety were expressed, which supports other studies that have revealed that the mere presence of green spaces might not always be viewed or experienced positively by residents (Battaglia et al., 2014; Martens et al., 2011).

However, it is worth noting that the Hilltop community saw more significant improvements in greening perceptions from 2013 to 2016 compared to Middlebay. One possible explanation is the different baselines between the two neighborhoods – Middlebay respondents reported higher levels of agreement with all of the greening questions in 2013 compared to Hilltop respondents, leaving Hilltop respondents with much more room for improvement. This can be partially attributed to: (1) Middlebay's involvement in other greening initiatives prior to this study period, and (2) The addition of an urban farm in Hilltop during the study period.

Study limitations

While the evaluation described here certainly helped the community foundation and CBOs "tell the story" of their impact, it experienced many of the challenges and limitations described by others in the literature, most importantly the inability to demonstrate a causal connection between the efforts of the CBOs and changes in outcomes. Beyond being able to document the exact number of trees they each planted, the evaluation could not help the CBOs claim that any change in resident perceptions was tied specifically to their efforts.

Our study also speaks to the notion that physical improvements do not necessarily equate to long-term environmental benefits. In a recent article examining biases in environmental impact estimates, Holmgren, Andersson, and Sorqvist (2018) explain how psychological processes such as the averaging bias, or the tendency to average behaviors rather than sum them, can lead to more environmentally damaging than friendly behaviors. For instance, when one engages in pro-environmental behaviors (e.g., recycling), moral licensing gives one permission to engage in less environmentally friendly behaviors, which can offset the benefits from the initial pro-environmental behavior. This suggests that merely planting more trees or cleaning the neighborhood are insufficient to conclude long-term environmental health benefits for residents.

The study design presents a number of challenges that limit generalizability of the findings. The use of convenience samples, as well as different data collection procedures at wave 1 and 2, introduce a number of potentially confounding factors in our study findings. For example, in order to achieve a more representative sample in wave 2, we targeted specific demographic groups such as Hispanic/Latino individuals in Middlebay and more heavily canvased particular sections of the neighborhood in Hilltop, which resulted in significantly different proportions of racial and ethnic groups from wave 1 to wave 2 for both neighborhoods. Thus, while achieving greater equity in participation, some of our findings might be a reflection of racial and ethnic differences. Additionally, we are not able to assess change over time, but rather compare the differences between the two samples within each neighborhood. Another limitation is the use of anonymous surveys, which precludes us from determining whether some respondents completed the survey at both time points, potentially violating the assumption of independent samples.

Other limitations pertain to our selection of measures and data availability. During the study period, this evaluation had access to limited objective neighborhood-level green and clean indicators. Other types of data have become available since the conclusion of our study period (e.g., tree canopy coverage), and their inclusion would have enriched the objective picture of change over time. Additionally, based on data availability, numerous confounding factors were not accounted for in our analyses (e.g. building renovations, transportation improvements), which could partially explain changes in neighborhood perceptions. Furthermore, the two survey questions which measured perceived changes in cleaning and greening (e.g., "Have you seen improvement ... over the last few years?") were admittedly vague, and may have captured a time frame inconsistent with the study period.

Implications

Given the inherent limitations with neighborhood studies such as ours, future evaluation efforts could consider supplementing resident perception data with analysis of "big data" (twitter, Facebook, Instagram) to identify the number of times residents mention cleaning and greening efforts in their communities. Neighborhood audits could be used to capture more fine-grained data (e.g., litter, broken windows, conditions of gardens/tree wells) at specific intervals to assess clean and green conditions in real-time. A truly comprehensive neighborhood audit would need to address the averaging bias

(Holmgren et al., 2018), by taking into account behaviors that benefit and harm environmental health. Additionally, residents could be trained to conduct these systematic observations on their block, to gather ongoing data as well as generate a deeper sense of ownership in their neighborhood. Such methods would likely require fewer resources than the survey methods used in this evaluation, and therefore, might be a more sustainable evaluation plan for CBOs.

In conclusion, this evaluation begins to demonstrate some ways in which CBOs can use both resident perception and objective indicator data to tell the story of neighborhood changes. The methods used in this evaluation, along with the additional ones mentioned above, align with the call to build the necessary evaluation capacity of communities that aim to improve well-being outcomes for urban residents.

ACKNOWLEDGMENT

We wish to thank the Baltimore Community Foundation for their support of this research, and gratefully acknowledge the work and partnership of the lead community organizations in each neighborhood who worked hand in hand with us to collect surveys and process survey results.

Disclosure statement

No potential conflict of interest was reported by the authors.

ORCID

Nicole Mattocks ⓘ http://orcid.org/0000-0002-4935-0859

References

Balram, S., & Dragićević, S. (2005). Attitudes toward urban green spaces: Integrating questionnaire survey and collaborative GIS techniques to improve attitude measurements. *Landscape and Urban Planning*, *71*(2), 147–162. doi:10.1016/j.landurbplan.2004.02.007

Baltimore Office of Sustainability. (2013). *Baltimore climate action plan*. Retrieved from http://www.baltimoresustainability.org/wp-content/uploads/2015/12/BaltimoreClimateActionPlan.pdf

Battaglia, M., Buckley, G. L., Galvin, M., & Grove, M. (2014). It's not easy going green: Obstacles to tree-planting programs in East Baltimore. *Cities and the Environment (CATE)*, *7*(2), 1–19.

Boone, C. G., Fragkias, M., Buckley, G. L., & Grove, J. M. (2014). A long view of polluting industry and environmental justice in Baltimore. *Cities*, *36*, 41–49. doi:10.1016/j.cities.2013.09.004

Buckley, G. L., Boone, C. G., & Grove, J. M. (2017). The greening of Baltimore's asphalt schoolyards. *The Geographical Review*, *107*(3), 516–535. doi:10.1111/j.1931-0846.2016.12213.x

Charmaz, K. (2006). *Constructing grounded theory*. Thousand Oaks, CA: Sage.

Donovan, G. H., & Prestemon, J. P. (2012). The effect of trees on crime in Portland, Oregon. *Environment and Behavior, 44*(1), 3–30. doi:10.1177/0013916510383238

Elo, I. T., Mykyta, L., Margolis, R., & Culhane, J. F. (2009). Perceptions of neighborhood disorder: The role of individual and neighborhood characteristics. *Social Science Quarterly, 90*(5), 1298–1320. doi: 10.1111%2Fj.1540-6237.2009.00657.x

Fone, D., Dunstan, F., Lloyd, K., Williams, G., Watkins, J., & Palmer, S. (2014). Does social cohesion modify the association between area income deprivation and mental health? A multilevel analysis. *International Journal of Epidemiology, 36*, 338–345. doi:10.1093/ije/dym004

Forests, A. (2012). *Urban forests case studies: Challenges, potential and success in a dozen cities*. Retrieved from http://www.americanforests.org/wp-content/uploads/2012/11/AF-CS -Baltimore.pdf

Franklin, T. W., Franklin, C. A., & Fearn, N. E. (2008). A multilevel analysis of the vulnerability, disorder, and social integration models of fear of crime. *Social Justice Research, 21*, 204–227. doi:10.1007/s11211-008-0069-9

Gatersleben, B., & Andrews, M. (2013). When walking in nature is not restorative – The role of prospect and refuge. *Health & Place, 20*, 91–101. doi:10.1016/j.healthplace.2013.01.001

Holmgren, M., Andersson, H., & Sorqvist, P. (2018). Averaging bias in environmental impact estimates: Evidence from the negative footprint illusion. *Journal of Environmental Psychology, 55*, 48–52. doi:10.1016/j.jenvp.2017.12.005

Jim, C. Y. (2013). Sustainable urban greening strategies for compact cities in developing and developed economies. *Urban Ecosystems, 16*(4), 741–761. doi:10.1007/s11252-012-0268-x

Kabisch, N., Qureshi, S., & Haase, D. (2015). Human-environment interactions in urban green spaces – A systematic review of contemporary issues and prospects for future research. *Environmental Impact Assessment Review, 50*, 25–34. doi:10.1016/j. eiar.2014.08.007

Kemp, S. P., & Palinkas, L. A. (with Wong, M., Wagner, K., Mason, L. R., Chi, I., Nurius, P., Floersch, J., & Rechkemmer, A.). (2015). *Strengthening the social response to the human impacts of environmental change (Grand challenges for social work initiative working paper no. 5)*. Cleveland, OH: American Academy of Social Work and Social Welfare. Retrieved from http://grandchallengesforsocialwork.org/wp-content/uploads/2015/12/WP5-with-cover.pdf

Kuo, F. E., & Sullivan, W. C. (2001). Environment and crime in the inner city: Does vegetation reduce crime? *Environment & Behavior, 33*(3), 343–367. doi: 10.1177% 2F0013916501333002

Leventhal, T., & Brooks-Gunn, J. (2003). Moving to opportunity: An experimental study of neighborhood effects on mental health. *American Journal of Public Health, 93*(9), 1576–1582. doi:10.2105/ajph.93.9.1576

Martens, D., Gutscher, H., & Bauer, N. (2011). Walking in "wild" and "tended" urban forests: The impact on psychological well-being. *Journal of Environmental Psychology, 31*(1), 36–44. doi:10.1016/j.jenvp.2010.11.001

Office of Disease Prevention and Health Promotion. (2018). *Healthy People 2020: Social determinants of health*. Retrieved from https://www.healthypeople.gov/2020/topics-objectives/topic/social-determinants-of-health

Organization, W. H. (2016). *World health statistics 2016: Monitoring health for the sustainable development goals (SDGs)*. Retrieved from https://www.who.int/gho/publications/world_ health_statistics/2016/en/

Padgett, D. (2008). *Qualitative methods in social work research* (2nd ed. ed.). Thousand Oaks, CA: Sage.

Parkman, J. (2016). *6 urban green space projects that are revitalizing U.S. Cities*. Retrieved from https://www.care2.com/causes/6-urban-green-space-projects-that-are-revitalizing-u-s-cities. html

Sampson, R. J., & Groves, W. (1989). Community structure and crime: Testing social-disorganization theory. *American Journal of Sociology, 94*, 774–802. doi:10.1086/229068

Sampson, R. J., & Raudenbush, S. W. (1999). Systematic social observation of public spaces: A new look at disorder in urban neighborhoods. *American Journal of Sociology, 105*(3), 603–651. doi:10.1086/210356

Tzoulas, K., Korpela, K., Venn, S., Yli-Pelkonen, V., Kazmierczak, A., Niemela, J., & James, P. (2007). Promoting ecosystem and human health in urban areas using Green Infrastructure: A literature review. *Landscape and Urban Planning, 81*, 167–178. doi:10.1016/j. landurbplan.2007.02.001

van Den Berg, A. E., Wendel-Vos, W., Van Poppel, M., Kemper, H., Van Mechelen, W., & Maas, J. (2015). Health benefits of green spaces in the living environment: A systematic review of epidemiological studies. *Urban Forestry & Urban Greening, 14*, 806–816. doi:10.1016/j.ufug.2015.07.008

Part III

Contradictions, Connections, and Challenges between the Global and Local Communities

Local–global linkages: Challenges in organizing functional communities for ecosocial justice

Joel Izlar

ABSTRACT
Communities face "glocalized" ecosocial problems. Functional Community Organization bridges local problems with globalized issues, organizes community, and meets need. Models describe glocal linkages and their outcomes, but little is known of processes and challenges in organizing. This article qualitatively explores ecosocial organizing challenges in a Community Technology Center in a US city, which organized around e-waste and digital inequality. Findings indicate that Functional Communities may face challenges in organizing aims due to complexities in balancing need while concurrently addressing global problems and issues in structure, funding, and process. This may be mitigated through communication, focus, self-awareness, and reflexivity.

Introduction

Communities face global ecosocial problems complicated by existential ecosocial threats. In response to these challenges, informal social welfare networks that provide direct services, nurture community cohesion, and challenge structures through direct action have developed (Shepard, 2014). Such efforts bridge globalized problems with localized issues (Shepard, 2008, 2014). These "glocal" influences continue to shape community organizing in a hyper-connected world (Moxley, Alvarez, Johnson, & Gutiérrez, 2005).

A current model of community organization that embodies glocalized action is *Functional Community Organization* (FCO) and communities that emerge from it, *Functional Communities* (Gamble & Weil, 2010; Weil & Gamble, 1995). Through qualitative meta-observation, this article examines the processes and challenges of organizing around *digital justice* and *environmental justice* in a midwestern-based Functional Community, a Community Technology Center (CTC). Existential ecosocial threats such as climate change, ecological collapse, and austerity paint a grim future but show the need to highlight practices that combine "direct action and direct services" (Shepard, 2014) and a "middle way" between reliance on the market or on the state (Breuggemann, 2012, p. 42). In other words, social services that function as social action are needed. There is little literature concerning FCO theory and practice in general, and this study seeks to expand the model by analyzing organizing contexts and challenges within an ecosocial context. Examining how Functional Communities organize glocalized problems, and by highlighting their processes, conditions, and operational complications, may help shape theory, practice, and inspire ecosocial action in new and creative ways.

The first part of the article discusses how globalization has made decentralized community organizing more relevant than centralized practices for its focus on linking local problems with global issues while concurrently meeting need. This section also builds upon the case for decentralized models by examining FCO and how it relates to glocalization. The second section discusses the glocalized ecosocial problems of digital justice and environmental justice. The third section reviews CTCs and their role in glocalized action toward the ecosocial issues of *e-waste* (*electronic waste*), community disempowerment, and digital inequality. After the methods section, findings include four major organizing challenges in the midwestern US, grassroots CTC, and how these issues affected ecosocial outcomes and organizing. The article concludes with an examination of these challenges and thoughts for future action.

The new community organizing

Globalization has influenced organizing in the US, particularly ecosocial-focused social work (Dominelli, 2013; Knight, 2006; Nöjd, 2016). It has eroded the authority of centralized organizing models in favor of decentralized models that link local problems with global issues. Shepard (2005) refers to this as "The New Community Organizing," which is distinguished by "play, creativity, joy, peer-based popular education, cultural activism, and a healthy dose of experimentation" (p. 47). Citing popular struggle, Shepard (2005) suggests social currents have synced organizing with social change. The New Community Organizing has emerged as public sphere resistance and community projects that jointly operate as forms of protest, organizing, and social care (Shepard, 2014). Shepard (2014) indicates these changes provide a link between "direct action and direct services," which suggests organizing that builds community, questions centralized leadership, and focuses on capacity and autonomy is more relevant than short-term, conflict-oriented methods.

The "new" in the New Community Organizing refers to organizing that (1) rejects centralized leadership in favor of horizontal power; (2) fuses the public and private spheres; (3) sees social services as organizing and organizing as social services; (4) emphasizes prefigurative politics (i.e., living the world as you want to see); (5) focuses on direct action; and (6) builds alternative systems outside of established structures. The "new" is differentiated from the "old" (Alinsky, 1971) in that it does not focus on centralized leadership, self-interest, short-term public sphere "battles" and "wins," the pressuring of politicians, landlords, corporations, and so on. It instead focuses on "organizing community" (Stall & Stoecker, 1998) which melds the public and privates spheres, as well as short-term and long-term organizing, through collective-interest, consensus, mutual aid, and a rejection of centralized leadership. A model that embodies these practices, and is able to link glocalized ecosocial justice issues, is FCO (Weil, 1996).

A Functional Community is a community that has formed to "commit positive change in a specific area of concern" (Weil, 1996, p. 47). Organizers are often "people who have a common interest about something they would like to change, but may not live in close proximity to one another" (Gamble & Weil, 2010, p. 174). The model stresses (a) a deep understanding of issue(s); (b) strategies for change; and (c) communication that promotes "inclusive networking" (Gamble & Weil, 2010, p. 182). Here, organizing is often an effort to craft social change around a concern, and this process empowers people to advocate for issues that affect themselves and others (Weil, 1996). By focusing upon a concern, interest, or function, the goal is direct action that forges links between, and makes changes within, ecological systems (Weil & Gamble, 1995). In other words, organizing around a specific issue that directly affects people – while providing services (if needed) – concurrently draws attention to, and directly addresses, glocal issues. The model is distinguished by activities that draw services users into organizing and organizers into service provision. In this sense, there is often little difference or hierarchy between *the organizer* and *the organized*, and these actions become forms of empowerment on their own. Functional Communities may replace larger institutions, making them more relevant to glocalized problems (Breuggemann, 2012). Current examples are community gardens, solidarity networks, and CTCs. These aspects are strengthened or lessened based upon inclusion and focus and can be areas that foster severe challenges in organizing multi-issue ecosocial issues.

Intersecting ecosocial problems: e-waste and digital justice

Language often prefigures our practice (Dominelli & Campling, 2002; Reines & Prinz, 2009), and because the challenges of *e-waste* (*electronic waste*) and digital justice are global problems with local consequences, it is important to understand their definitions. Current concepts of environmental justice emphasize (a) definitional nuance and elasticity; (b) autonomy over knowledge and narrative experiences from those affected; and (c) non-human-centered views that are ecologically inclusive of all life forms (Schlosberg, 1999, 2007). Environmental justice is a diverse set of views that refer to the just distribution of ecosocial burdens and benefits, as well as theories, laws, policies, practices, and governance (Schlosberg, 2007). The *digital divide* has shifted from ideas of digital inequality as problems of access toward social justice issues that transcend equality of access to include equity of access, autonomy in, and common ownership and control of, Information and Communications Technologies (ICTs) (*digital justice*). These concepts are the bedrock of CTCs and pose a challenge in organizing them. Because these problems are interlinked, it is necessary to examine them in detail, how they relate to one another, and how their complexity may facilitate organizing dilemmas.

The e-waste problem

The material prosperity of consumer capitalism brings luxury to many living in high-income nations and is a major environmental justice issue (Peet, Robbins, & Watts, 2011), such as the mass production and worldwide disposal of toxic e-waste (Giusti, 2009). High-tech industry plays a large role in e-waste accumulation and disposal, as well as its negative outcomes (Robinson, 2009). E-waste is electronics that no longer have "any value to [their] owne[rs]" (Widmer, Oswald-Krapf, Sinha-Khetriwal, Schnellmann, & Böni, 2005, p. 438) and consists of computers, printers, televisions, appliances, and mobile devices. The prevailing method of e-waste disposal is through landfilling, the bulk of which is produced in the Global North and sent to the Global South for processing (Pellow, 2007).

Most e-waste is either dumped directly into local landfills or smuggled through quasi-legal recycling operations that skirt international law (Pellow, 2007). Nations often lack recycling infrastructure that protects human and environmental health (Olds, 2012). E-waste contains a number of precious metals, and mining is a lucrative and hazardous industry (Kumar, Holuszko, & Espinosa, 2017) that exposes communities to highly toxic substances (Labunska, 2017).

According to the United Nations Environmental Programme [UNEP] (2015), up to 90% of the world's e-waste is "illegally traded or dumped," with Europe and North America its largest producers. Despite global treaties (UNEP, 1992), electronic tracking (Lee, Offenhuber, Duarte, Biderman, & Ratti, 2018), and third sector regulation such as *e-Stewards* and *R2* (Pickren, 2014), the problem persists. Shipments have also been difficult to quantify. While conflicting definitions of e-waste, inconsistent product classifications, poor record keeping, and the illegality of trade contribute to unreliable information (Collins, Kuehr, Kandil, & Linnell, 2013), some studies provide clarity. In 2013, Massachusetts Institute of Technology researchers collected data from 184 countries and made an interactive map of the transboundary movements of electronics. According to Collins et al. (2013), in 2012, the US generated 9.4 million tons of e-waste per year, more than any other country, most of which was illegally exported. Despite not ratifying the United Nations' 1992 regulatory treaty, the *Basel Convention on the Control of Transboundary Movements of Hazardous Wastes and their Disposal*, the US has made steps toward dealing with e-waste. In 2011, the US began encouraging the prevention of "discarded electronics from ending up in our landfills" and to "recycle used electronics for the betterment of our economy, health, and environment" (Interagency Task Force on Electronics Stewardship, 2011, p. 21). While reusable electronics are trashed for new devices, people glocally experience ecosocial problems from e-waste disposal and a lack of consistent access to, and control of, ICTs.

Digital justice

Because the limits and definitions of communities are molded by technological trends, the ability for Functional Communities to effectively balance complexities inherent in organizing globalized problems with localized issues is aggravated. In the Global North, the shift of social reality to cyberspace has created a privileged access chasm that is commonly known as the *digital divide* (Norris, 2001). This divide refers to geographic, social, economic, political, and cultural inequality, and inequity linked to a lack of access to ICTs (Norris, 2001).

Understanding this divide as limited to access and use is short-sighted, as it does not address people's relationships to one another, and how interaction with others and technology relates to power structures (Eubanks, 2011). In line with this, *digital justice* is having ICT "access, participation, common ownership" and community health as central components (Detroit Digital Justice Coalition, 2009, p. 1). It is the ensured, fair, just, and equitable relations between individuals, groups, and communities and their access to, participation in, and common ownership and control of, ICTs.

Though access is common for many in the Global North, forms of digital exclusion and *information poverty* (Bach, Shaffer, & Wolfson, 2013), such as control, autonomy, location, knowledge, politics, and culture, exist. In the Global North, gaps fall along categories of traditionally marginalized populations (Norris, 2001). These challenges mirror the injustices, inequities, and inequalities of a globalized world and place digital justice as an important social justice issue for community work. CTCs bridge these ecosocial views and issues together, which spawn successes and challenges.

Community Technology Centers: Silicon community gardens?

The contemporary role of FCO is to bridge global issues with localized problems, organize community, educate and empower participants, focus on problems, and make social change. The issues of e-waste and digital justice are more interconnected than they may appear, and a model for addressing glocalized problems is in CTCs. A CTC is an organization and space located in an urban, suburban, or rural environment that reduces the glocal ecosocial impacts of e-waste by promoting technology reuse, education, empowerment, and social inclusion that benefits individuals, organizations, and communities.

Many Functional Communities operate under *franchise activism*, which refers to applying organizing methods from one community to another. Many CTCs in the Global North have organized under the *Free Geek* model, which aims to reuse discarded e-waste and get it to people in need and, in the process of this, build community, empower participants, prefigure reuse, link ecosocial issues, and fight e-waste. Through direct action, glocalized issues of environmental justice and digital justice are channeled through an awareness of (a) ecosocial problems and their glocally negative effects; (b) feasible models for change; and (c) the need for policy change and direct action.

In the mid-2000s, the Portland, Oregon-based Free Geek, began reusing computers and getting them to people in need, which sparked the Free Geek movement in the US.

The literature on Free Geeks and their impacts are limited, and current information is in non-scholarly literature. Wikipedia ("Free Geek," 2019) reports that there are currently 13 Free Geek-modeled organizations in the Global North, with most in North America.

Studies of non-Free Geek-like organizations in the US note that centers may act as hubs of social activity for marginalized neighborhoods and that they may foster positive social outcomes such as community empowerment, community activism, race and class consciousness building, workforce development, and social change (Davies, Wiley-Schwartz, Pinkett, & Servon, 2003; Gismondi & Cannon, 2012).

Although the information on CTC social benefits and outcomes are limited, what is known about them correlates with similar Functional Communities such as community gardens. For example, like CTCs, community gardens have shown to facilitate social ties and community interaction, health and well-being, individual and collective self-efficacy, a sense of purpose, education on ecosocial problems, and the empowerment of participants to get involved in the organizing (Draper & Freedman, 2010; Ohmer, Meadowcroft, Freed, & Lewis, 2009; Shepard, 2013). In the ways that community gardens provide localized social benefits – while highlighting and challenging the ecosocial justice issues of industrialized food systems, food waste, and inequality – CTCs provide localized social benefits while linking and challenging the ecosocial justice issues of digital inequality, disempowerment, and the high-tech trashing of the planet. In line with this, the CTC in this study set out to address the local ecosocial issues of community disempowerment, e-waste, and information poverty with the global ecosocial problems of e-waste disposal and throwaway culture. By organizing around local problems using the functions of reuse, education, and empowerment as "social lubricants," e-waste is (a) directly prevented from being dumped locally and abroad; (b) awareness is raised concerning the glocalized connections between these ecosocial issues; and (c) the CTC's community is empowered by organizing community and meeting direct need. In other words, by organizing locally, glocally interlinked ecosocial problems are taken head on, and organizing processes make impacts locally *and* globally. Continued organizing around these functions causes a ripple effect through glocally interlinked feedback loops. It is through these linkages and feedback loops where FCO shows the possibility to link local problems with global issues (Shepard, 2005), and the potential for Free Geek-modeled CTCs to make change, as well as to incur significant organizing challenges.

Building upon community strengths is a central method in community work (Itzhaky & Bustin, 2002); however, balancing strengths with glocalized problems presents organizing complications that should be viewed alongside positive footholds. For example, complications such as volunteer retention and a need for better community partnerships have affected a community garden's ability to expand (Ohmer et al., 2009), and the multiple functions of a community garden have facilitated personal individuation (Booth, Chapman, Ohmer, & Wei, 2018). While the CTC in this study experienced some similar challenges to those found in community gardens, studies of garden challenges have mostly focused on the local without discussion of complications linked to balancing the local with the global, such as organizer roles, organizational structure, perspective, funding, and autonomy.

Methods

Because of the incipient nature of the research, this study used exploratory qualitative case study analysis (Yin, 2009). Exploratory case study methodology is a useful method of inquiry for emerging and unexplored topics that lack detail, description, or hypotheses, which, compared to other methods, allows for a more detailed look into subjects that have no real preliminary explanations (Streb, 2010). The following research questions guided this inquiry: (1) How does the CTC foster and facilitate individual, collective, and community empowerment? (2) How does the CTC foster and facilitate community organization? (3) How, and in what ways, does the CTC address issues of the digital inequality and the glocal e-waste problem via community organization and empowerment? and (4) How, in what ways, do CTC members think of the successes, challenges, and contributions of the CTC? The case was the center, bounded by the contexts of time, city, and neighborhood. Single, embedded case design was used, and embedded cases consisted of the organization and community. In an effort to protect the confidentiality of all participants, descriptions and titles are pseudonymous. From January to March of 2018, I conducted semi-structured interviews with 23 participants that ranged from 30 minutes to 2 hours, as well as participant observation, photographic inquiry, and a review of documents at a CTC in the midwestern US. Article findings are not based directly on these methods but meta-observations through the research process. Participants were defined as "volunteer," "staff," "service user," and "community partner" and chose what they best identified with. I spent 40 hours over 2 months at the center and participated in and observed the areas of e-waste disassembly, recycling, computer reuse and distribution, donations, meetings, community outreach, interpersonal communication, and organizing. I set out to research the CTC's operations and effects at the individual, organizational, community, and global levels.

Table 1 displays interviewee racial-ethnic, age, and gender demographic information. The demographics of participants were diverse and were recruited through snowball sampling methods. For example, I would get to know someone through a shared activity, a reference, or from observation and would invite them to participate in the study. Participants were not compensated for their time and were required to read and sign consent forms. All protocols and forms were approved by an Institutional Review Board of a Southeastern-based US University. My relation to participants was that of an outside observer and I had no affinity with anyone prior to the

Table 1. Descriptive characteristics of CTC interview participants.

Participant	Role	Race/ethnicity/heritage	Age	Gender
1	Volunteer	White/Caucasian-American	40s	Cisgender man
2	Volunteer	Black/African-American	60s	Cisgender woman
3	Volunteer	White/Caucasian-American	30s	Cisgender man
4	Volunteer	Asian/Filipino-American	60s	Cisgender man
5	Volunteer	Black/African-American	70s	Cisgender man
6	Volunteer	Black/African-American	40s	Cisgender woman
7	Volunteer	White/Caucasian-American	60s	Cisgender woman
8	Volunteer	White/Caucasian-American	50s	Cisgender man
9	Volunteer	White/Jewish-American	60s	Cisgender man
10	Volunteer	Latino/Salvadoran-American	40s	Cisgender man
11	Volunteer	Black/African-American	50s	Cisgender man
12	Volunteer	Black/African-American	50s	Cisgender man
13	Volunteer	Black/African-American	60s	Cisgender woman
14	Volunteer	Black/African-American	40s	Cisgender woman
15	Volunteer	Black/African-American	60s	Cisgender man
16	Staff	Latina/Puerto Rican	30s	Cisgender woman
17	Staff	White/Caucasian-American	50s	Cisgender man
18	Staff	Black/African-American	20s	Cisgender man
19	Service user	Black/African-American	60s	Cisgender woman
20	Service user	Black/African-American	70s	Cisgender man
21	Community partner	Latino/American	40s	Cisgender man
22	Community partner	Latino/American	50s	Cisgender man
23	Community partner	White/Caucasian-American	30s	Cisgender woman

study. I ensured my credibility through prolonged engagement, persistent observation, data triangulation, peer debriefing (Creswell, 2013), and curbed my assumptions and biases by looking for misinformation through memoing and member checking, as well as building the trust of participants, the host organization, and the community through continued dialog and interaction. Data analyses began as soon as data were collected and continued after my stay. I used the qualitative data analysis package QualCoder (Curtain, 2018) to tabulate, code, and analyze data.

Findings

The Community Technology Center and the organizing process

Research questions placed emphasis on organizing processes and conditions, as well as exploratory design, which allowed challenges within the CTC's operations to emerge clearly. Although observing challenges within the CTC was not an overarching goal of the research, it did surface throughout the research process and became an important meta-observational finding related to understanding the processes and conditions in organizing glocal ecosocial problems (of which these findings are based). The CTC operated in a middle-to-low income, ethnically and racially diverse neighborhood of roughly 80,000 residents in a large midwestern US city. It resided in a gentrifying neighborhood and met the needs of the city regarding affordable technology, recycling, training, and community empowerment. It was founded in the mid-2000s from combined community efforts to reuse technology to make social change.

The community created a CTC with a central location, where anyone regardless of skill could help convert e-waste into working computers, gain skills, help the environment, and organize community – these functions addressed localized problems, met need, and linked them to the greater e-waste problem. Although they maintained a grassroots structure over time, it grew in complexity and reach due to community demand. The main activities can be seen in Table 2.

The center was structured around a number of *functions* that expanded into what I refer to as *subfunctions*, which are a combination of organizing subprocesses that are in sync with primary functions. The primary functions around, and through which, the organization was configured were computer reuse, e-waste reduction, popular education, and community organization (i.e., the center's mission and vision). Within the organizing, primary functions were broken into subfunctions of *need* and *interest*. That is to say, people's motivations for involvement were due to having a need (e.g., a computer or skill) or an interest (e.g., wanting to help out). Primary functions were guided and influenced by subfunctions of need and interest and which, in turn, fed back to the goals and outcomes of the main functions. Table 3 illustrates these relationships.

Table 2. Descriptive information on Community Technology Center activities.

	Type of activity	Description of activity	Organizational focus on activity
Administration	Explicit	Organization administration has been weak, but still functions enough to keep activities afloat. Such work entails nonprofit administration, operations administration, and legal compliance administration.	Moderate to great
Community outreach	Explicit	Community outreach involves maintaining and growing community relationships through constant communication; and partnership and relationship building with outside organizations, individuals, and community members.	Low to moderate
Community organization	Explicit/ implicit	Community organization occurs at all levels *within* the organization and the Community Technology Center space and is effective. However, community organization into the greater community (i.e., neighborhood and city) is inadequate compared to the levels of organizing occurring within the organization.	Moderate to great
Donations	Explicit	Donations (physical and monetary) were the lifeblood of the organization, and the CTC did well with ethically accepting refurbishable materials and getting them back into the community. However, the organization was weak in their outreach *for donations* – something reflected in general community outreach.	Great
Education	Explicit/ implicit	Education mostly occurs in the Teardown and Build areas, where participants learn about the dangers of e-waste, how to recycle it properly, and to refurbish technology for the community. There are no explicit educational guidelines for these areas, and the organization depends heavily on volunteers that mutually share knowledge and learn together – there is no formal educational structure, nor a teacher. A positive aspect of this is that people learn *from each other*, build community, and work toward ecosocial problems *together*. These areas are some of the most potent for individual and collective empowerment, as well as *organizing community*. Topical classes on technical and entry-level themes are offered from time-to-time, but not consistently, nor are they advertised within the organization (for those without technology and Internet access).	Low to moderate
Recycling	Implicit/ explicit	The recycling program is also a large component of the CTC; however, it is mostly run by staff with respect to pick-ups. It could be improved by encouraging organizational participants to get involved with pick-ups, which require a good bit of manual labor. It is implicitly conducted through the prefigurative reuse of not only just old technology, but office supplies, desks, etc. Reuse breathes through the organization – this CTC lives its mission and vision.	Great
Refurbishing	Explicit	Refurbishing, like recycling, is a major component of the organization. And if it were to be compared to an organ in the human body, it would be the heart of the operation. Refurbishing builds friendships and community, teaches skills, informs of the ecosocial problems of digital inequality and the e-waste problem, provides working computers that are needed in the community, reduces e-waste abroad, and provides revenue that goes back into the organization's administrative costs.	Great

Table 3. Organizational functions and subfunctions: An example.

Primary functions	Technology reuse	
	Reuse technology and get it to those in need.	
	Need	Interest
Subfunctions	Technology due to lack of affordability, knowledge of how something works, or some other structural constraint.	Have an interest in technology, tinkering with technology, or helping the environment.
	Help with existing technology, skill development, or as a way out of poverty.	Have a want to "give back" the privilege of having high levels of technological know-how.
	Community, friendship, or a sense of belonging. Lonely and wanting something to do.	Community, friendship, or a sense of belonging. Lonely and wanting something to do.
Subfunctionally mediated outcomes	Without a subfunctional focus on maintaining mission and vision, those that participate based on need alone have the potential to:	Without a subfunctional focus on maintaining mission and vision, those that participate based on need alone have the potential to:
	Gain a computer and move on, never gaining skills, empowerment, or community and friendship.	Reinforce privileged hierarchies, classes, and position(s) of technological knowledge without sharing information with other participants (and learning racial, ethnic, social, etc., things about them)
	Knowledge of the eco-environmental aims of the organization because of the sole focus on gaining technology or skills.	Lose sight of the ecosocial mission of the organization.

Participants were involved for unique reasons, which were complex, overlapping, and not mutually exclusive. For those involved because of need, many participated because they lived in poverty. Some simply could not afford computer equipment, some did not have the knowledge of how to use computers, and others were unemployed and needed equipment or knowledge to find employment. Others participated due to emotional need. People were involved because they were bored, socially isolated, looking for activity, friendship, and community. These needs were interlinked and could not be parsed out, but those that were involved in one area often crossed over into another. For example, an African-American woman in her 50s came to learn how to start a website for her business. She did not expect to come in longer than the time to learn this skill but became a key part in the organization, working for 10 years in ecosocial education.

For those involved based on interest, many participated because of an interest in technology. Opportunities to refurbish and recycle components were appealing, and for some, this was a primary motive for engagement. Participants also became involved because they were interested in ecosocial issues. Opportunities to promote reuse and recycling were cited as a reason for involvement. Others participated due to an interest in "giving back." Because some participants were technologically proficient, many wanted to share knowledge and skills. For example, an Asian-American man that had worked a number of years in ICTs understood knowledge as a privilege and that it was a social duty to share with others that did not have such access, understanding, or autonomy. He viewed participation as a privilege itself and sought to spread this view. Even so, the organization experienced four challenges in consistency of processes and outcomes.

Challenge 1: need vs. interest

Functional Communities are fused by a harmony between functions and subfunctions. Though subfunctional outcomes and crossovers between need and interest were generally balanced, they also created dysfunction. The subfunctions of need and interest frequently complemented each other but created unneeded hierarchies that countered empowerment processes. For those involved based on interest, many were technologically knowledgeable and willing to share information with others. However, despite this willingness, knowledge was not always shared equally or equitably, and some organizers did not have the proper training to deal with understanding hierarchical differences or working with marginalized populations.

Challenge 2: structure

The center operated by community consensus, which was a democratic, cooperative meeting and decision-making process where a council made of participants made decisions about operations. According to some, this was effective for a number of years; however, procedural problems were ignored by lead organizers or not seen as such. The main challenges identified by participants concerning the community consensus model were (a) privacy; (b) autonomy; and (c) effectiveness. After over 10 years, some felt that it was problematic for non-paid staff and non-board members to make decisions about sensitive issues concerning internal personnel operations. This called into question power dynamics between community members. The effectiveness of meetings was also called into question, with many participants expressing concern with the length of meetings, issues presented, and member commitment(s) to follow-through. It appeared that there was a low level of accountability in the organization. Why the model was abandoned is unclear, but the organization later transitioned to an advisory model.

Challenge 3: perspective

In theory, every problem that affects a community is within the grasp of that community, and organizing is seen as a way to address complex issues. In practice, models are used to craft social change (Weil & Gamble, 1995), with problems an intrinsic characteristic. Organizers today struggle with a complexity in their work, and many struggle with tensions between *action* and *services* (Shepard, 2014). Though glocal organizing is a way to bridge these, it is not immune to challenges. The model is susceptible to hyper-focusing on singular issues while sidelining others – which may occur concurrently, over periods of time, or statically. These foci not only have the potential to create hierarchies of function but hierarchies of individuals *within* functions.

The center was formed around ecosocial justice issues such as technology reuse, e-waste reduction, popular education, and community building, but meta-observational findings indicate these foci were not always consistent, and the lack of focus was due to complexities in the organization and its organizing. Inconsistencies may be related to the subfunctions of need and interest, but the data show that it may have been a result of structure and a lack of mission-focus. For example, people that participated based on need may have not seen ecological angles, and those that participated based on interest may not have seen social aspects, and so on. To put it simply, each intersection or interaction between subfunctions and functions had the potential to divert efforts almost entirely toward a particular subfunction. The possibility of meeting primary functions (mission and vision) fell to those active in these subfunctions and the organization at large. From this, there was great potential to shift goal-oriented processes from primary functions to subfunctions – which could impact the center's ability to meet its mission.

Challenge 4: funding and autonomy

Currently, community organizations struggle with complex funding sources, and many are forced to accept money from sources that cause mission drift (INCITE! Women of Color Against Violence [INCITE], 2017). The center started with a philosophy of refusing funding from sources that may divert its mission. Throughout its life course, programs were funded by donations and sales of refurbished equipment. This proved to be a good way to avoid the *Nonprofit Industrial Complex* (INCITE, 2017), but balancing internal complications with greater demands of the community – and striking a balance between these tensions with glocal ecosocial problems – proved to be a great challenge. Many expressed a concern with the lack of funding and that it was preventing the center from achieving its mission and expanding its reach. Participants were also timid about looking for funding. This tension between needing more funding and not wanting to be absorbed into greater structures of power and control was a legitimate enough concern for the organization to continually depend on a fee-for-service model. In fact, a dependence on the fee-for-service model diverted attention away from the organization's primary functions into the subfunction of technology sales. Nonetheless, a lack of outside funding helped maintain autonomy, but at a cost to the community. Operating on less than $100,000 per year affected the ability to reach out to the neighborhood, build capacity, grant equipment, recycle, and maintain more consistent hours of operation.

Discussion and implications

Although the "new" in the New Community Organizing shows potential for timely, decentralized responses to glocalized existential ecosocial threats, it is not immune to organizing difficulties. This is particularly clear in FCO, where there are numerous internal and external forces that make it difficult to accomplish goals, meet community needs, intersect issues, and challenge greater systems. Ecosocial organizing compounds these problems by adding greater complexity to organizing, primarily through attempts to meet need while linking worldwide problems. FCO faces similar challenges to multi-issue organizing (Shepard, 2010); in that, actions have a multitude of processes and subprocesses that may push and pull organizing from larger goals into subgoals, ineffectiveness, and even failure. This is aggravated by contexts of communities in a glocalized society, wherein local issues are worsened by global currents, or local issues may prevent a community from making global impacts. These complexities and contradictions are further strained with the urgency of addressing lived ecosocial conditions such as austerity, climate change, mass species extinction, and ecological collapse. This calls into question how to balance these seemingly contending goals, currents, needs, interests, processes, and structures.

Hierarchy, structure, and environment appear to have facilitated a number of the challenges experienced in organizing at the center. Shepard (2008) contends that a way to avoid pressures found in organizing is to (a) not accept funds that control service provision; (b) be service user-led; and (c) emphasize mission over funding. These challenges may create opportunities for an infusion of organizing into an agenda that reflects mission and vision and individual, organizational, community, and global need (Arches, 1999). For example, because the center "recruited" people based on needs and interests, participants should be better educated and trained on the organizations' goals (e.g., reuse, e-waste reduction, education, and community organization), how subfunctions fit into the overall mission and vision of the organizing, and how this contributes to overall aims. This could be done by lead organizers ensuring participants understand *why* they are involved in *each and every step* of a project. Here, the critical work will be interlinking need, interest, and psycho-social energy toward a more inclusive empowerment process – which may also prevent subfunction "siloing," a process that sidetracks a Functional Community's energy away from issues such as environmental justice and digital justice, into unimportant, nuanced technicalities.

Structure is difficult to change and the center functioned for over a decade on a community consensus model, which had issues due to hierarchies created by funding and a lack of care toward *process* by lead organizers. This caused the center to lose sight of its mission and vision. It is possible that if much of what was being done in different areas (such as subfunctions) were federated – with a focus on inclusive networking – hierarchies may be lessened and communication and effectiveness strengthened. Consistent training and reflexive practices on ways to resist hierarchy and foster communication may impact flow between functions and subfunctions. It is possible that the center could continue to organize under the FCO model if certain changes were made. When examining practice models, Weil (1997) states that it is "critical to carefully analyze the particular action group (or groups) and the salient issues related to desired outcomes" (p. 2) and that models are influenced by economic, political, and social structures. Organizing is not done in isolation and models that manifest in reality as they do in theory are rare, which is why some advocate "mixing and phasing" (Rothman, 1996). While the want to combine models and tactics is great, such practices lack clarity and lead to underestimations of process (Hyde, 1996). It is important that affected communities lead the organizing. Lastly, the refusal to take funding from sources that may control is laudable, but is also a stubborn view given current trends that force communities to take money from sources they once denied. Although this helped maintain autonomy, it also affected the ability to reach the neighborhood. Neighborhood members had not heard of the center, whereas people in the city had – which suggests that although this autonomy resisted control, it lost opportunities for neighborhood empowerment.

Given the glocalized state of the world, study findings have far-reaching implications for not only ecosocial justice issues but for organizers and organizing practices that seek new ways of organizing under complex and delicately interconnected social conditions. Organizing that seeks to address short-term and long-term issues at the same time is notably challenging. Study findings are concurrent with typical challenges found in organizing community; however, challenges in ecosocial organizing are differentiated from these problems as complexities in organizing are local *and* global, and inclusive of all lifeforms. While all communities are unique, it is unwise to assume that what works in one community will work in another. Even so, findings such as these may be a useful guide for those utilizing "new" methods in the context of addressing ecosocial justice issues.

A way to avoid or mitigate some of the problems found in this study may be through (1) consistent training on organizational mission and vision, organizing practices and their complexities, and how they relate to overall goals; (2) consistent reflexive practices (e.g., meetings, inclusive networking practices, interorganizational practices) that pay attention to contradictions and complements within roles, functions and subfunctions, goals, and process; and (3) emphasizing the connection between impacts of internal (e.g., structure and perspective) conditions and external conditions (funding) on goals and operations.

Conclusion

These challenges are a reminder that the myth of "if you build it they will come" remains so. The lesson here is that communities must actively ensure that processes and outcomes are the same in relation to localized issues with global effects. The hands of the doomsday Clock are now weighted and guided by global existential ecosocial threats, which adds a tremendous amount of pressure to craft solutions that meet need while ensuring expedited planetary ecosocial justice. Collective experience is often the basis of organizing, and the glocalization of social problems brings shared experiences to the fore, which necessitates organizing practices based on experimentation, mutual aid, and fun. Although there is not one singular, all-encompassing organizing model or practice that will address the greatest existential threats of our time, there is potential in new forms of organizing, such as FCO. If attention and efforts are made toward analyzing and changing organizing practices and how they relate to meeting immediate need while addressing larger issues, and the internal and external conditions that color and influence these problems, the potential for CTCs and other ecosocial community projects to make glocalized change is great.

Disclosure statement

No potential conflict of interest was reported by the author.

References

Alinsky, S. (1971). *Rules for radicals: A practical primer for realistic radicals*. New York, NY: Vintage.

Arches, J. L. (1999). Challenges and dilemmas in community development. *Journal of Community Practice, 6*(4), 37–55. doi:10.1300/J125v06n04_03

Bach, A., Shaffer, G., & Wolfson, T. (2013). Digital human capital: Developing a framework for understanding the economic impact of digital exclusion in low-income communities. *Journal of Information Policy, 3*, 247–266. doi:10.5325/jinfopoli.3.2013.fm

Booth, J. M., Chapman, D., Ohmer, M. L., & Wei, K. (2018). Examining the relationship between level of participation in community gardens and their multiple functions. *Journal of Community Practice, 26*(1), 5–22. doi:10.1080/10705422.2017.1413024

Breuggemann, W. G. (2012). Community-based social organizations. In M. Weil, M. Reisch, & M. L. Ohmer (Eds.), *The handbook of community practice* (2nd ed., pp. 29–33). Thousand Oaks, CA: Sage.

Collins, T., Kuehr, R., Kandil, S., & Linnell, J. (2013). *World e-waste map reveals national volumes, international flows*. Retrieved from https://i.unu.edu/media/unu.edu/news/41225/World-E-Waste-Map-Reveals-National-Volumes-International-Flows.pdf

Creswell, J. W. (2013). *Qualitative inquiry and research design: Choosing among the five approaches* (3rd ed.). Thousand Oaks, CA: Sage.

Curtain, C. (2018). *QualCoder (Version 1.3)* [Software]. Retrieved from https://github.com/ccbogel/QualCoder

Davies, S., Wiley-Schwartz, A., Pinkett, R. D., & Servon, L. J. (2003). *Community technology centers as catalysts for community change: A report to the Ford foundation*. New York, NY. (n.p.).

Detroit Digital Justice Coalition. (2009). *Communication is a fundamental human right.* [Brochure]. Retrieved from http://detroitdjc.org/wp-content/uploads/2010/09/ddjc_1_2009.pdf

Dominelli, L. (2013). Environmental justice at the heart of social work practice: Greening the profession. *International Journal of Social Welfare, 22*(4), 431–439. doi:10.1111/ijsw.12024

Dominelli, L., & Campling, J. (2002). *Anti oppressive social work theory and practice.* London, UK: Palgrave Macmillan.

Draper, C., & Freedman, D. (2010). Review and analysis of the benefits, purposes, and motivations associated with community gardening in the United States. *Journal of Community Practice, 18*(4), 458–492. doi:10.1080/10705422.2010.519682

Eubanks, V. (2011). *Digital dead end: Fighting for social justice in the information age.* Cambridge, MA: The MIT Press.

Free Geek. (2019, August 8). *Wikipedia.* Retrieved from https://en.wikipedia.org/wiki/Free_Geek

Gamble, D. N., & Weil, M. (2010). *Community practice skills: Local to global perspectives.* New York, NY: Columbia University Press.

Gismondi, M., & Cannon, K. (2012). Beyond policy "lock-in?" The social economy and bottom-up sustainability. *Canadian Review of Social Policy, 67*, 58–73.

Giusti, L. (2009). A review of waste management practices and their impact on human health. *Waste Management, 29*(8), 2227–2239. doi:10.1016/j.wasman.2009.03.028

Hyde, C. A. (1996). A feminist response to Rothman's "The interweaving of community intervention approaches". *Journal of Community Practice, 3*(3–4), 127–145. doi:10.1300/J125v03n03_05

INCITE! Women of Color Against Violence. (Eds.). (2017). *The revolution will not be funded: Beyond the non-profit industrial complex* (2nd ed.). Durham, NC: Duke University Press.

Interagency Task Force on Electronics Stewardship. (2011). *National strategy for electronics stewardship.* Retrieved from https://www.epa.gov/sites/production/files/2015-09/documents/national_strategy_for_electronic_stewardship_0.pdf

Itzhaky, H., & Bustin, E. (2002). Strengths and pathological perspectives in community social work. *Journal of Community Practice, 10*(3), 61–73. doi:10.1300/J125v10n03_04

Knight, L. (2006). Garbage and democracy: The Chicago community organizing campaign of the 1890s. *Journal of Community Practice, 14*(3), 7–27. doi:10.1300/J125v14n03_02

Kumar, A., Holuszko, M., & Espinosa, D. C. R. (2017). E-waste: An overview on generation, collection, legislation and recycling practices. *Resources, Conservation and Recycling, 122*, 32–42. doi:10.1016/j.resconrec.2017.01.018

Labunska, I. (2017). *Environmental contamination and human exposure to PBDEs and other hazardous chemicals arising from informal e-waste handling* (Doctoral dissertation). Retrieved from http://etheses.bham.ac.uk/7549

Lee, D., Offenhuber, D., Duarte, F., Biderman, A., & Ratti, C. (2018). Monitour: Tracking global routes of electronic waste. *Waste Management, 72*, 362–370. doi:10.1016/j.wasman.2017.11.014

Moxley, D. R., Alvarez, A., Johnson, A., & Gutiérrez, L. (2005). Appreciating the glocal in community practice. *Journal of Community Practice, 13*(3), 1–7. doi:10.1300/J125v13n03_01

Nöjd, T. (2016). *A systematic literature review on social work considering environmental issues and sustainable development* (Master's thesis). Retrieved from https://jyx.jyu.fi/bitstream/handle/123456789/52488/URN:NBN:fi:jyu-201612205206.pdf?sequence=1

Norris, P. (2001). *Digital divide: Civic engagement, information poverty, and the internet worldwide.* Cambridge, MA: Cambridge University Press.

Ohmer, M. L., Meadowcroft, P., Freed, K., & Lewis, E. (2009). Community gardening and community development: Individual, social and community benefits of a community conservation program. *Journal of Community Practice, 17*, 377–399. doi:10.1080/10705420903299961

Olds, L. (2012). Curb your e-waste: Why the United States should control its electronic exports. *Cardozo Journal of International & Comparative Law, 20*, 827–872.

Peet, R., Robbins, P., & Watts, M. (Eds.). (2011). *Global political ecology*. New York, NY: Routledge.

Pellow, D. N. (2007). *Resisting global toxics: Transnational movements for environmental justice*. Cambridge, MA: The MIT Press.

Pickren, G. (2014). Political ecologies of electronic waste: Uncertainty and legitimacy in the governance of e-waste geographies. *Environment and Planning A: Economy and Space, 46* (1), 26–45. doi:10.1068/a45728

Reines, M. F., & Prinz, J. (2009). Reviving Whorf: The return of linguistic relativity. *Philosophy Compass, 4*(6), 1022–1032. doi:10.1111/j.1747-9991.2009.00260.x

Robinson, B. H. (2009). E-waste: An assessment of global production and environmental impacts. *Science of the Total Environment, 408*(2), 183–191. doi:10.1016/j.scitotenv.2009.09.044

Rothman, J. (1996). The interweaving of community intervention approaches. *Journal of Community Practice, 3*(3/4), 69–99. doi:10.1300/J125v03n03_03

Schlosberg, D. (1999). *Environmental justice and the new pluralism: The challenge of difference for environmentalism*. Oxford, UK: Oxford University Press.

Schlosberg, D. (2007). *Defining environmental justice: Theories, movements, and nature*. Oxford, UK: Oxford University Press.

Shepard, B. (2005). Play, creativity, and the new community organizing. *Journal of Progressive Human Services, 16*(2), 47–69. doi:10.1300/J059v16n02_04

Shepard, B. (2008). Anti-authoritarian mutual aid and radical social work. *NYC Anarchist Bookfair Collective*. Retrieved from https://archive.org/details/NycAnarchistBookfair2008Anti-authoritarianMutualAidAndRadicalSocial

Shepard, B. (2010). Lessons for multi-issue organizing: From the women's movement to struggles for global justice. *Social Justice in Context, 5*(1), 36–55.

Shepard, B. (2013). Community gardens, creative community organizing, and environmental activism. In M. Gray, J. Coates, & T. Hetherington (Eds.), *Environmental social work* (pp. 121–134). New York, NY: Routledge.

Shepard, B. (2014). *Community projects as social activism: From direction action to direct services*. Thousand Oaks, CA: Sage.

Stall, S., & Stoecker, R. (1998). Community organizing or organizing community? Gender and the crafts of empowerment. *Gender & Society, 12*(6), 729–756. doi:10.1177/089124398012006008

Streb, C. K. (2010). Exploratory case study. In A. J. Mills, G. Eurepos, & E. Wiebe (Eds.), *Encyclopedia of case study research, volume 1&2* (pp. 372–373). Thousand Oaks, CA: Sage.

United Nations Environmental Programme. (1992, March 22). *The basel convention on the control of transboundary movements of hazardous wastes and their disposal* [Basel Convention]. Retrieved from http://www.basel.int/Portals/4/Basel%20Convention/docs/text/BaselConventionText-e.pdf

United Nations Environmental Programme. (2015, May 12). *Illegally traded and dumped e-waste worth up to $19 billion annually poses risks to health, deprives countries of resources, says UNEP* [Press release]. Retrieved from https://www.unenvironment.org/news-and-stories/press-release/illegally-traded-and-dumped-e-waste-worth-19-billion-annually-poses

Weil, M. (1996). Model development in community practice: An historical perspective. *Journal of Community Practice, 3*(3–4), 5–67. doi:10.1300/J125v03n03_02

Weil, M. (1997). Introduction: Models of community practice in action. *Journal of Community Practice, 4*(1), 1–9. doi:10.1300/J125v04n01_01

Weil, M., & Gamble, D. N. (1995). Community practice models. In *Encyclopedia of social work* (19th ed., pp. 577–594). Washington, DC: NASW Press.

Widmer, R., Oswald-Krapf, H., Sinha-Khetriwal, D., Schnellmann, M., & Böni, H. (2005). Global perspectives on e-waste. *Environmental Impact Assessment Review, 25*, 436–458. doi:10.1016/j.eiar.2005.04.001

Yin, R. K. (2009). *Case study research: Design and methods* (5th ed.). Thousand Oaks, CA: Sage.

"Mining is like a search and destroy mission": The case of Silver City

August Kvam and Jennifer Willett ⓘ

> **ABSTRACT**
> While mines are often thought of as a driving force for development, this may not be the case due to power discrepancies between companies and local communities, as well as lack of protection provided by the government. In response, communities have begun to challenge mining companies. The industry itself has countered by developing negotiation techniques to gain local support. This study contributes to the literature on mining and ecosocial work practice, by drawing on the case of Silver City Nevada, where the broad consensus in the community is that the positive local-level impact of mining activities is negligible.

Introduction

In the early 1850s, the Comstock Lode, a series of natural mineral veins including gold and silver in Northwest Nevada, was discovered. This led to mass migration to the area for prospectors hoping to strike it rich (Green, 2015). For the next 30 years, millions of dollars of gold and silver were mined from the region. This contributed to Nevada's statehood in 1864, created internationally recognized mining technology, and, for a short period, gave Nevada more foreign-born residents per capita than any other state in the country (Nevada Humanities, n.d.). As many mining areas tend to do, the boom ended up a bust around 1880 when the natural minerals of the area were largely exhausted.

Although mining has declined in state since its boom days, Nevada remains a friendly environment for the industry and there are still 48 active mines (Nevada Mining Association, n.d.). The Nevada Constitution currently caps the taxes mines pay at five percent tax of the net proceeds only (Robison, 2014). This is the lowest taxation rate of mining across the United States, Canada, and many other places in the world (Nevada Business Magazine, 2012). Federal taxes paid by the mining industry are also low or non-existent; the federal government owns 85 percent of land in Nevada and hardrock mining, which includes common Nevada mining resources like gold and silver, on federal land remains royalty free. The permitting processes in Nevada are also weak and often not locally managed (Nevada Division of Environmental Protection [NDEP], n.d.). Many active and potential mines in Nevada are located in unincorporated rural areas, meaning there is no local municipal government. Therefore, decision-makers that approve local mining activities may live hundreds of miles away from the mining site and local community.

Social workers in the state regularly practice in communities affected by mines and use their positions to advocate for change. For example, in 2014, a social worker was one of the leaders of a campaign to increase state mining taxes; the referendum failed the popular vote by less than 5,000 votes. Because social workers are practicing in these areas, exploring the impacts of mining is analytically productive to advancing ecosocial work practice particularly in Nevada. In this paper, we analyze the case of a small Nevadan town that is fighting to close the local mine.

Literature review

While the mining industry has benefits like employment and infrastructure development (Cavaye, 2001; Wolf-Powers, 2014), welcoming a mine into a local town is not without significant environmental and economic risks. The mining industry is inherently not environmentally healthy. It is not sustainable per the United Nations' sustainable development goals: minerals are not renewable, substitutes cannot be developed in the local area, and the environmental risks related to mining are considerable (Griggs et al., 2013). Mining changes geological landscapes due to current mining processes that tend to favor surface mining (i.e., strip mining, mountaintop removal, and open-pit mining) (Bridge, 2004; Darling, 2011). Common pollutants from mining are harmful to human health and include mercury, lead, and arsenic; these can be ingested through air and water contamination when in relative proximity to mining operations (Bridge, 2004).

The boom and bust cycle of mining also creates economic instability for local communities rather than long-term development (Browne, Stehlik, & Buckley, 2011). Mining towns tend to alter their economy and infrastructure to accommodate the mining industry, rather than save their wealth earned from mining to plan for when the minerals are exhausted (Banks, Kuir-Ayius, Kombako, & Sagir, 2013; Browne et al., 2011; Darling, 2011). When mining industries leave the town, community members can become economically destitute with few other opportunities (Prno, 2013). Additionally, other industries which rely on environmental health, such as tourism, can be permanently damaged or destroyed due to modern mining techniques and their adverse impacts on the ecological landscape of a region (Banks et al., 2013; Darling, 2011).

The intersecting environmental and economic effects of mining can be long term and can have irreversible impacts on its residents including displacement, natural resource scarcity, and adverse health conditions (Banks et al., 2013; Darling, 2011). Therefore, there is increasing pushback against mining activities. Local communities have been able to pause mining activities for negotiations and stop mining operations completely (Browne et al., 2011). Indeed, local communities are emerging as significant "governance actors" in the operations of various mining industry projects that are demanding a fairer relationship (Darling, 2011; Prno & Slocombe, 2012). Mining industries may not have the greater social or environmental good at heart, but they have an incentive to listen to community requests and find mutually agreeable solutions to move their business forward. Because of the environmental and economic risks, and the trend of negotiations between mining industries, local communities, and local power actors, is a prime area of research and practice for ecosocial work.

Three strategies are emerging for mining companies to work with local communities: social license to operate (SLO), community development, and corporate social responsibility. These strategies can be related and interdependent (Ofori & Ofori, 2019). For example, obtaining a social license to operate is a common goal for mining companies, which allows them to operate within a local community without significant opposition. To do this, mining companies commonly utilize a corporate social responsibility strategy and/or a community development strategy. When synergized, the underlying objectives and outputs can be the same, such as an economic development goal (community development), employment training programs funded by the mining company (corporate social responsibility), and community support for the mine to be involved in achieving these goals (social license to operate). These concepts will be explained further in this section.

Earning a SLO occurs when a mine (or other industry) has ongoing informal approval from the local community (Browne et al., 2011; Darling, 2011; Kemp & Owen, 2013; Prno, 2013). This approval is not official governmental approval through a licensing process but frequently occurs when mining industries go above and beyond the regulatory requirements set by the government to achieve broad societal acceptance of its activities (Prno & Slocombe, 2012). Credibility and trust with the community are built, which takes time and significant ongoing investment by the mining company (Prno & Slocombe, 2012). While a SLO is difficult to define and contextually specific, it essentially means that the industry is accepted by the local community and is allowed to operate. In contrast, industries without a SLO may be forced to operate through the backing of force, may be sued by the local community, may not find local people who are willing to work at the industry, or may be forced to shut down.

Newmont's mining operations in Ghana are often held up as a successful SLO (Ofori & Ofori, 2019). The SLO was negotiated across the stages of the mine's life cycle. Before mining began, mining officials met with local farmers to determine compensation for their land, resettlement needs, and whether the local community members expected to be employed at the mine, which they did. After negotiating in these areas, Newmont earned a SLO and broke ground. Through continuous dialogs with the local community, Newmont also engaged in several development projects that the community identified as needing. Even in this "success" though, at the conclusion of this case study, Newmont had not upheld their employment promises and thus the community support appeared to be decreasing (Ofori & Ofori, 2019). SLO relationships are fragile and trust is easily broken when promises are not kept.

In this example, Newmont used two recognized strategies to earn a SLO: community development and corporate social responsibility. Community development is a common construct within social work community practice through which local involvement is utilized to design systems to create tailored solutions to community needs (Green & Haines, 2015; Midgley & Ochoa-Arias, 2012). The process is interdisciplinary and privileges indigenous and local knowledge (Lathouras, 2016). Such an approach can be empowering, inclusive, practical, resourceful, and long-lasting. The community development literature on mining frequently addresses the need for communities to have an active role in the decision-making process to share in the benefits (Kemp & Owen, 2013; Prno, 2013; Prno & Slocombe, 2012). Because mining extracts a community asset (minerals), local community members must benefit from the industry in ways that are of value to them (Midgley & Ochoa-Arias, 2012). Relatedly, the community development process can also identify gaps in local assets, which development can fill, such as a need for local employment. A simplified example of utilizing the community development framework within the mining context occurs when a mining company approaches a community with a plan for a mine. The community determines that to make the mine work, the industry must agree to hire 40 percent of the workforce from the local community, which will also require the mine to fund a continuing education and training center.

Corporate social responsibility (CSR) is another common strategy to earn a SLO across various industries and is commonly used by mining companies (Ofori & Ofori, 2019). In contrast to community development plans that are community-driven, CSR is self-regulated and driven by the industry (Wilson, 2015). Social good is, essentially, written into the business plan in order to reduce potential costs of community opposition (Frederiksen, 2018; Wilson, 2015). A simplified example of CSR is when the mining company approaches a community with a plan for a mine, as well as plans for future remediation and ongoing philanthropy.

While CSR is centered with the industry and community development is centered with the community, the lines are becoming blurred within the scholarship. Scholars that work to develop CSR best practices are now arguing that CSR strategies must include opportunities for community-based communication, resident participation, stakeholder engagement, and rapport building (Ross, 2017; Wilson, 2015). Therefore, strong CSR strategies tend to be aligned with local community development goals.

While operating a mine with community support is generally a preferable outcome, these strategies are critiqued. CSR was not born out of goodwill between mining companies and local communities. Rather, the emergence of this concept within the mining context is attributed to recent examples of community opposition to mining projects that have resulted in adverse operational, economic, and social consequences for mining companies (Frederiksen, 2018). Therefore, while mining industries have recently prioritized CSR, the strategies tend to be related to risk management that focuses on the greatest threats to the mining company and not on the greatest needs of the local community (Frederiksen, 2018). In contrast, community development projects that are often identified by the local community are those that support the long-term benefit of the town such as housing, infrastructure, public services, and attracting new/diverse businesses in the area (Fernando & Cooley, 2016). However, as SLO efforts by mining companies are typically guided by cost analysis principles, these actions are often not deemed cost essential by the mining company and thus not supported (Bridge, 2004).

Understanding the disagreements within the scholarship is critical to framing an investigation of a mining community in Nevada. This study explores mining, community development, and corporate responsibility within a mining community in Nevada utilizing the firsthand experiences of local community members.

Context: Silver City, Nevada

Silver City is an unincorporated rural community of about 170 individuals (U. S. Census Bureau, 2016). The town has several unique and contradictory classifications. It is within the federally designated Carson River Mercury Superfund Site due to the high levels of mercury contamination that remain from nineteenth-century mining processes (U. S. Environmental Protection Agency [EPA], n.d.). It is also a federally recognized historic district due to the numerous historical structures that still stand and attracts visitors from across the world (National Park Service, 2018). Other visitors tour Silver City because the community sits in the lower part of the Virginia Range, which is a collection of mineral-rich mountains that contribute to a visually stunning landscape. The area also has unique wildlife such as the Pronghorn Antelope and the endangered Sage-grouse, which have attracted environmental researchers to the area (Nevada Department of Wildlife, 2019).

The history of Silver City is equally unique. The population of Silver City peaked in 1861 and declined with the end of the Comstock Lode mining rush, becoming a ghost town with a rich collection of archeological monuments. During the 1970s, Silver City experienced a community revitalization with the relocation of numerous young recent college graduates from the nearby San Francisco Bay area. As described by study participants, the community of Silver City developed into a bedroom community (i.e., commuter town with little industry) with many young families. Residents recalled that they considered mining to be a historic industry of the past. This changed in the 1980s. In 1986, Nevex Gold Company purchased land within the Silver City community and applied to the County Commission for permits to conduct mining operations in the region. In response, Silver City residents formed the Silver City Residents Association, hired legal representation, and successfully stopped the planned mining activities for several decades.

However, in 2011, Comstock Mining Incorporated (CMI) purchased the same land and submitted new permit requests to the board of County Commissioners, which is located 60 miles away in the city of Yerington. These new re-zoning permits and amendments to the county's Comstock Master Plan would allow the company to conduct extensive mining activities in the region (Trout, 2013). To influence the makeup of the County Commission, CMI made a sizable campaign contribution to County Commissioner candidate, Bob Hastings during the county's 2012 elections (Office of the Nevada Secretary of State, 2012). Hastings was elected to the board and has since voted in favor of all CMI's applications (Trout, 2013).

In protest of CMI's recent re-zoning and permit application, Silver City residents organized against opening new mining activities again. However, despite these efforts, the mining company's requests were approved (Lyon County, Nevada, 2012). Consequently, mining and drilling activities are currently being conducted in close proximity to the community, including local businesses and residences. The residents have filed suit and are currently seeking remediation through the Nevada Court system. This study focuses on the experiences of Silver City residents related to CMI mining activities.

Methodology

This study explores one environmental injustice: mining against community wishes. Because environmental injustice is grounded in critical analysis of power relationships, we chose to intentionally lower the power discrepancy associated with traditional top-down research methodologies by utilizing a community-based participatory research (CBPR) orientation (Lincoln, Lynham, & Guba, 2011). We partnered with a local non-profit organization that has been working across the state on environmental and social issues for

25 years. The non-profit organization's staff members facilitated much of the community contacts for recruitment. They also helped write interview questions that supported their work and assisted in collecting the data after appropriate training from the researchers. The intention behind these decisions was to develop solutions rooted in grassroots knowledge. In addition to the CBPR orientation of the study, we chose to follow a phenomenological approach to understand the firsthand experience of living near an unwanted mine (Padgett, 2016).

Participants were recruited using the snowball sampling method. The non-profit organization's staff connected to the first participant. Subsequent participants were recruited through referrals. Because of the phenomenological orientation of the study, the inclusion criterion for participation was firsthand experience with a local environmental injustice/the mine in Silver City, which we assessed at first contact. Nine participants were recruited from a population of about 170 people (U. S. Census Bureau, 2016). The average age of the participants is 73 and most are retired, with one participant working part-time and two participants who are local small business owners. All of the participants are local homeowners. Five of the participants are women. All participants are white, as are all residents in Silver City.

The interviews explored several domains including the experience of environmental problem, context, coping mechanisms, needs, and ideal responses. Importantly, the interview guide asked participants to identify both positive and negative impacts of the mine. This was needed data for the non-profit organization as they could use it to create change by praising the positives while identifying solutions to the negatives (i.e., the residents are thankful for the good jobs, but request the mine to move the waste pit further from their water source). Participants were interviewed in 2017. Supplemental data came from sources including documents from CMI summaries of meetings, and community reports. These sources were primarily used to triangulate findings.

Data were analyzed thematically in NVivo through multiple cycles of coding and analysis by two researchers to support trustworthiness (Padgett, 2016). First, we inductively developed our codebook through open-coding the data, chunking passages into themes, and developing a codebook from these themes (Corbin & Strauss, 2008). This resulted in a codebook with 28 codes such as impacts, leadership, and coping mechanisms. Second, we established coding rules to support consistency of coding across our coding process. Third, we coded the interviews and checked each other's codes. Fourth, we thematically analyzed these codes to have a baseline understanding. Fifth, we applied a second coding scheme to the interviews that was related to the theoretical framework. This included codes such as ideal response from government, ideal response from mining company, accountability, and community inclusion. Finally, we analyzed this second coding scheme thematically.

Thematic saturation was reached within the interviews from the nine participants, in which additional data were offering few new insights (Padgett, 2016). Because these findings were all uniformly against the mine, we attempted to recruit participants that could give other viewpoints about the mine, including explicitly attempting to recruit local individuals that were in favor of the mine. We were unsuccessful in recruiting alternative opinions. While this could been because of many reasons, this lack of diversity in opinion is triangulated by other sources. Media sources stated that "the community" opposes the mine (Margiott, 2019) and community pages state they are "united under assault" (Savesilvercity.org, 2019). This stands in contrast to CMI public relations that promotes the mine as a positive force for rural community development. We explored this case due to these contradictions and focused on issues related to SLO, community development, and CSR. To understand the participants' firsthand experiences in this case, we focused on exploring two main themes, impacts and responses.

Findings

Impacts

Participants described their experiences living in a mining town and detailed the impacts of CMI's activities. These included direct impacts, such as environmental degradation, and secondary effects, such as the impacts on tourism, economic distress, and health impacts. Many of these concerns overlap and bleed into each other, making the impacts complicated to resolve. In this section, we detail these impacts.

In the simplest terms, mining operations strip layers of rock with heavy machinery to reach valued minerals. Environmental degradation in a nearly universal side effect of mining operations as the area is excavated. However, Silver City was unique because the destruction was so close to town and their houses, which created a new environment that was unhealthy and uncomfortable for residents. Participant 2 described her life as, "I can't sit outside. The fumes, and the dust, and the noise, the rattling and blasting, it's just horrible." Similarly, participant 3 described the area around his house as, "They bring in heavy equipment and they grade roads all over the place and they drill for core samples. The drilling generates dust like you wouldn't believe and it generates terrible noise. Because sometimes they drill twelve hours or eighteen hours a day." In addition to living in a degraded environment, participants were concerned about long-term environmental damage, particularly as Silver City is located in an environmental fragile ecosystem. Participant 1 said, "The environmental results have yet to be seen … .Know your watershed and be kind to it because after you're done, somebody else is gonna need it." This concern was notable as often long-term environmental degradation is difficult to identify but these participants could and they feared it would worsen over time.

Environmental concerns were often linked to the secondary impacts on the tourism industry that combined the local arts scene with local outdoor activities. For example, participants often described CMI's decision to sit an open-pit mine near a unique geological feature known as Devil's Gate which drastically changed the landscape. Participant 3 said, "They took the whole top off of that mountain." Participant 4 characterized this mining activity as a "humongous pit ... They dug it and abandoned it." As no reclamation efforts are mandated by state laws, CMI was under no obligation to restore the area to its former condition, which angered residents. While these actions negatively affected the local environment for residents, participants stated that Devil's Gate previously drew tourists to the region and with the changes in the landscape, they assumed the tourist flow had been reduced. In addition, participants feared more of these actions, which would further reduce the tourism industry. Their fears are not unfounded: CMI has expressed intentions to conduct similar activities across the area, which they are legally allowed to do regardless of the consequences for local residents and other industries.

Relatedly, CMI activities also impacted specific tourist ventures and the local infrastructure. CMI mining activities necessitate driving heavy mining trucks and equipment through town on small roads. This resulted in the collapse of the main road through Silver City. While bothersome for residents, traffic had to be re-routed, which limited the flow of outsiders into the community and several tourism-related businesses closed. Participant 1 summarized the problem as, "Everything has closed down because the mining has destroyed the county."

While damage to the tourism industry economically impacted residents, many participants also described personal economic instability due to a widespread decrease in property values. Participant 3 explained that because of the drilling, noise, and operation of heavy machinery, "Houses on both sides of the hill and our property values, along with the dump that everybody else in the country took, that our property values took, an unbelievable dump." This is a critical point when combined with the environmental degradation. Participants explained that much of their financial stability was in their property values. Because their property was decreasing and they had no other source of wealth, no matter how bad their local environmental became because of the mining activities, they could not leave the community and move elsewhere. They were stuck.

Having to stay in Silver City is particularly important to understanding their discussions of health impacts, which they felt were dire. Participants were extremely concerned they were actively being poisoned through stirring up historic mining waste into the air and water through CMI activities. Silver City is located on an EPA Superfund site due to historic mining processes that discarded toxic levels of mercury into nearby communities. While not ideal, local residents had long taken recommended actions to protect themselves, such as not disturbing the polluted land. However, participants felt that CMI's activities went against these recommended protections for residents living in this area. Participant 1, a woman in her 60s, explained that, "When you dig and the wind blows, [mercury is] there. You can't get away from it. So the mining all around here has toxified everyone." Participant 3 echoed these concerns and stated, "There's been no study to see what putting all this dust in the air for us to breath, how that arsenic would affect us." These are not unfounded fears for Silver City residents. In the 1980s, many tested positive for heavy metal poisoning from similar mining activities, for which they received no compensation.

Health impacts were not limited to physical health. Because of their concerns for the environment, their community, their finances, and their health, participants regularly described significant psychological distress due to the mining activities and the secondary effects. Participant 2, a woman in her 70s, described the "wear and tear on your body and mind from constantly being worried."

Responses

Government processes

Silver City participants described fights with other mining industries for decades, most of which they won. Therefore, they attempted to fight back against CMI and halt mining activities in their town. While a lawsuit is presently ongoing, they have currently lost and CMI has proceeded with legal mining activities that have been approved by the levels of government involved. Therefore, Silver City residents are extremely upset with government processes. Participant 5, an 80-year-old male, summarized the situation as "One of the big negatives from all of this is that it has destroyed confidence in the government. It has really eroded trust."

Indeed, participants blamed all levels of government for lack of environmental protection. Participants described the local government, which is sat 60 miles away, as "corrupt" and "bought" due to CMI's donations into the political process. At minimum, Silver City residents do not have an ally or representative in the local government where the permitting decisions are being made. Participants also felt that the state overvalued industry and undervaluing the local people. For example, participant 1 said, "There's the mining and the agriculture and industrial things that are going on that Nevada has embraced and is not maintaining a healthy environment in the doing of it. Those things bug me, I'm not good with that." This view is arguably true. CMI's activities are causing widespread negative impacts in Silver City but Nevadan regulatory laws are weak. Therefore, even though CMI has created damage to Silver City, CMI is acting lawfully and Silver City residents have little legal basis for complaint at the state level.

Negotiations with CMI

As it became clear that Silver City residents would likely not be able to block CMI's activities and government officials would not protect them, residents attempted to negotiate with CMI to reach a compromise. CMI initially engaged with the community and held multiple community meetings during which they committed to providing jobs and other benefits to the community. CMI also initiated a historical restoration foundation to rehabilitate aged and dilapidated structures with historical relevance within the Silver City community. While seemingly positive, these benefits were not what the community wanted. Regarding jobs, participant 2 explained, "Most of the people in this community are retired. I don't want a job." The historical structures that were identified for restoration were also not deemed valuable by the local community, particularly when their property values were damaged by mining activities.

Instead of these actions by CMI, community members wanted commitment to eco-sustainability of their community and less risk related to property values, tourism, and community health. These concerns went unaddressed. Participant 2 explained, "They keep floating this idea that this (sustainability) is something that they could do. But they never came out and say that this is something that they will do though." Because CMI was not willing to address community-identified needs, participants explained that they perceived the efforts of shared benefits from the mining company to be a means of coercion, rather than developing a means to truly work with the local community. The situation was summed up by participant 1 as, "We don't need a new billboard or a new park, or whatever. They put money into things that aren't important and then when it comes to cleaning up the environmental impact there may not be any money left for that."

CMI continued to hold recurring meetings with local residents at the community's request. During this time, residents aimed to reach a compromise on only one point: reducing the noise pollution from the mining activities that was often occurring 12–18 hours per day, most days per week. Participant 6, a woman in her 70s, described what happened, "The mining company said 'Okay, we are only going to blast on two or three days a week and it will be at such and such a time.' Well, they did not adhere to that schedule." Further distrust of CMI developed rapidly from this particular broken promise. In addition, while community members did not want the promised jobs, the jobs also did not materialize, which also contributed to the growing distrust.

Shortly after, CMI unilaterally decided to stop meeting with local community members. Participant 3 concluded, "They don't give a damn what we think. They're going to do what they want to do. They made it really clear and now the head of CMI is always describing the mining company as a responsible mining company and they're not."

Discussion

Earning a SLO is a common goal for mining companies to support cooperation from local communities. However, while local cooperation is positive for the mining industry, strategies to earn a SLO may not lead to a fair and equitable partnership for the local community. The case of Silver City helps explore these issues.

Within this case, we see problematic strategies of attempting to earn a SLO. CMI did not attempt to earn a SLO before beginning mining activities, as is suggested as a best practice. Instead, the industry received approval from the County Commission to conduct proposed mining activities so they began their work and adhered to the minimum governmental regulations, an entirely legal process. When Silver City residents began to fight against the mine, CMI responded by holding community meetings, promising employment, and funding a philanthropy arm to support the historical restoration of Silver City. This case is an example of a reactionary SLO with an industry-driven CSR strategy (Ofori & Ofori, 2019). While not inherently problematic, conflict arose because CMI's offer was not aligned with needs that were identified by the community in response to the impacts of CMI's mining activities: sustainability, remediation, support for tourism, and fewer negative impacts on local residents. Instead of negotiating with the community, CMI moved forward on remediating a historic water tower, a cost-efficient action but a "solution" to a non-problem. At minimum, this case provides an example for mining companies on how not to earn a SLO. Indeed, CMI and Silver City residents remain in a court battle.

However, this case highlights concerns with the current focus in the scholarship on earning a SLO. First, SLOs frame the mining industry, and other industries, as an unavoidable activity which will inevitably exist regardless of contextual factors (Lacey, Parsons, & Moffat, 2012; Prno & Slocombe, 2012). Because of this inevitability, local communities should use their power to form a relationship with the mine and gain what they need. Community members essentially cannot refuse a mine within the SLO model; the best-case scenario is an happy partnership between the industry and the community. This is problematic, as exemplified in this case. While participants in Silver City attempted to negotiate with CMI after the mining activities were approved, it was clear what Silver City residents actually wanted: no mine. However, the appropriateness of this mine seemed to have never been seriously considered at any level – by CMI, the County Commission, or the State regulatory agencies. Focusing on earning a SLO narrows possible outcomes and choices for a community where mining operations have been proposed.

Secondly, SLOs do not address the underlying issue of environmental injustice: power inequities. CMI's power was never reduced in their strategies to implement their mining activities. Rather, they pursued different avenues in response to contextual changes to keep their power. CMI first utilized their power from the top-down by making a sizeable contribution to Commissioner Hastings during the 2012 elections, who approved all CMI applications in the following years. This utilization of power was successful until the Silver City residents fought back, upon which time CMI engaged in several community meetings to negotiate. These talks ended as CMI removed the community members from the meetings after failed negotiations between what Silver City wanted (sustainability and tourism) and what CMI was willing to offer (historic restoration). This exemplifies that even though CMI was attempting to earn a SLO at one point in the process, all of the power remained with CMI. Silver City resident could never blanketly decided that CMI would have to leave their town. However, CMI could decide to stop working with the community at any point and they did so when it became too challenging.

As is shown in this case, responsibility for ensuring environmental protection and equity is not clear when the environmental hazard or industry is following the law, as CMI was. CMI followed the minimum government regulations for mining but because Nevadan laws are weak, community members felt unsafe. Earning a SLO is not a formal agreement so when CMI offered benefits that the community did not want (e.g., restoration of a water tower) or compromises were not adhered to (e.g., reduced operating times), Silver City residents had no recourse. In addition, the ideal solution from Silver City residents is for CMI not to operate a mine they lawfully bought, which may not be an achievable goal. While these intersecting issues make solutions difficult to develop, the case of Silver City supports skepticism that SLOs are a productive strategy for the development and wellbeing of communities. Another avenue must be developed for addressing mining operations in communities.

Conclusion

The goal of this study was the explore and document the experiences of people in a mining town that could not identify benefits from the local industry. This case is not generalizable to other communities due to its unique context and history but we conclude that these specific experiences of the mine in Silver City were very poor, with little chance at benefiting the community. While CMI attempted to earn a SLO and may even be held up as a model due to their community meetings, a SLO was never earned. CMI only offered benefits to the community that were of low cost and of little benefit to the community in an attempt to earn goodwill. Silver City participants felt that CMI's mining activities were simply too harmful to their other community assets. We see this in their concerns for their health, other economic ventures of the area, their property values, and the local environment. There was no way to reach a middle ground.

As community practitioners that are concerned with sustainability and ecosocial work practice, we must be vigilant to remain open to the possibility of this conclusion in other communities – that an industry does not belong in a community. We are trained to negotiate with different powers from the community to achieve a suitable outcome for all involved. However, this supports the assumption that mining companies can operate safely in communities and middle ground can be reached. Our clients may be better served in some instances if we do not negotiate but we pick their side and we support their fight without compromise. The findings in this paper point to no easy solutions but may offer a reality that we must contend with while working in ecosocial work practice.

Disclosure statement

No potential conflict of interest was reported by the authors.

ORCID

Jennifer Willett (iD) http://orcid.org/0000-0003-0156-6826

References

Banks, G., Kuir-Ayius, D., Kombako, D., & Sagir, B. (2013). Conceptualizing mining impacts, livelihoods and corporate community development in Melanesia. *Community Development Journal*, *48*(3), 484–500. doi:10.1093/cdj/bst025

Bridge, G. (2004). Contested terrain: Mining and the environment. *Annual Review of Environmental Resources*, *29*, 205–259. doi:10.1146/annurev.energy.28.011503.163434

Browne, A. L., Stehlik, D., & Buckley, A. (2011). Social licenses to operate: For better not for worse; for richer not for poorer? The impacts of unplanned mining closure for "fence line" residential communities. *Local Environment*, *16*(7), 707–725. doi:10.1080/13549839.2011.592183

Cavaye, J. (2001). Rural community development: New challenges and enduring dilemmas. *Journal of Regional Analysis and Policy*, *31*(2), 109–124.

Corbin, J., & Strauss, A. (2008). *Basics of qualitative research* (3rd ed.). Thousand Oaks, CA: SAGE.

Darling, P. (Ed.). (2011). *SME mining engineering handbook* (Vol. 1). Englewood, CO: Society for Mining, Metallurgy, and Exploration.

Fernando, F. N., & Cooley, D. R. (2016). Socioeconomic system of the oil boom and rural community development in Western North Dakota. *Rural Sociology*, *81*(3), 407–444. doi:10.1111/ruso.12100

Frederiksen, T. (2018). Corporate social responsibility, risk and development in the mining industry. *Resources Policy*, *59*(495), 495–505. doi:10.1016/j.resourpol.2018.09.004

Green, G. P., & Haines, A. (2015). *Asset building & community development*. Los Angeles, CA: Sage Press.

Green, M. (2015). *Nevada: A history of the Silver State*. Reno, NV: University of Nevada Press.

Griggs, D., Stafford-Smith, M., Gaffney, O., Rockström, J., Öhman, M. C., Shyamsundar, P., & Noble, I. (2013). Policy: Sustainable development goals for people and planet. *Nature, 495*(7441), 305–307. doi:10.1038/495305a

Kemp, D., & Owen, J. R. (2013). Community relations and mining: Core to business but not "core business". *Resources Policy, 38*(4), 523–531. doi:10.1016/j.resourpol.2013.08.003

Lacey, J., Parsons, R., & Moffat, K. (2012). *Exploring the concept of a Social License to Operate in the Australian minerals industry: Results from interviews with industry representatives.* EP125553. Brisbane, AU: CSIRO.

Lathouras, A. (2016). A critical approach to citizen-led social work: Putting the political back into community development practice. *Social Alternatives, 35*(4), 32.

Lincoln, Y. S., Lynham, S. A., & Guba, E. G. (2011). Paradigmatic controversies, contradictions, and emerging confluences, revisited. In N. K. Denzin & Y. S. Lincoln (Eds.), *The Sage handbook of qualitative research* (4th ed., pp. 97–128). Thousand Oaks, CA: Sage Publications.

Lyon County, Nevada. (2012). *Board of commissioner meeting minutes.* Retrieved from https://www.lyon-county.org/archive.aspx

Margiott, B. (2019, April 16). On your side: Tiny Nevada town fights proposed open pit gold mine. *News 4 On Your Side.* Retrieved from https://mynews4.com/on-your-side/tiny-nevada-town-fights-proposed-open-pit-gold-mine

Midgley, G., & Ochoa-Arias, A. (Eds.). (2012). *Community operational research: OR and systems thinking for community development.* New York, NY: Springer Science & Business Media.

National Park Service. (2018). *Virginia historic district: Three historic Nevada cities: Carson City, Reno and Virginia City: A national register of historic places travel itinerary.* Retrieved from https://www.nps.gov/nr/travel/nevada/vhd.htm

Nevada Business Magazine. (2012, April 2). Does the mining industry pay its fair share? Monte Miller vs. Tim Crowley. *Nevada Business Magazine.* Retrieved from https://www.nevadabusiness.com/2012/04/is-the-mining-industry-paying-its-fair-share-monte-miller-vs-tim-crowley/

Nevada Department of Wildlife. (2019). *Pronghorned antelope.* Retrieved from http://www.ndow.org/Species/Furbearer/Pronghorn_Antelope/

Nevada Division of Environmental Protection. (n.d.). *Mining, regulation branch.* Retrieved from https://ndep.nv.gov/land/mining/regulation

Nevada Humanities. (n.d.). Virginia city and early Nevada mining. *Online Nevada Encyclopedia.* Retrieved from http://www.onlinenevada.org/articles/virginia-city-and-early-nevada-mining

Nevada Mining Association. (n.d.). *Minerals in Nevada.* Retrieved from https://www.nevadamining.org/minerals-in-nevada/

Office of the Nevada Secretary of State. (2012). *Bob hastings.* Retrieved from https://www.nvsos.gov/SOSCandidateServices/AnonymousAccess/CEFDSearchUU/CandidateDetails.aspx?o=MaVvHHJ0luv1k0Epo9dM4w==

Ofori, J., & Ofori, D. (2019). Earning a social license to operate: Perspectives of mining communities in Ghana. *The Extractive Industries and Society, 6*(2), 531–541. doi:10.1016/j.exis.2018.11.005

Padgett, D. K. (2016). *Qualitative methods in social work research* (Vol. 36). Thousand Oaks, CA: Sage Publications.

Prno, J. (2013). An analysis of factors leading to the establishment of a social license to operate in the mining industry. *Resources Policy, 38*(4), 577–590. doi:10.1016/j.resourpol.2013.09.010

Prno, J., & Slocombe, D. S. (2012). Exploring the origins of 'social license to operate' in the mining sector: Perspectives from governance and sustainability theories. *Resources Policy*, *37*(3), 346–357. doi:10.1016/j.resourpol.2012.04.002

Robison, M. (2014, October 18). Election 2014: 'Sky's the limit' on mining tax. *Reno Gazette Journal*. Retrieved from https://www.rgj.com/story/news/politics/2014/10/19/election-skys-limit-mining-tax/17395637/

Ross, D. (2017). A research-informed model for corporate social responsibility: Towards accountability to impacted stakeholders. *International Journal of Corporate Social Responsibility*, *2*(8), 1–11. doi:10.1186/s40991-017-0019-7

Savesilvercity.org. (2019). *Save Silver City*. Retrieved from https://www.savesilvercity.org/

Trout, K. (2013, December 24). Conflicts surface for commissioners ahead of Comstock Mining vote. *Reno Gazette Journal*. Retrieved from https://www.rgj.com/story/news/2013/12/25/conflicts-surface-for-commissioners-ahead-of-comstock-mining-vote/4194907/

U. S. Census Bureau. (2016, October 05). *Community facts – Nevada*. Retrieved from https://factfinder.census.gov/bkmk/cf/1.0/en/state/Nevada/POPULATION/DECENNIAL_CNT

U. S. Environmental Protection Agency. (n.d.). *Carson river mercury site profile*. Retrieved from https://cumulis.epa.gov/supercpad/cursites/csitinfo.cfm?id=0903020

Wilson, S. (2015). Corporate social responsibility and power relations: Impediments to community development in post-war Sierra Leone diamond and rutile mining areas. *The Extractive Industry and Society*, *2*(4), 704–713. doi:10.1016/j.exis.2015.09.002

Wolf-Powers, L. (2014). Understanding community development in a "theory of action" framework: Norms, markets, justice. *Planning Theory & Practice*, *15*(2), 202–219. doi:10.1080/14649357.2014.905621

Amassing rural power in the fight against fracking in Maryland: A report from the field

Kathleen H. Powell, Ann Bristow, and Francis L. Precht

ABSTRACT
Social workers can mobilize vulnerable populations to shape policy decisions about industrial practices that could have adverse impacts on their wellbeing. One such practice is hydraulic fracturing or "fracking" to extract oil and natural gas from shale rock deposits. There is scant social work literature on mobilizing opposition to fracking despite a proliferation of literature from other disciplines. This article documents the campaign in Maryland that led to the adoption of the first legislative ban on fracking in a U.S. state with shale gas reserves, using social movement theory to identify factors that led to this successful outcome.

New technologies have enabled energy companies to harvest oil and natural gas from shale rock, a practice known as unconventional natural gas development (UNGD) or "fracking." The development of UNGD combined with the decline of global coal markets prompted some states in the Marcellus Shale region of the U.S. (Pennsylvania, West Virginia, and Ohio) to embrace the practice while others (Maryland and New York) have been more cautious.

This report arose from the authors' involvement as activists in a campaign to ban fracking in the largest municipality in the Marcellus Shale region of Maryland, part of a statewide effort to ban fracking. We were inspired by similar reports by activists chronicling localized anti-fracking efforts in the U.S. (Briggle, 2015; Staggenborg, 2018). This article applies a social movement framework to the Maryland campaign to consider factors that contributed to passage of the first U.S. legislative ban on fracking in a state with shale gas reserves (Wood, 2017, March 27).

Ecosocial work and fracking

The social work profession has only recently focused on the natural environment (Gray, Coates, & Hetherington, 2013) and adopted *grand challenges* that include the creation of social responses to a changing environment (American Academy of Social Work and Social Welfare, 2018). While social workers have a long history of political advocacy supporting the wellbeing of vulnerable populations, fracking presents a new issue around which social workers need to organize (van Wormer & Link, 2018).

Analytical framework of civic mobilization

McAdam and Boudet (2012) compared 20 communities across the U.S. and identified six structural or community-contextual factors (outlined in the following sections) that influence whether or not a community would mobilize in opposition to liquefied natural gas (LNG) projects. Carter and Fusco (2017) applied this framework to an anti-fracking campaign in western Newfoundland and found that it was helpful in explaining contextual variables rooted to place, but did not account for dynamic interactions between local and non-local activists and local interpretation of global debates. Maryland's ban presents another opportunity to apply this framework and Carter and Fusco's (2017) analysis of local and broader connections.

Level of threat and perceived risk

McAdam and Boudet (2012) found that the presence of a perceived threat to the environment, the community's safety, and/or property values prompted citizens to oppose a proposed LNG project. Maryland contains little more than 1% of the Marcellus Shale region with the shale play concentrated in Garrett County on the state's westernmost border with a small portion extending into Allegany County to the east ("Western Maryland Fracking Fight," 2017). This area also constitutes the coal-mining region of Maryland. Although this small shale reserve may have created few statewide concerns about fracking, Western Marylanders were particularly concerned about risks to water resources and were aware of water contamination caused by coal mine runoff and the money spent on reclamation (Pelton, 2006).

Frostburg, the largest municipality in Maryland's Marcellus Shale region, operates a regional water system serving smaller communities in western Allegany County, many with water supplies impacted by coal-mining operations (Blaisdell, 2011). Garrett Countians' concerns about water were linked to agriculture and the growth of eco-tourism dependent on higher quality water supplies ("Western Maryland Fracking Fight," 2017).

The Frostburg city council's 2009 decision to sell raw water to a fracking operation in nearby Pennsylvania heightened awareness of the potential adverse effects on the region's water. A former city mayor, who also served in the Maryland Senate, publicized the sale after the fact, which angered local residents who were previously unaware of the decision (Blaisdell, 2011).

In anticipation of permitting fracking in Maryland, land speculators began signing leases with property owners in 2006 (Masters, 2011), with many of these leases contiguous to municipal and private water supplies as mapped in Figure 1 using a Geographic Information System (GIS). Activists shared this map with residents, local businesses, and legislators, which intensified concerns about potential threats to water supplies. As with western Newfoundland, local threats to water were of great public concern (Carter & Fusco, 2017).

In 2011, Democratic Governor Martin O'Malley issued an Executive Order establishing the Marcellus Shale Safe Drilling Initiative Commission to study UNGD's economic, social, and environmental impacts, which created a de facto moratorium (Masters, 2011). Commission meetings were held in Western Maryland over a three-year period, and many Western Marylanders attended and learned of potential harms associated with fracking including to their nearby neighbors in Pennsylvania and West Virginia. Particularly persuasive was the Maryland Institute for Applied Environmental Health (2014) health impact assessment, which raised concerns about harms that would not be mitigated by proposed best practice regulations.

Civic capacity

A critical factor predicting mobilization of citizen opposition to energy projects is the presence of organizational and civic capacity (McAdam & Boudet, 2012). Maryland has a strong tradition of environmental activism and resource allocation for Chesapeake Bay preservation, according to Paul Roberts, President of Citizen Shale and former Commission member (personal communication, January 23, 2019). Thus, there has been a historic commitment to environmental activism and knowledge about organizing in the face of perceived threats. Western Maryland activists formed new organizations to oppose fracking, notably Citizen Shale. They partnered with regional and national organizations to form the Don't Frack Maryland (DFMD) Coalition in December 2014, which eventually totaled 140 member organizations (http://www.dontfrackmd.org/who-we-are). In the year leading up to introduction of the legislative ban, Food & Water Watch and Chesapeake Climate Action Network assigned experienced organizers in western Maryland, further building capacity. Organizing was bi-directional, with both local and state actors steering legislative and communications teams, creating a shared leadership also present in western Newfoundland (Carter & Fusco, 2017).

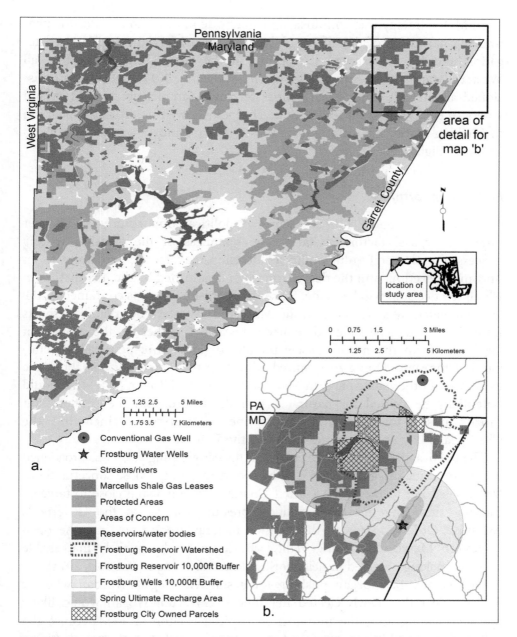

Figure 1. Marcellus Shale Gas Leases and Potentially Impacted Environmental Features in Garrett County, Maryland (a) and Surrounding the City of Frostburg, Maryland's Municipal Water Supply (b). This map should not be used for navigation or legal purposes since it is intended for general reference use only. There are no warranties, expressed or implied, including the warranty of merchantability or fitness for a particular purpose accompanying this map. All information was assembled from publicly available sources and is not endorsed nor does it represent the opinion or policy of Frostburg State University, the University System of Maryland, or the state of Maryland. Source Materials and Additional Notes about Methodology may be found at https://www.frostburg.edu/academics/colleges-and-departments/geography/precht/precht-materials.php

DFMD's strategy was both local and statewide in order to counter the pro-fracking narratives of the all-Republican Western Maryland legislative delegation and the widespread perception in the General Assembly that all Western Marylanders supported fracking (Wheeler, 2017). DFMD commissioned a statewide poll, which deliberately over-sampled western Maryland voters to ensure their representation. The poll showed bipartisan opposition to fracking across the state and in Western Maryland ("Western Maryland Fracking Fight," 2017).

Political opportunity

McAdam and Boudet (2012) identified political opportunity as another important causal factor, including the openness of the decision-making process, the electoral vulnerability of decision-makers, the proximity to an upcoming election, and the degree of influence afforded by the jurisdiction in which the decision will be made. Since the Marcellus Shale is contained in the less-populated western portion of Maryland, Western Maryland activists framed the issue as a statewide concern because they needed the support of legislators from the more densely populated (and more politically liberal) parts of the state. Doing so required educating the state's citizens about the existence of other shale plays in Maryland (Utica and Taylorsville) that could potentially be tapped for natural gas in the future, and the concomitant threats posed to the state's interconnected waterways, including the Chesapeake Bay and the Nation's River, the Potomac.

The political decision-making process in the early leasing years was broadened by a Democratic delegate from a wealthy suburban county whose concerns about fracking led her to meet with Garrett County residents living close to targeted fracking sites. She marshaled political pressure leading to the Governor's Executive Order and forced the decision-making process out into the open ("Western Maryland Fracking Fight," 2017), unlike the publicly inaccessible decision-making observed in neighboring states (cf. Hudgins & Poole, 2014).

DFMD members began pushing for a statewide legislative ban when it became clear that newly-elected Republican Governor Hogan would likely approve drilling after the moratorium expired (Pelton, 2014). Because the debate about fracking in Maryland was taking place between state elections, DFMD decided to campaign for local fracking bans and stricter zoning ordinances, similar to the one adopted by Mountain Lake Park, Garrett County's largest municipality in 2011 ("Friendsville Bans Fracking," 2016). In total, there were 12 bans or ordinances enacted statewide (http://www.dontfrackmd.org/local-actions). This pressure provided evidence of citizen opposition to fracking and prompted some legislators to support a statewide ban. This strategy capitalized on the political realities in Maryland, a state where both General Assembly chambers, the governor's office, and the federal legislative delegation have been consistently controlled by Democrats and where the few Republicans in high office are moderates by necessity (Willis & Smith, 2012).

Economic hardships

McAdam and Boudet (2012) contend that regions in economic decline are more likely to embrace LNG projects for their perceived economic benefits. In Maryland, the Western Maryland legislative delegation put forth this argument, and initially their colleagues in the General Assembly assumed that the vast majority of Western Marylanders supported fracking on this basis as well (Wood, 2017 March 2). The median income of the two westernmost counties is almost half of the state's median income, and the poverty rate is nearly double (U.S. Census Bureau, 2018). Among Western Maryland residents and business owners, however, concern grew that fracking would negatively impact tourism, a growth sector in the region's economy ("Western Maryland Fracking Fight," 2017). For these reasons, the campaign included a business petition, and Western Maryland business owners lobbied and testified about how their businesses would be harmed by fracking (Blaisdell, 2015).

One group supporting fracking in Western Maryland was the Garrett County Farm Bureau, whose support was largely based on saving small family farms (Hicks, 2017 February 26). A newspaper exposé of a Garrett County delegate's conflicts of interest effectively challenged this position (Hicks, 2017 March 8). This delegate is from a farming background and owns significant farmland in Garrett County. The exposé suggested that he would benefit financially if fracking were to be permitted and raised doubts about the ethics of his stance on the matter.

Experience with prior land-use issues

Communities that have experienced prior land-use issues are more likely to mobilize in opposition to LNG projects according to McAdam and Boudet (2012), and in Western Maryland, this was indeed the case. Residents had previously organized opposition to proposed landfill uses in Allegany County (Loverro, 1991) and to the siting of wind turbines in state forests in Garrett County (Pelton, 2008). Single issue-based organizations developed in response to these proposals in addition to pressure applied by existing environmental conservation groups including two local watershed associations and a local chapter of the Sierra Club. This experience proved useful in the fight against fracking and included many of the same activists.

Prior experience with a similar industry

McAdam and Boudet (2012) postulated that communities that experienced similar industries were more likely to embrace a proposed LNG project, although they did not assess citizens' perceptions of these projects. As noted earlier, many residents of Western Maryland either remembered or continued to experience adverse effects of mining on water quality and raised concerns about proposed fracking operations. These concerns existed in spite of Western Marylanders' pride in their coal-mining past and celebration of the contributions and sacrifices that coal miners have made to the local, state, and national economy (Larry, 2014). Fracking also raised concerns about surface property rights vs. mineral rights, an issue reminiscent of the heyday of coal mining in the region (Sangaramoorthy et al., 2016).

Conclusion

Maryland's experience supports three factors in McAdam and Boudet's (2012) framework: a clearly perceived threat, primarily to water quality; experience in opposing prior land-use issues; and experience with a similar extractive industry, although, in Western Maryland, familiarity fueled opposition to fracking. The lack of coherence with the three other factors, however, challenges this framework. First, there were few organizational structures in Western Maryland to lead the opposition; however, experienced activists created organizations and forged a co-equal partnership with larger state, regional, and national organizations to develop mutually reinforcing strategies. Maryland's rural activists were not "quiet" as described in other rural communities (Eaton & Kinchy, 2016). Rather, they provided leadership within the statewide campaign, supporting Carter and Fusco's (2017) analysis of dynamic networking.

Second, the political environment in Maryland was complex, and the decision on fracking could easily have gone either way. Had there not been a pause in the rush to frack created by the moratorium, which gave activists time to mobilize, and had local activists not framed fracking as a statewide issue, it is likely that legislators would have supported the pro-fracking stance of the Western Maryland delegation and the newly-elected governor who campaigned in support of fracking (Hicks, 2015). Instead, the election of a pro-fracking governor greatly heightened the level of risk and perceived threat (Emily Wurth, Co-Organizing Director, Food and Water Watch, personal communication, January 24, 2019).

Finally, Western Maryland is economically distressed, which could have led the majority of residents to support fracking. However, activists countered economic arguments by linking public health harms to existing economic sectors, notably water-dependent agriculture and eco-tourism. This public health focus gave anti-fracking legislators a politically viable way to oppose fracking (Emily Wurth, personal communication, January 24, 2019).

The rich and growing literature of community-based fracking opposition can inform social work activists' support of local residents in successfully opposing oil and gas projects that threaten the health and wellbeing of vulnerable populations. Social workers have a great deal of experience mobilizing populations exploited by industrial practices, experiences they can apply in anti-fracking campaigns. Social workers could be especially valuable working within communities with little to no prior organizing experience and by facilitating networking with non-local organizations. Their community-based work, grounded in knowledge of local public health issues and political realities, could facilitate the dynamic networking that appears to maximize the structural and community contextual opportunities associated with social change.

Disclosure statement

Kathleen H. Powell served as a lead local organizer for Frack-Free Frostburg; Ann Bristow represented the Savage River Watershed Association on the Marcellus Shale Safe Drilling Initiative Commission in Maryland and was a member of the Don't Frack Maryland Coalition, and Francis L. Precht served as a technical advisor to Frack-Free Frostburg.

References

American Academy of Social Work and Social Welfare. (2018). Grand challenges for social work. Create social responses to a changing environment. *Fact Sheet*. Retrieved from http://aaswsw.org/wp-content/uploads/2015/12/180604-GC-Environment.pdf

Blaisdell, E. (2011, January 9). Frostburg selling untreated water for natural gas fracking. *Cumberland Times-News*, p. 1A.

Blaisdell, E. (2015, April 1). Garrett residents to support fracking moratorium. *Cumberland Times-News*. Retrieved from https://www.times-news.com/news/garrett-residents-to-support-fracking-moratorium/article_2d856f96-d89c-11e4-8e0d-67012fdb85f0.html

Briggle, A. (2015). *A field philosopher's guide to fracking: How one Texas town stood up to big oil and gas*. New York, NY: W. W. Norton & Company.

Carter, A. V., & Fusco, L. M. (2017). Western Newfoundland's anti-fracking campaign: Exploring the rise of unexpected community mobilization. *Journal of Rural and Community Development*, *12*(1), 98–120. Retrieved from http://journals.brandonu.ca/jrcd.

Eaton, E., & Kinchy, A. (2016). Quiet voices in the fracking debate: Ambivalence, nonmobilization, and individual action in two extractive communities (Saskatchewan and Pennsylvania). *Energy Research & Social Science*, *20*, 22–30. doi:10.1016/j.erss.2016.05.005

Friendsville bans fracking within its borders. (2016, July 6). *Cumberland Times-News*. Retrieved from https://www.times-news.com/news/local_news/friendsville-bans-fracking-within-its-borders/article_c2f9c618-be9f-5165-b59a-034bb040f06f.html

Gray, M., Coates, J., & Hetherington, T. (2013). Introduction: Overview of the last ten years and typology of ESW. In M. Gray, J. Coates, & T. Hetherington (Eds.), *Environmental social work* (pp. 1–28). New York, NY: Routledge.

Hicks, J. (2015, May 29). Md. fracking moratorium to become law without Hogan's signature. *Washington Post*. Retrieved from https://www.washingtonpost.com/local/md-politics/md-fracking-moratorium-to-become-law-without-hogans-signature/2015/05/29/e1d10434-062c-11e5-a428-c984eb077d4e_story.html?noredirect=on

Hicks, J. (2017, February 26). In rural western Maryland, fracking divisions run deep. *Washington Post*. Retrieved from https://www.washingtonpost.com/local/md-politics/in-rural-western-maryland-fracking-divisions-run-deep/2017/02/26/3dc0c0d4-f791-11e6-bf01-d47f8cf9b643_story.html?utm_term=.235e10ad9059

Hicks, J. (2017, March 8). Pro-fracking Md. lawmaker criticized for potential personal financial stake in drilling. *Washington Post*. Retrieved from https://www.washingtonpost.com/local/md-politics/2017/03/08/3c1d51e6-fe0a-11e6-99b4-9e613afeb09f_story.html?utm_term=.9798365bfc1e

Hudgins, A., & Poole, A. (2014). Framing fracking: Private property, common resources, and regimes of governance. *Journal of Political Ecology, 21*(1), 303–319. doi:10.2458/v21i1.21138

Larry, G. (2014, February 9). Group hoping to bring coal miner statue to Frostburg. *Cumberland Times-News*. Retrieved from https://www.times-news.com/news/local_news/group-hoping-to-bring-coal-miner-statue-to-frostburg/article_f2245685-a5c8-55df-b797-b6dba5946312.html

Loverro, T. (1991, February 6). Allegany landfill gets state permit. *Baltimore Sun*. Retrieved from https://www.baltimoresun.com/news/bs-xpm-1991-02-06-1991037015-story.html

Maryland Institute for Applied Environmental Health. (2014). *Potential public health impacts of natural gas development and production in the Marcellus shale in western Maryland.* Retrieved from http://www.marcellushealth.org/final-report.html

Masters, G. (2011, November 28). Fracking debate hits home in western Md. *The Star Democrat*. Retrieved from https://www.stardem.com/news/state_news/fracking-debate-hits-home-in-western-md/article_f00cb389-2599-5ec1-990f-1181b7c039b7.html

McAdam, D., & Boudet, H. S. (2012). *Putting social movements in their place: Explaining opposition to energy projects in the United States, 2000–2005.* New York, NY: Cambridge University Press.

Pelton, T. (2006, December 8). Md. coal mining's toxic legacy. *Baltimore* Sun. Retrieved from https://www.baltimoresun.com/news/bs-xpm-2006-12-08-0612080028-story.html

Pelton, T. (2008, January 29). Wind farms hit opposition. *Baltimore Sun*. Retrieved from https://www.baltimoresun.com/news/bs-xpm-2008-01-29-0801290041-story.html

Pelton, T. (2014, November 11). New governor may open western Maryland to fracking. *WYPR*. Retrieved from http://www.wypr.org/post/new-governor-may-open-western-maryland-fracking

Sangaramoorthy, T., Jamison, A. M., Boyle, M. D., Payne-Sturges, D. C., Sapkota, A., Milton, D. K., & Wilson, S. M. (2016). Place-based perceptions of the impacts of fracking along the Marcellus shale. *Social Science & Medicine, 151*, 27–37. doi:10.1016/j.socscimed.2016.01.002

Staggenborg, S. (2018). Mobilizing against fracking: Marcellus shale protest in Pittsburgh. In A. E. Ladd (Ed.), *Fractured communities: Risk, impacts, and protest against hydraulic fracking in U.S. shale regions* (pp. 107–127). New Brunswick, NJ: Rutgers University Press.

U.S. Census Bureau. (2018, July). *Quick facts*. Retrieved from https://www.census.gov/quickfacts/fact/table/MD,garrettcountymaryland,alleganycountymaryland/PST045218

van Wormer, K., & Link, R. J. (2018). *Social work and social welfare: A human rights foundation.* New York, NY: Oxford University Press.

Western Maryland fracking fight reveals differences. (2017, June 2). *WJZ TV, CBS Baltimore*. Retrieved from https://baltimore.cbslocal.com/2017/06/02/western-maryland-fracking-fight-reveals-differences

Wheeler, T. B. (2017, March 17). Maryland governor throws support behind permanent fracking ban. *Bay Journal*. Retrieved from https://www.bayjournal.com/article/maryland_governor_throws_support_behind_permanent_fracking_ban

Willis, J. T., & Smith, H. C. (2012). *Maryland politics and government: Democratic dominance*. Lincoln: University of Nebraska Press.

Wood, P. (2017, March 2). Activists push for ban on fracking in Maryland. *Baltimore Sun*. Retrieved from http://www.baltimoresun.com/news/maryland/politics/bs-md-fracking-rally-20170302-story.html+&cd=1&hl=en&ct=clnk&gl=us

Wood, P. (2017, March 27). Maryland General Assembly approves fracking ban. *Baltimore Sun*. Retrieved from https://www.baltimoresun.com/news/maryland/politics/bs-md-fracking-ban-passes-20170327-story.html

The future of environmental social work: Looking to community initiatives for models of prevention

Samantha Teixeira ⓘ, John Mathias ⓘ, and Amy Krings ⓘ

ABSTRACT
Social work responses to environmental degradation have sought to mitigate harm that has already occurred and create strategies to respond or adapt to environmental hazards. Despite a good deal of literature suggesting the promise of prevention-focused models, social workers have less frequently considered prevention models to address environmental issues. In this manuscript, we consider how communities engaged in environmentally-based prevention work might inform the development of ecosocial work practice. We describe how a prevention-focused agenda, in partnership with communities, can be a promising avenue for ecosocial work practice to address the root causes of environmental degradation and its social impacts.

Social workers have proposed a number of avenues through which to contribute to addressing the root causes as well as the social and ecological effects of environmental degradation (Ramsay & Boddy, 2017). The majority of social work responses to environmental degradation and its disparate social impacts have sought to mitigate harm that has already occurred and to create strategies to respond or adapt to disasters (Kemp et al., 2015; Ramsay & Boddy, 2017). Despite a good deal of social work literature that finds that a focus on prevention is an important component of interventions, social workers have less frequently considered prevention-based practice as a model to address environmental issues. A recent literature review on the state of scholarship in environmental social work identified a strong literature base relating to responses to natural disasters, but limited research on "interventions that can mitigate or prevent crises, such as macro-level sustainable development and conservation" (Krings, Victor, Mathias, & Perron, 2018, p. 12). In this manuscript, we consider how communities engaged in environmentally-based prevention work might inform the development of ecosocial work practice.

Ecosocial work attends to social and structural inequalities and emphasizes the linkages between social work and ecological issues (Matthies, Närhi, & Ward, 2001). Scholars of ecosocial work stress the importance of privileging voices outside of the dominant, Western perspective and voices of those who are not traditionally considered to be experts to address social and environmental inequalities. Ecosocial work is rooted in viewing social problems with an ecological lens and promotes addressing environmental and social issues holistically (Matthies et al., 2001). It provides a useful backdrop for contextualizing renewed scholarly interest in environmental social work.

The resurgence in interest in environmental social work is still nascent (Gray, Coates, & Hetherington, 2013; Ramsay & Boddy, 2017). Ramsay and Boddy (2017) note that, "The mandate to be environmentally pro-active may be clear, yet application of environmental social work in practice is limited" (p. 69). In fact, much of social work, by design, is reactive. Typical clinical social work interventions are designed to, for example, react to reports of abuse or treat diagnosed mental health issues. At the community level, social work advocates often mobilize in reaction to threats or in response to existing social and structural issues. Resource constraints often preclude adding a proactive strategy to the standard reactive approach. In environmental social work, some have posited that the lack of a proactive approach may also be due to disciplinary norms and boundaries that relegate preventative environmental work to the natural sciences, while making reactive work the domain of the social sciences (Krings et al., 2018).

Yet the need for a preventative social responses to the inequitable impacts of environmental crises such as industrial pollution, deforestation, fresh water scarcity, and climate change could not be more apparent. If prevention guards against the crises of the future, it is nonetheless motivated by the "urgency of now." To that end, we consider the ways in which social workers can act today with "conscientious foresight" to mitigate or prevent future environmental injustices, with a focus on community-based prevention efforts (Alston, 2015). We begin by providing background on the concept of prevention and its application to solving complex social problems, as well as two current initiatives that provide useful jumping off points from which to explore prevention-focused community practice. We then present three brief case examples that illustrate community practice approaches to prevention in ecosocial work. Finally, we discuss key takeaways from the approaches and conclude with implications for community practice.

Background

Early scholarly discussions of the promise of prevention-focused interventions for social work described it as "early discovery, control, and elimination of conditions which potentially could hamper social functioning" (Rapoport, 1961). A prevention focus affirms core social work values; prevention models are woven into the history of social work, from the Settlement House movement to adolescent problem behavior prevention (Rishel, 2015). This natural fit has led to a robust prevention-focused body of research and practice in some arenas of social work, like adolescent development (see for example, Hawkins, 2006).

A prevention focus is also common in community-centered health promotion aimed at chronic conditions like obesity, and health damaging behaviors like substance use (Wandersman & Florin, 2003). Likewise, prevention science frameworks focus on going from epidemiology, that is, studies of the prevalence and predictors of problems, to testing preventive interventions and diffusing findings (Hawkins, 2006). While we do not want to overemphasize a medical approach, these concepts may be valuable to community practitioners and inform a more holistic view in line with the ecosocial work focus on the interplay between the social environment, the natural environment and well-being (Närhi & Matthies, 2018). The Communities that Care Model, which illustrates prevention science in a social work context, helps community coalitions identify prevention needs specific to youth and implement locally-relevant community-based prevention strategies (Hawkins, Shapiro, & Fagan, 2010). These models may provide lessons for ecosocial work.

Although not directly focused on prevention, two influential proposals for addressing environmental change bear discussion. One, within social work, aims to address the social response to the human impacts of environmental change through the Grand Challenges for Social Work initiative. The other is the UN Sustainable Development Goals (SDGs) adopted in 2015 by global leaders in an effort to end poverty, protect the planet from degradation, and form global partnerships to ensure peace and prosperity (United Nations General Assembly, 2015).

The Grand Challenges for Social Work encourage social workers and allied disciplines to address pressing social problems through partnerships, innovation, and scientific inquiry. A policy brief written by the group tasked with the Grand Challenge of "creating social responses to a changing environment" highlights the unique position of social workers as potential change-makers and innovators "at the human-environment nexus" (Kemp, Reyes Mason, Palinkas, Rechkemmer, & Teixeira, 2016, p. 1).

The working paper outlining the agenda for this Grand Challenge focuses on policies and practices in three areas: mitigation, adaptation, and treatment. According to Kemp et al. (2015), these concepts stem from the public health prevention model which includes primary, secondary, and tertiary prevention. Mitigation, or primary prevention, aims to stop environmental changes and limit the degree of change. Adaptation or secondary prevention is focused on addressing the consequences of existing hazards and preventing further consequences in areas of known risk. Treatment, or tertiary prevention, works to alleviate and treat the consequences of problems after they occur (Kemp et al., 2015).

The preventative approaches outlined in the Grand Challenges working paper (Kemp, et al. 2015) and associated policy brief primarily focus on the individual level (e.g., trauma response to prepare for intervention after natural disasters) and the structural level (e.g., advocating for policies and allocating resources to promote equity). The suggestions at the community practice level (e.g., community organizing) are largely reactive. Thus, the community-based prevention approaches we discuss here could fill in gaps in these recommendations.

The UN Sustainable Development Goals (SDGs) focus on ending poverty, protecting the planet, and ensuring prosperity. The SDGs embed relevant ecosocial work themes, connecting economic, social, and ecological aspects of sustainability (Närhi & Matthies, 2018). For example, SDG Goal 13 warns that climate change and associated natural disasters are occurring and that irreparable damage has already been done, while putting forward a mandate to prevent further harm. These multi-level, preventative measures provide opportunities for social workers to take a lead in establishing scalable interventions that incorporate the multiple actors (e.g., government, private sector, community) necessary to address climate change.

Drawing on these frameworks, and highlighting the role of community-level practice, we discuss how a prevention-focused, proactive agenda for ecosocial work will provide a role for social workers in collaborative partnerships, and allow us to learn from grassroots groups that have been working to prevent environmental change and its social impacts.

Method

To better understand how communities engaged in environmentally-based prevention work might inform the development of ecosocial work practice, we employed an instrumental case study method. We present three instrumental case studies that aim to describe the phenomenon of community engaged environmental prevention in the real life context in which it occurs (Baxter & Jack, 2008). Instrumental case studies are used when the goal of inquiry is to provide insight into an issue and/or help refine a theory (Baxter & Jack, 2008; Stake, 1995). In instrumental case studies, a case is examined in depth; the goal is not to generalize or compare it to others but to illuminate one case and come to know it in detail (Stake, 1995).

The authors drew on their collective experience and expertise in environmental justice-focused scholarship to select instrumental cases. These cases were selected because of their utility for illustrating and better understanding how community groups undertake environmental prevention work. The first (Approach 1) presents a historical account of a classic environmental justice case. The authors reviewed each instrumental case and interrogated them for lessons specific to understanding how communities can inform the development of ecosocial work practice. Our second case (Approach 2) introduces the Flint Water Study (http://flintwaterstudy.org/about-page/about-us/) as an illustration of how citizen science can prevent environmental health impacts. It draws on data collected through interviews with civic leaders as well as archives of newspaper articles that describe the Flint Water Crisis (see Krings, Kornberg, & Lane, 2018) for a detailed methodological description). Our third case (Approach 3) describes how community organizers in Kerala, India imagine and put into practice alternative practices with the aim of supplanting the systems that produce environmental injustices. The case is based on two years of ethnographic fieldwork including participant observation and interviews in the local language of Malayalam (see Mathias, 2017 for a detailed description of methods and limitations).

Because these three cases draw on different empirical materials, we have opted to present each individually. Across all three, we briefly describe and contextualize the case before analyzing it as an approach to prevention. In the discussion and conclusion, we compare these approaches and offer an analysis of prevention as a paradigm for community practice. There are several notable limitations to this method of analysis and presentation. First, we intend these cases to be illustrative and generative of creative thought. While we situate them in relation to broader literatures and social patterns, we do not attempt to determine generalizability. Second, these cases should be viewed in light of the authors' positionality. While we each have unique identities, we all are faculty at schools of social work in the United States which is the main lens through which we interpreted the cases.

Community approaches to prevention

Approach 1: community practice shaping policy in Warren County, North Carolina

Places inhabited by poor people of color are not protected from environmental harm to the same degree as places inhabited by predominantly white and more affluent people (Mohai, Pellow, & Roberts, 2009). As a result, environmental justice campaigns have emerged to address the practices, policies, and conditions that shape disparities including; unequal enforcement, disparate exposure to harm, and discriminatory and exclusionary practices (Bullard & Johnson, 2000, p. 557–558). A brief historical example is instructive in our discussion of how community practice skills can be engaged to not only mitigate and adapt to environmental degradation (and root causes of degradation such as racism), but also to further community-based prevention.[1]

In 1978, employees of the Ward Transformer Company traveled rural roads across North Carolina, secretly dumping a chemical mixture containing polychlorinated biphenyl (PCB) to avoid paying to properly dispose of it (McGurty, 1997). Because this dumping occurred along state roads, North Carolina was responsible for remediating the contamination (McGurty, 1997). The state identified a farm in Warren County, a rural county populated predominantly by poor, black residents, on which to dispose of the PCB-contaminated soil. Residents resisted vigorously, but after three years of unsuccessfully trying to block the site through the courts, permits were granted for the Warren County dump site (McGurty, 1997).

At this stage, Warren County resident advocates reframed the movement with the support of prominent civil rights leaders. McGurty (2000) notes that the initial strategy, used for the first years of the resistance between 1978 and 1979, was to frame the argument against the dumpsite using a "Not in My Backyard" argument, citing threats to local economic development and stigma associated with hosting a toxic waste site. Seeing that the initial strategy was failing, in 1982, the Warren County Citizens Concerned about PCB shifted to frame the dumpsite as an example of environmental racism which attracted substantial support from the civil rights movement, sparked direct action, and connected their experience of disparate environmental harm directly to racism and political powerlessness among the poor (McGurty, 2000, p. 376). The Warren County Citizens Concerned about PCB, who led the initial legal battles, were comprised largely of white landowners without direct action experience. When they joined forces with a local black Baptist church affiliated with the United Church of Christ (UCC), they gained support from powerful black leaders with experience in community organizing.

The reframing and coalition with the UCC marked a transition to a more disruptive community organizing strategy. In late 1982, mirroring the civil rights march at Selma, organizers staged a 60 mile march from Warren County to the state capital and EPA offices in Raleigh (McGurty, 1997). Protesters intervened, lying down and blocking the roads as trucks came to dump the PCB-contaminated soil. These direct actions drew national attention and, despite failing to protect Warren County residents, shifted the movement's aims and eventual impacts from local resistance to national policy change.

The aftermath of Warren County protests included further organizing efforts, a surge of academic research, and federal legislative action (Agyeman, Schlosberg, Craven, & Matthews, 2016). The protests led members of Congress to request an analysis at the national level of the relationship between hazardous waste dump site locations and the demographics of area communities, published in 1983 (Agyeman et al., 2016). It also prompted a report, "Toxic Wastes and Race in the United States" (1987) which set the stage for the development of the fundamental principles of environmental justice created at the First National People of Color Environmental Leadership Summit. These reports, along with the attention at the government level, initiated academic research to empirically test environmental racism in facility siting, which continues to be a robust area of work today. Perhaps most importantly, Environmental Justice Executive Order 12250 was signed in February 1994, mandating that the mission of every federal agency include environmental justice.

This example provides a sense of how, historically, the environmental justice movement was shaped by community practice and how a community went from a reactive local agenda to stop an undesirable land use to a national policy that aims to prevent harm caused by environmental racism. Bullard, Mohai, Saha, and Wright (2008) note that the local struggles "blossomed into a multi-issue, multi-ethnic, and multi-regional movement" (p. 376). The history of the environmental justice movement shows how integral community residents have been in sparking policies aimed at preventing environmental harm.

Approach 2: street science and the Flint Water Crisis

To prevent environmental injustices, there is a need for social workers to advocate for proactive environmental regulations, monitoring, and enforcement. In a political climate where environmental regulations are being reduced or eliminated (consider the US departure from the Paris Climate Accords), when a community is contaminated, the burden of proof is often pushed to those who are harmed. This presents an important intervention point for ecosocial workers. By partnering with communities to rigorously document impacts, local concerns can be leveraged to gain the attention of media and enforcement agencies. The importance of this sort of partnership, known as "street science" (Corburn, 2005), can be demonstrated through an examination of the Flint water crisis.

Decades of divestment in Flint, Michigan were caused by a combination of economic and political forces including closure of auto plants, a decline in urban investment by the federal government, and racial segregation (Highsmith, 2009). Consequently, when the City was faced with bankruptcy, the Michigan Governor appointed a receiver (known as an emergency manager) whose job was to balance the city's budget without raising taxes, securing funding from state or national government, or negotiating with creditors. This context created an environment in which city services were eliminated or reduced. Decisions were made to provide and monitor the quality of Flint's drinking water in the least expensive manner possible.

Soon after the City shifted its water source to the local Flint River, residents began to notice health impacts including skin rashes, burning eyes, and hair falling out. Representatives from the State Department of Environmental Quality responded that these problems were exaggerated, and any problems with the drinking water were short-term. Despite assurances, residents reported that their health problems were growing worse and some even died from Legionnaire's disease. Later, it was discovered that Flint residents had been exposed to lead due to deteriorating water pipes.

The Flint water crisis reveals multiple points in which decisions that were made in the name of fiscal austerity resulted in public health crises. Yet, to a degree, residents and grassroots community organizations were able to prevent a crisis that could have been even larger in scope if not for local pressure to change the water source (Krings et al., 2018). These groups used many tactics familiar to community practitioners. They asked questions and pressured officials in public meetings, organized protests, pursued a class action lawsuit, educated neighbors, and distributed bottled water and filters. Additionally, they sought out and partnered with scientists who were able to validate local claims in a way that was viewed to be "credible" by external groups including funders and media. The Flint Water Study, for example, was a partnership between researchers at Virginia Tech and a grassroots coalition of residents and community organizations (http://flintwaterstudy. org/about-page/about-us/). The group collected and analyzed its own water samples, discovering that the water was, indeed, not safe to drink. Further, the Study suggested the City had been cutting corners, with the knowledge of the State Department of Environmental Quality, to test the water in the least rigorous way possible. While the Flint Water Study alone did not lead the City of Flint to switch back to the safer and more expensive water provided through the City of Detroit, pressure from the media and foundations, who were more inclined to believe the Study's report than residents' complaints, ultimately did.

The street science approach, and the Flint case in particular, shed light on ways that community practitioners can support the advancement of environmental justice. Not all residents of marginalized communities can access researchers and therefore it is likely that many communities that would benefit from such partnerships will fall through the cracks. Similarly, there is a danger that researchers will only partner with community groups in response to visible health impacts as opposed to slow-onset disasters that are less visible. This reactive approach has been common within environmental social work interventions (Krings et al., 2018; Mason, Shires, Arwood, & Borst, 2017). Community practitioners are thus positioned to extend the use and efficacy of street science by assisting civic groups in locating and developing on-going relationships with academic partners. Furthermore, community practitioners are needed to develop inclusive decision-making processes that attend to power imbalances between residents and researchers. Finally, community practitioners can recruit, train, and support residents who might not otherwise have the skills or confidence to engage in street science.

Additionally, the Flint case reveals opportunities for community practitioners to increase the political power of residents and communities – goals that are central to the mission and ethics of the social work profession. Examining the role (and lack thereof) of national media in the Flint Water Crisis, Jackson (2017) notes that reporters did not "credential" residents, that is, they did not give credence to their complaints and instead focused on the voices of Flint leaders who defended and justified the shift in the city's water source. Jackson argues that if reporters had deemed residents to be credible before researchers stepped in, then the crisis could have been curtailed. Thus, beyond partnering with local groups, ecosocial community practitioners and scholars can work with communities to counter classist and racial bias embedded in conceptions of expertise and authority. This includes the development of institutions that are accountable to residents, providing information in a transparent and timely way, and including public participation in the design and implementation of environmental policy.

Approach 3: experiments with alternatives in Kerala, India and Detroit, USA

Environmental injustices are not only caused by inequitable policies and hierarchies of expertise; they are also deeply rooted in ordinary social practices like shopping, eating, or inhabiting. As such, those pursuing environmental justice have sought to develop alternative practices that transform humans' relations to nature and to one another. For example, for environmental activists in Kerala, India imagining and experimenting with "alternatives" (*badal*) is crucial to the pursuit of environmental justice and can inform ecosocial work practice.

As the second author of this manuscript found during ethnographic research on environmental justice organizing in Kerala (Mathias, 2017), the logic of such alternatives can be vividly seen in activists' efforts to develop and promote new methods of organic farming. In visiting the experimental farm of a farmer/activist named Peter, for example, Mathias (2017) noticed how different it looked from other farms he had seen in either India or the US. Rather than even rows of crops in an open field, this farm was more like a meadow of pumpkin and other vegetables, growing amidst banana and jackfruit trees, with plenty of weeds mixed in as well. Peter explained that his approach to farming is to let the weeds grow and avoid putting too much work into tending the plants. Instead, he said, he just planted things, let them grow, and picked whatever came.

Peter's non-intensive approach to farming was not born of laziness. Rather, he was frugal with his time because he hoped to show others that organic farming can be a practical, profitable activity. For several decades, agrarian livelihoods have become increasingly precarious in India, with farmers often trapped in downward spirals of debts for seed, pesticide, and fertilizer (Deshpande & Nagesh, 2005; Mohanty, 2005; Walker, 2008). Food security has become a major concern, particularly in urbanizing regions like Kerala (Kannan, 2000; Kumar, 2017). Peter and others like him see organic farming as the cornerstone of a more just social order – a mechanism for liberating India's lower classes from exploitative economic structures. Thus, alternative agriculture is as much about community organizing as farming. Though it often begins with experiments on activists' own land, it is only successful insofar as it is taken up by a community. To that end, Peter holds educational programs for teenagers who live nearby and talks with his neighbors about the income he is making from his farming. The real fruits of his labor are not the vegetables in his own garden, but the cultural and socio-economic changes he hopes alternative approaches to farming will bring for his community. Aside from organic farming, Indian activists are developing other alternatives such as building homes out of earth instead of concrete, selling cloth alternatives to the plastic shopping bag, or drinking an herbal preparation called *jappi* instead of coffee or tea. Though these practices vary with regard to both the means and desired ends of social change, the logic of such alternatives as an approach to prevention can be roughly compared with the notion of "alternative energy." Just as alternative energy attempts to prevent climate change by supplanting the carbon dioxide-producing fossil fuels that contribute to it, so earth homes supplant mining industries that chew up forests and poison rivers, and herbs supplant tea leaves grown on exploitative plantations.

Globally, a wide range of initiatives share a similar logic of developing alternatives to prevent future environmental injustices. Närhi and Matthies (2018) describe a range of "ecosocial transition" projects such as communal housing, through which "local communities develop new kinds of living models that aim at self-sufficiency and social justice" (p. 496). Similarly, Loh and Agyeman (2017) describe how "solidarity economy" movements are using participatory budgeting, land trusts, and other alternative practices that make "serving people and ecological sustainability … the goal of economic activity, rather than maximization of profits (p. 261, quoting Quinones 2008, 13). White's (2011) study of women farmers in the Detroit Black Community Food Security Network (DBCFSN) offers an example that parallels the alternative agriculture practices of activists in Kerala. For these women, White (2011) argues, urban farming differs from protests because it is not a reaction to environmental destruction but a proactive assertion of control over the food supply and, more generally, over their relation to the earth. Such initiatives vary widely in how they theorize the problems to which they are developing alternatives. However, they share an appreciation for how environmental injustices are entangled with economic systems as well as a belief that systemic change can be achieved by re-inventing everyday social practices.

The latter notion – that neighborhood groups, for example, can produce more just economic systems – raises one of the chief challenges for the pursuit of environmental justice alternatives. Often, environmental justice movements have been approached as locally bounded, to specific geographic sites of pollution (Mathias, 2017). Even if it is easy to see the roots of such problems in geographically-dispersed social systems, it can be difficult to imagine how localized organizations can challenge these systems. Perhaps one reason that urban gardening seems a particularly promising alternative is that it shows how global food systems can, within a limited domain, be supplanted by a small number people and an empty lot. But other environmental justice problems, like climate change, appear less amenable to local alternatives.

Such challenges of scale point to the need for creativity in this approach to preventing environmental injustice. Social workers can be a resource for such creative thinking. For example, they can mediate knowledge sharing between, for example, activist farmers in the US and India. Cross-national and cross-cultural knowledge sharing will be vital to developing alternatives because encounters with difference stimulate the imagination of new possibilities. Thus, by facilitating knowledge sharing, social workers can help develop new social systems that promote environmental justice.

Discussion

Ecosocial workers need to engage at the community level, with a prevention focus, to effectively promote social and environmental justice. Yet, social workers tend to be reactive when addressing environmental issues (Krings et al., 2018). Thus, this manuscript aims to articulate opportunities for ecosocial workers, in partnership with community and grassroots groups, to prevent environmental change and its social impacts. The three approaches demonstrate how prevention-focused work has been enacted by communities over time and across the globe to prevent environmental degradation and its root causes.

While policy advocacy, street science, and community development alternatives can all contribute to preventing environmental injustice, they do so in different ways. Organizing in Warren County was initially aimed at preventing toxic waste from being dumped on a specific site. However, the policy advocacy inspired by this organizing was aimed further upstream, at preventing the racist siting of toxic industries from happening again.

In the context of inadequate policy and chronic failures of enforcement, the Flint Water Study took a different tack. Residents sought out and partnered with researchers to examine the quality of Flint's drinking water. These findings were able to prevent the spread of a public health crisis by convincing external allies, such as media and foundations, to pressure regulators and elected officials to change the City's water supply. This approach mixed immediate downstream interventions, such as providing bottled water to residents, with long-term upstream strategies aimed to address the root causes of the crisis (Braveman, Egerter, & Williams, 2011). Like street science, urban gardening can increase community control; these kinds of alternatives aim at the roots of environmental injustice, attempting to prevent inequities by supplanting the systems that produce these inequities.

Kemp et al. (2015) conceptualize mitigation, adaptation, and treatment (or primary, secondary, and tertiary levels of prevention), as potentially useful organizing heuristics rather than immutable categories. Considering primary, secondary, and tertiary levels of prevention can be useful for analyzing and planning community-based approaches to preventing environmental injustice. Both policy advocacy and developing alternative social systems might be considered primary in the public health idiom as both intervene to prevent harm from happening at all. However, at least some alternatives might be considered *more* primary insofar as they seek to root out injustices prior to state oversight and regulation. Street science, by contrast, can be likened to secondary or tertiary levels of prevention, aiming to affect those known to be at elevated risk for harm and to mitigate harm that has already occurred. While we have contrasted such approaches with more "reactive" work like providing resources and mental health treatment in the aftermath of natural disasters, the latter might also be thought of as tertiary prevention to the extent that they attempt to ameliorate the long-term impacts of harm for those at highest risk.

These distinctions of degree can help to clarify what we mean by prevention, but it should be noted that aims of community interventions are often multiple. For example, Flint residents' use of street science has been the basis for calls to ameliorate the long-term impacts of lead poisoning as well as calls for stronger regulation. In practice, these different aims and activities will often co-occur. Holding them apart analytically is useful, however, when it facilitates strategic thinking and shows the many roles community practitioners can play.

Across each of the case approaches, and in the existing literature, the challenge of scale is a cross-cutting theme. Issues of environmental degradation are daunting challenges because they typically begin with powerful actors or forces seemingly well-beyond the control of community-based groups, which exert their effects from afar (Freudenberg, 2004). Prevention-focused work requires us to think creatively about how communities, and community practitioners in a supporting role, can work across different scales to identify points of disruption in the root causes of environmental change (Ramsay & Boddy, 2017). Though organizing in Warren County and Flint did not immediately succeed in preventing harm locally, each incrementally advanced prevention objectives and raised awareness of environmental injustices, eventually leading to work that may prevent such harms in the future.

Limits of time and resources also pose practical challenges for preventative approaches. Reactive interventions like the Warren County protests tend to be the norm in environmental movements because acute situations require immediate solutions. As in much of social work practice, reactive solutions tend to get the lion's share of resources while proactive solutions take so much time and effort to develop that individuals and communities simply might not have capacity for both. However, balancing reactive and preventative work need not be a zero-sum game. Community practitioners may find ways to integrate prevention by looking for points where responses to current crises can catalyze action for enacting new policy, bolstering community control, or creating partnerships that can more effectively guard against future injustices.

Despite these challenges, we see great promise in the community initiatives described here as models for prevention in community practice and ecosocial work. A combination of macro social work practices like learning from partner organizations, coalition building, and policy advocacy, combined with the lessons learned from community initiatives will be necessary to mitigate and prevent future harm from large-scale environmental problems.

Conclusion

An orientation toward prevention in ecosocial work means that "social workers are viewed as political actors working toward social change rather than adjusting to current conditions of society" (Närhi & Matthies, 2018, p. 32). We acknowledge that much environmentally-focused community practice work, particularly in the environmental justice arena, has been carried out by community leaders and groups outside of social work. Nonetheless, social work practitioners have skillsets that make us uniquely situated to support these practitioners and begin setting the stage for preventing future harm from environmental issues (Teixeira & Krings, 2015). Social work scholars can support community groups and practitioners in advancing environmental justice by approaching environmental degradation with an eye toward being proactive. In practice, this means partnering with local groups and pressing for change in the root causes of environmental problems, fighting for racial and income equity, developing institutions that are accountable to marginalized communities, and improving public participation in the design of environmental policy. It also requires thinking creatively about how communities can work across different scales and where the points of disruption may lie.

We present a case for approaching prevention as an essential part of community practice for ecosocial work. Though there are challenges inherent in such an approach, community practice already includes many models for preventing environmental degradation and promoting environmental justice. Community practitioners have much to learn from community-based prevention initiatives like those described in this manuscript and, in partnership with community groups and scholars, can address root causes of environmental degradation and build more environmentally just global futures.

Note

1. It should be noted that the definition of environmental justice has been expanded since these early efforts focused on race and class-based disparities in the United States. Research and practice has since developed to begin to understand the intersectional impacts of environmental injustices incorporating, for example, gender, geographic location, historic and social context (Malin & Ryder, 2018).

Disclosure statement

No potential conflict of interest was reported by the authors.

Funding

This work was supported by the Fulbright Hays Doctoral Dissertation Research Award grant # P022A120002-002.

ORCID

Samantha Teixeira ⓘ http://orcid.org/0000-0003-0219-848X
John Mathias ⓘ http://orcid.org/0000-0001-8372-0078
Amy Krings ⓘ http://orcid.org/0000-0001-5499-5101

References

Agyeman, J., Schlosberg, D., Craven, L., & Matthews, C. (2016). Trends and directions in environmental justice: From inequity to everyday life, community, and just sustainabilities. *Annual Review of Environment and Resources, 41*, 321–340. doi:10.1146/annurev-environ-110615-090052

Alston, M. (2015). Social work, climate change and global cooperation. *International Social Work, 58*(3), 355–363. doi:10.1177/0020872814556824

Baxter, P., & Jack, S. (2008). Qualitative case study methodology: Study design and implementation for novice researchers. *The Qualitative Report, 13*(4), 544–559.

Braveman, P., Egerter, S., & Williams, D. R. (2011). The social determinants of health: Coming of age. *Annual Review of Public Health, 32*, 381–398. doi:10.1146/annurev-publhealth-031210-101218

Bullard, R. D., & Johnson, G. S. (2000). Environmentalism and public policy: Environmental justice: Grassroots activism and its impact on public policy decision making. *Journal of Social Issues, 56*(3), 555–578. doi:10.1111/0022-4537.00184

Bullard, R. D., Mohai, P., Saha, R., & Wright, B. (2008). Toxic wastes and race at twenty: Why race still matters after all of these years. *Environmental Law, 38*, 371–411.

Corburn, J. (2005). *Street science: Community knowledge and environmental health justice.* Cambridge, MA: MIT Press.

Deshpande, R. S., & Nagesh, P. (2005). Farmers' distress: Proof beyond question. *Economic and Political Weekly, 40*(44/45), 4663–4665.

Freudenberg, N. (2004). Community capacity for environmental health promotion: Determinants and implications for practice. *Health Education & Behavior, 31*(4), 472–490. doi:10.1177/1090198104265599

Gray, M., Coates, J., & Hetherington, T. (Eds.). (2013). *Environmental social work.* New York, NY: Routledge.

Hawkins, J. D. (2006). Science, social work, prevention: Finding the intersections. *Social Work Research, 30*(3), 137–152. doi:10.1093/swr/30.3.137

Hawkins, J. D., Shapiro, V. B., & Fagan, A. A. (2010). Disseminating effective community prevention practices: Opportunities for social work education. *Research on Social Work Practice, 20*(5), 518–527. doi:10.1177/1049731509359919

Highsmith, A. R. (2009). Demolition means progress: Urban renewal, local politics, and state sanctioned ghetto formation in Flint, Michigan. *Journal of Urban History, 35*(3), 348–368. doi:10.1177/0096144208330403

Jackson, D. Z. (2017) Environmental justice? Unjust coverage of the Flint water crisis. *Shorenstein center on media, politics and public policy.* Retrieved from https://shorenstein center.org/wp-content/uploads/2017/07/Flint-Water-Crisis-Derrick-Z-Jackson-1.pdf

Kannan, K. P. (2000). *Food security in a regional perspective: A view from 'food deficit' Kerala* (CDS Working Paper 304). Thiruvananthapuram, India: Centre for Development Studies.

Kemp, S. P., Palinkas, L. A., Wong, M., Wagner, K., Reyes Mason, L., Chi, I., ... Rechkemmer, A. (2015). *Strengthening the social response to the human impacts of environmental change.* Cleveland, OH: American Academy of Social Work and Social Welfare. Retrieved from http://grandchallengesforsocialwork.org/grand-challenges-initiative/12-challenges/create-social-responses-to-a-changing-environment/

Kemp, S. P., Reyes Mason, L., Palinkas, L. A., Rechkemmer, A., & Teixeira, S. (2016, September). *Policy recommendations for meeting the grand challenge to create social responses to a changing environment* (Policy Brief No. 7). Cleveland, OH: American Academy of Social Work and Social Welfare. Retrieved from: https://openscholarship. wustl.edu/cgi/viewcontent.cgi?article=1787&context=csd_research

Krings, A., Kornberg, D., & Lane, E. (2018). Organizing under austerity: How residents' concerns became the Flint water crisis. *Critical Sociology, 45*(4–5), 583–597. doi:10.1177/0896920518757053

Krings, A., Victor, B. G., Mathias, J., & Perron, B. E. (2018). Environmental social work in the disciplinary literature, 1991–2015. *International Social Work,* 002087281878839. doi:10.1177/0020872818788397

Kumar, P. (2017). Food and nutrition security in India: The way forward. *Agricultural Economics Research Review, 30*(1), 1–21. doi:10.5958/0974-0279.2017.00001.5

Loh, P., & Agyeman, J. (2017). Boston's emerging food solidarity economy. In A. Alkon & J. Guthman (Eds.), *The new food activism: Opposition, cooperation, and collective action* (pp. 257–283). Berkeley, CA: University of California Press.

Malin, S. A., & Ryder, S. S. (2018). Developing deeply intersectional environmental justice scholarship. *Environmental Sociology, 4*(1), 1–7. doi:10.1080/23251042.2018.1446711

Mason, L. R., Shires, M. K., Arwood, C., & Borst, A. (2017). Social work research and global environmental change. *Journal of the Society for Social Work and Research, 8*(4), 645–672. doi:10.1086/694789

Mathias, J. (2017). Scales of value: Insiders and outsiders in environmental organizing in South India. *Social Service Review, 91*(4), 621–651. doi:10.1086/695352

Matthies, A., Närhi, K., & Ward, D. (2001). Taking the eco-social approach to social work. Reflections on three European countries. In A. Matthies, K. Närhi, & D. Ward (Eds.), *The eco-social approach in social work*. (p. 5–15). Jyväskylä, Finland: Sophi. Retrieved from https://jyx.jyu.fi/bitstream/handle/123456789/48562/SoPhi58_978-951-39-6497-9.pdf?sequence=1

McGurty, E. M. (1997). From NIMBY to civil rights: The origins of the environmental justice movement. *Environmental History*, *2*(3), 301–323. doi:10.2307/3985352

McGurty, E. M. (2000). Warren County, NC, and the emergence of the environmental justice movement: Unlikely coalitions and shared meanings in local collective action. *Society & Natural Resources*, *13*(4), 373–387. doi:10.1080/089419200279027

Mohai, P., Pellow, D., & Roberts, J. T. (2009). Environmental justice. *Annual Review of Environment and Resources*, *34*(1), 405–430. doi:10.1146/annurev-environ-082508-094348

Mohanty, B. B. (2005). 'We are like the living dead': Farmer suicides in Maharashtra, Western India. *The Journal of Peasant Studies*, *32*(2), 243–276. doi:10.1080/03066150500094485

Närhi, K., & Matthies, A. (2018). The ecosocial approach in social work as a framework for structural social work. *International Social Work*, *61*(4), 490–502. doi:10.1177/0020872816644663

Ramsay, S., & Boddy, J. (2017). Environmental social work: A concept analysis. *The British Journal of Social Work*, *47*(1), 68–86.

Rapoport, L. (1961). The concept of prevention in social work. *Social Work*, *6*, 3–12. doi:10.1093/sw/6.1.3

Rishel, C. (2015). Establishing a prevention-focused integrative approach to social work practice. *Families in Society: The Journal of Contemporary Social Services*, *96*, 125–132. doi:10.1606/1044-3894.2015.96.15

Stake, R. E. (1995). *The art of case study research*. Thousand Oaks, CA: Sage.

Teixeira, S., & Krings, A. (2015). Sustainable social work: An environmental justice framework for social work education. *Social Work Education*, *34*(5), 513–527. doi:10.1080/02615479.2015.1063601

United Nations General Assembly (2015, October 21). *Transforming our world: The 2030 agenda for sustainable development*. A/RES/70/1. Retrieved from https://sustainabledevelopment.un.org/post2015/transformingourworld

Walker, K. L. M. (2008). Neoliberalism on the ground in rural India: Predatory growth, agrarian crisis, internal colonization, and the intensification of class struggle. *The Journal of Peasant Studies*, *35*(4), 557–620. doi:10.1080/03066150802681963

Wandersman, A., & Florin, P. (2003). Community interventions and effective prevention. *American Psychologist*, *58*(6–7), 441. doi:10.1037/0003-066X.58.6-7.441

White, M. (2011). Environmental reviews & case studies: D-Town farm: African American resistance to food insecurity and the transformation of Detroit. *Environmental Practice*, *13*(4), 406–417. doi:10.1017/S1466046611000408

Green grey hairs: A life course perspective on environmental engagement

Mary Kate Dennis and Paul Stock ⓘ

ABSTRACT
Older adults provide a long view of understanding environmental engagement from their early beginnings to their current community activities. This study draws on interviews with self-described environmentalists and follows a life course analysis that employs social work values and practice skills as they work towards environmental justice in their Midwestern communities. We conclude that the older adults of this second generation of environmentalists offer valuable lessons for social workers with regard to environmental justice, while at the same time contributing insights into older adult volunteering and addressing the challenge of a generational gap in participation in their community organizations.

Introduction

Pope Francis released an encyclical entitled *Laudato Si: On care for our common home* in June of 2015. This was the first papal encyclical to focus solely on environmental issues with a hope to "enter into dialogue with all people about our common home" and the future of the planet (Francis, 2015). Furthermore, he recommends a new conversation that includes everyone while also acknowledging the tireless work of the ecological movement to create organizations committed to raising awareness and working tirelessly on environmental issues. One of these organizations hosted a public conversation on the encyclical, where we facilitated small group discussions. From our discussions with the older adults, in majority attendance, we learned of their longstanding engagement in Earth Care. We developed an interdisciplinary study that explored the intersection of environmental engagement, faith, and spirituality over the life course of older adults living in Kansas and how environmental social work practice can be informed by their work in this community. For this special issue advocating for ecosocial work, this cohort, not social workers themselves, work for social change in their community, showing the multidisciplinary nature of ecojustice activism,

Literature review

Revisiting the "second" generation of American environmentalists

Most narratives of the US environmental movement read something like this:

The US helped win WWII, which then led to a unique expansion of wealth and the middle class. We then turned some of those tools developed during the war into consumer products, like DDT, that made everyday life easier, except that DDT, it turns out, is quite dangerous, and to people, too. So, Carson, (1962) wrote *Silent Spring* so that we would know about DDT and the predicament for the global community. The book's success galvanized the frustration and anger over the lack of planetary stewardship into the American environmental movement through organizations like Greenpeace, the Audubon Society, and the Sierra Club. With these groups at the forefront and the emergence and growth of the Civil Rights, feminist, and farmworkers movements, the US took major steps to turn the post-war growth into planetary care indicated by Earth Day, the formation of the EPA, and major environmental legislation.

It is slightly more complicated than that, in part, because there is a paucity of literature on the recollections of the activists from that era.

American environmental efforts began in earnest in the late nineteenth and early twentieth centuries; these characterized by competing ideologies between economic use and wilderness and species protection. In the 1960s, there was a distinct difference in environmental activism sparked by the other emergent movements around Civil Rights and Black Power, feminism, and the American Farmworkers Union.

> Within a decade, the old conservationist-inspired environmental movement was displaced by a 'new' or 'second generation' environmentalism (Brulle, 2000; Dunlap & Mertig, 2014; Gottlieb, 2005) ... By 1970, progressive-era conservationist discourse and organizations were subsumed within a much larger and far more diverse environmental movement. (Johnson & Frickel, 2011, pp. 307–308)

That diversity in the environmental movement included the rise of environmental justice (Taylor, 2000), an expansion of global environmental activism, and the formation of the Intergovernmental Panel on Climate Change (Klein, 2015). The research herein examines the evolution of the environmental movement through the experiences of some who were a part of it.

Older adults and environmental volunteering

The generations born after WWII, the Baby Boomers, are now reaching older adulthood, resulting in the long-awaited global demographic shift. With regard to environmentalism, they are thought to have been socialized differently because they were active in a culture that had a new ecological paradigm (Johnson & Schwadel, 2018). Despite this, there is a perception that older adults do not express pro-environmentalist attitudes (Johnson & Schwadel, 2018). Contextual variables must be examined in relation to the age/cohort influences on environmental concerns because it does not reflect fully older adults' views on the environment. For example, the Cornell National Social Survey indicated older adults believe that climate change is a serious problem, but only 12% participated in environmental organizations and only 15% reported engaging in environmental activities. Additionally, 80% of respondents said they would spend additional time and money towards doing what is right for the environment and 97% felt it was important to maintain the environment for future generations (Bushway, Dickinson, Stedman, Wagenet, & Weinstein, 2011; Frumkin, Fried, & Moody, 2012). In order to bridge the gap between concern and action, there is a large pool of older adults who currently do not volunteer for environmental organizations but might if there were efforts to recruit them (Pillemer, Wagenet, Goldman, Bushway, & Meador, 2009). Baby Boomers will spend more years post-career than any generation preceding them, thereby creating an opportunity to create new social roles for older adults (Binstock, Sykes, & Reilly, 2009; Bushway et al., 2011).

The literature is limited on insights of older adults and *environmental* volunteering. First, benefits from environmental, or green engagement, can include: an increase of physical activity, exposure to nature, increasing social supports, and offering a fulfillment of the need for leaving a legacy for the future generations (Pillemer et al., 2009). Green volunteering is broadly more age-integrated compared to senior-focused facilities and activities (Formosa, 2012). Second, green volunteerism must be more inclusive to older adults, with efforts to do their part by working hard to become more "age-friendly" in order to meet the needs of older adults (Formosa, 2012, p. 41). They can do so by having an accessible location, offering a variety of tasks for different interests and physical abilities, providing transportation, and offering daytime activities (Pillemer et al., 2009). The emergence of specific organizations to capitalize on such volunteerism offer compelling examples of older adults using their time, money, and energy towards helping the planet, often with intergenerational concern on their minds. Groups like *Gray Is Green* and the *Environmental Alliance for Senior Involvement* recruit older adults and help them partner in and across communities to work on common environmental issues.

Life course theory

The life course perspective focuses on how the time, period, and cohort shape individuals and social groups as they age (Bengtson, Burgess, & Parrott,

1997). Elder, Johnson, and Crosnoe (2003) offer five principles of the life course theory: 1) Human development and aging are a lifelong process and, therefore, the interplay of the individual and social change can be examined, 2) Individuals construct their life course through choices and actions constrained by history and social circumstance, 3) Time and place are embedded and shaped by the historical times and places they experience over their lifetime therefore meaning is shaped and differ in regions of the nation, 4) Timing of a person's life affect the experience depending on when they occur in the life course and 5) Linked lives, where the larger social changes can create "turning points" that lead to changes in behavior. Thus, the life course theory can offer explanations of the effects of history on the behaviors of cohorts of individuals (Bengtson et al., 1997).

Study purpose

Older adults living today experienced the activism of the 1960s and the start of the green movement of the 1970s. Little attention has been offered in capturing the participation across the life course of the second generation of environmentalists living today. In this study, we explore the origins of their interest in the environment, historical events that shaped their engagement, their lifelong community involvement, and challenges they face in intergenerational participation in their community groups and organizations. We address how their environmental activities can inform environmental social work practice because they have been organizing, advocating, facilitating, educating and negotiating on behalf of the environment.

Methods

Participant recruitment and data collection

We were invited to facilitate the community conversation on the papal encyclical. This activity inspired this study and through our relationship with one of the organization's leaders, we were able to introduce the study and the recruitment criteria. All of the research activities were conducted together, in tandem. We adopted a purposive sampling strategy to recruit participants (Creswell, 2013). We were primarily interested in people who identified as: a) 60 years and older, b) living in Kansas, c) engaged in environmental activities, and d) having religious or spiritual values that guide environmentalism. We intentionally chose Kansas because the authors both lived there and were drawn to the energy and involvement of environmental activism in this community. There are unique environmental issues rooted in this particular location, both positive (e.g., the most prairies) and challenging (e.g., water scarcity and contamination related to agriculture).

After receiving approval from the university IRB, we met with a node in the civic and faith-based environmental justice activities in this community. He networked on our behalf, introducing the study to community members. When they consented to be interviewed, they gave permission to have their contact information shared with us. We contacted directly an order of Catholic sisters known for being environmental activists. We conducted 20 exploratory, semi-structured interviews lasting between 60 and 140 minutes, averaging 94 minutes. We structured our interview schedule thematically around the ideas of their background (e.g., demographics, faith background and experiences), environmental engagement over time, motivations, and community/group engagement (benefits and challenges of working in groups). The interviews were digitally recorded and professionally transcribed.

The participants ranged in age from 60 to 88 years. The age cohorts revealed to be significant in terms of experience and, according to life course theory, how their position in historical time influenced their interest in environmental issues. There were six who were in their 60s, nine who were in their 70s and five who were in their 80s. Eleven participants were women. All but one of the older adults were white. All participants lived in Kansas at the time of the interview and most were born and raised in Kansas and those who were not had spent many years living and working in eastern Kansas.

Analysis

The authors employed thematic analysis (Braun & Clarke, 2006) to identify, analyze and report themes from the data. First, after each interview, we debriefed and assessed the interviews and the information shared by each participant. We took notes throughout the data collection and used these as initial descriptive codes and areas for additional exploration across the data. Once we received the transcripts, we read over them and clarified the list of codes that label and describe the data. We coded the data separately and met to resolve coding decisions through discussion and exploration of each other's perspectives. We sorted the coded data into broader themes and defined and named the themes and how these fit into broader understanding of older adults and environmental engagement.

Findings

We identified five themes that collectively describe the older adults' participation in environmental activism across their lives from their early beginnings to today. These themes include: a) origins outside on the farm, b) becoming an engaged environmentalist, c) contexts and zeitgeist through national and local movements, d) community and organizational activities, and e) challenges to intergenerational participation.

Origins outside on the farm

The older adults reflected on how they became interested in the environment. Nearly all of them grew up on a farm or out in the country, referred to by one man as "egg alumni," those who have ancestors or family who were farmers (E14, age 62). One participant shared,

> So growing up on that farm meant everything ... And my mother then, we had big gardens, my dad with the crops and the cattle ... So growing up with all that ... it forms you in every way I think. So I've always loved being outside and on the farm. And my mother would often talk about the beauty of the Earth, and the garden, and the rainbows, and rain. (E18, age 77)

Others grew up in the country and were exposed to farms and being outside. One woman offered:

> My roots go back to when I was a kid visiting an organic farm. They weren't known that way at the time, but it was a typical farm that had ducks, geese, and we were lucky enough to know him, so we had spent a lot of weekends out there. I grew up in town, but – I think those were the best days that I had, because I was free to roam, no restraints. You know, puddle and the creek, climbed the barns, did all kinds of fun things. And I really enjoyed it. I don't think I thought of it at that point of how refreshing and fulfilling it was, but it really and truly was, and I think that's what started me enjoying the outdoors. (E8, age 78)

For those that were not raised on a farm, they were raised in the country or with exposure to the outdoors, as one woman shared how the values of her family influenced her passion for the environment:

> We did things as a family together outdoors, walking, skiing, hanging out in the backyard, having a vegetable garden – a Victory Garden during World War II – which my dad, both my parents, both my parents worked really hard in it, and my brother and I helped. That was very important. (E6, age 88).

As a teenager during WWII and exploring the outdoors through the garden we see how the early influences of the farm and nature, which were also connected to global events, shaped these young people while providing a solid foundation for further exploration while in college.

Becoming an engaged environmentalist

The late 1960s and early 70s felt like a time of major generational divide between the optimism of a sort-of technological utopianism and a pessimism driven by constant roadblocks to major success in the converging social and environmental justice movements. The film *The Graduate* (1967) summed it up perfectly, as described by one of our participants:

> "Go plastics," ... I've always known, the whole society knows, plastics, the future's in plastics ... And I was aware that there was a camp that thought plastics were the future, and there was a camp that was skeptical of that. That it was kind of like a joke. "Oh yeah, like plastics is the future." (E3, age 62)

She then continued to make a connection between that optimism of the previous generation and the skepticism of the younger generation based on her mother's experience of work as a child.

> And, I certainly think that I respect my parents' generation for wanting things easy ... My mother is a living example of child labor laws. Her parents had a flower shop, and when she was entirely too young she was having to get up in the morning and fix flower arrangements ... And it's hard on your hands. You know, its work. And that's why it would take an atom bomb, now, to get my mom to work ... that's my observation of her. (E3)

As this participant explains, one of the generational divides revolves around the relationship of meaningful work and material comfort. For our participants, their views on this relationship were further forged in college. Dynamic teachers pushed them not just to learn about the Earth (including botany, biology and philosophy) that expanded their Earth Care commitment originally developed in childhood, but to do something about it. As one older adult shared,

> I had a wonderful history teacher ... in eighth and ninth grade ... He taught me about American imperialism. He probably mentioned the *Silent Spring* [by Rachel Carson], which was at that point was sort of the environmental manifesto. So we had an environmental club in the first Earth Day and we went out by the side of the road and picked up trash ... just something symbolic ... I was kind of plugged into that whole hippie environmental Back-to-the-Earth type thing ... but [my teacher] as a person, was a big influence in bringing it. (E14)

For those who lived through WWII and the Vietnam era, attending college was a time of exploration of ideas. For one sister, a theology professor exposed her to readings that expanded her consciousness:

> [I had a] very uninformed conscious. I had been through World War II. I wasn't there but I was in the seventh grade when it happened and heard about the Jews but didn't think a thing about it and felt that it was perfectly Okay. But I didn't know how many had been killed. When I learned that in a moral theology class, I was just struck dumb. How could we do that to people in the Holocaust? So I was developing some kind of a much broader moral consciousness in regard to relationships to people. And what the bomb had done to the Earth, there in Japan. (E17, age 88)

One participant said simply, "By the end of my freshman year at college I was fully immersed in [everything environmental]" (E15, age 60). These courses coupled with the local and political events related to Civil Rights and anti-war activism in Lawrence shaped how they carried these new commitments into their careers or communities. Education gave them the formal knowledge "because it gave me the names ... and really opened me up to the incredible diversity there was up in both the woodlands and the prairies, and ... it was a really important class for me" (E11, age 62). Some of these young environmentalists who were exploring topics came together through these courses and created a community group working on environmental issues:

> Met some really cool people and I decided to teach something called Appropriate Technology which was E.F. Schumacher and all those folks. And so I decided to do a free university class on that, and a group of people got together and we became super tight ... we would meet at each other's houses. We just kept meeting after the class was done, because it was a semester type of thing. And so we became – the general focus of the people that were involved – there was alternative energy, there was healing and holistic health, and then there was the environmental aspects. (E11)

By the early 1970s this cohort of activists joined not only the mainstream movements and protests (e.g., Greenpeace, Audubon, Sierra Club, progressive political campaigns, anti-nuke protests), but also started their own organizations to focus exclusively on issues marginalized by other community groups. The longevity and commitment afforded this kind of involvement varied by participant with some very specific events intersecting with personal biography.

The 1960s and '70s zeitgeist–national and local movements converge

Significant historical events were happening nationally and locally (Coen, 2001) which coincided with the first Earth Day and participation in environmental justice activities. As one man described, "I was in college from '65 to '69, a lot of protests related to Vietnam War, but also the awakening of the environmental movement in those days" (E16, age 69). For those living in Lawrence in 1970, there was civil unrest as described by a woman who knew the young black man in the event that affected the whole community (see Metz, 2010; Ranney, 2002).

> And then this horrible thing happened in the Union and all the unrest that was in Lawrence at that time was just unbelievable. One day when things were so bad on campus, I don't know. He was in an alleyway and he ran. He saw the police and he ran and he was shot dead. I'll never forget it. It's just awful. Just awful. (E10, age 77)

Another elder spoke to other events related to race relations in Lawrence at this time. He said,

Back in the first Earth Day, that was in 1970 … And the union was burning and there were [race] riots and so Earth Day was hardly a blip. At least the first Earth Day around here that I was aware of – because Lawrence High [School] made *Time Magazine* [May 4, 1970] because of the riots. (E11)

The question then centers on whether this cohort in Lawrence represents something unique or can we find some commonality with the "second generation" environmentalists (Johnson & Frickel, 2011)? While civil unrest related to race relations and anti-war activism Lawrence tended to obscure the emerging Earth Day-environmentalism overtaking the rest of the country, other trends of the second generation did impact our cohort.

Back-to-the-land

For the purposes of understanding this cohort of environmentalists, the back-to-the-land movement provided an out for many who maintained a Christian orientation who also found the existing power structures and community status quo oppressive without being involved in direct actions of protest. It is important to note that it was students from the University of Kansas that founded the first hippie commune in Trinidad, Colorado, known as Drop City (Matthews, 2012). Those in our cohort described much smaller and more local engagement with the back-to-the-land movement and self-sufficiency popular at the time. One woman offered:

> I was kind of a quasi-hippie. Graduating high school in' 73, I feel like I was a late hippie, because I was too young to do the 60s. But I was very involved with the back-to-nature movement, with the "Whole Earth News." (E3, age 62)

The "Whole Earth News" was a hippie bible, offering both goods for purchase as well as articles and how-to manuals for creating and maintaining a life of self-sufficiency on the land (Turner, 2010). Some of the participants had moved into their post-college years and, as young families, were negotiating the draft and embracing the back-to-the-land movement. One woman shared,

> We did a little, back-to-the-land farm … So, we had goats, and we had chickens, and butchered rabbits, and we had geese … It was just a community in St. George, Kansas, that knew how to do all that stuff. So, we kind of just moved into that community, and we always laughed about, well, how did you accept these hippies that are coming back? I don't know if we were really hippies. (E12, age 74)

Her husband then added,

> But you move back to the country because that's when the gas lines were happening. We were looking at a self-sufficient lifestyle, but not from an environmentalist perspective, but rather a teaching perspective for our kids … It's just a matter of, here's the gas lines; we move out to a small farm and do everything we can there to irritate our children so that they never want to be in a small farm situation again! … At least we were on the edge of environmentalism then. (E13, age 74)

While jesting about how their children experienced the back-to-the-land experiment, these participants, like others who tried to live rurally, embraced environmental activism out of necessity given the early 1970s gasoline shortages. But those experiences shaped a lifetime of environmental involvement.

Community and organizational activities

The older adults participated in environmental activism in various ways throughout their adult lives. Focusing on their community activities, they participated in formal organizations like the Audubon Society, the Sierra Club, their congregations' green teams, and informal organizations of like-minded people supporting one another in their work with environmental issues. Gathering together in one of their homes to discuss environmental issues created benefits both socially and emotionally, "Oh, very much so. Yes, [the gatherings are] very valuable to me, yeah" (E5, age 88). Another elder referred to these gatherings as their collective "support group" (E1, age 76). One woman participates in a women's environmental group that offers many modes of engagement.

> Because there's so much research and truth to "women can succeed only because there's other women that are supporting them" … Now it's acknowledged, and women are saying, "Yeah, I need other women around." The [group] is providing that kind of support. We meet four times a year … but then there's all these other splinter groups. There's a reading group … there's a walk and talk group that meets …, but it looks different for everybody that's in it … And yet there's this big Facebook group that hears about jobs, about conferences … I think that's the new model, maybe, of activism. (E12)

Like many in their generation, the older adults believe in the purpose of these organizations. As one environmentalist said,

> Oh yeah, they do a tremendous amount of educating other people, whether they're aware of it or not. And they have the ability to put on functions like an Earth Day. Both Sierra and Jayhawk Audubon have an impact there … . So they do have the ability to influence people whether or not they attend regular meetings. And protests at the steps of the capital, Sierra and Jayhawk Audubon certainly are involved in that … I think it's kind of immeasurable the impact it has on the people that attend. I think they go out as disciples and tell other people what they're passionate about. And I think quite often it gets them a reassurance that's needed, appropriate. If not them, who? kind of thing. I don't know how else the word would be put out there. Somebody's got to do it. (E16)

As this participant emphasizes, our cohort find value in the work of these pedigreed organizations in spite of declining involvement, membership, and cash flows. While our cohort see value in these organizations going forward there seems to be a declining interest in general to "belonging" to organizations as part of one's civic involvement.

Challenges of intergenerational participation

When asked about the greying of the organizations, the older adults shared the struggle of connecting to younger generations who are interested in Earth Care work. They stated simply, "across all of my groups is mostly older people" (E4, age 74) and we "can't get anybody young to go to any of that stuff" (E13), and "I think young people are allergic to meetings" (E2). While they are interested in younger people and their ideas there is a hope that the tactics and structures might remain the same. There then exists a contradiction between desiring the new blood and ideas younger activists can bring, but also a reluctance to cede control of these organizations that shape much of their own identities.

The older adults had various views on why this gap in participation exists. For one who is active in several organizations stated, "We grew up with having a monthly meeting. We had it in 4-H. In churches, we have regular meetings in churches" (E4). For these older adults, they were socialized to participate in groups even as they raised their own families. They were also living in activist times. One man argued: "Some of it may be the 60s. I was radicalized in the 60s. It was an interesting process" (E14). As one commented:

> But I just don't think there's a lot of young people that are willing to sign up for and participate in leadership which is what we really need to bring in their young ideas and their newer ideas and take an active part. It's hard for us to get young people involved. (E4)

Those involved in another organization added, "But to get people that would be actually willing to be leaders and commit to a monthly board meeting or something like that, it just seems like it is just really difficult" (E4).

The environmentalists themselves had criticisms of the groups with one wrestling with his own participation,

> I bailed out on all of them, because I lost interest in being in the group. The group was not functioning as – it was not giving me anything. But to be outside of a group and go to their meetings, I still think that's important. The Audubon Club, they have a speaker every meeting, and there's always a tidbit or two of information … I think just being there … networking … should be beneficial, I would think. (E13)

While not personally gaining anything from the groups, he also reflected on other challenges "Well it's hard to get them to talk to each other. The four groups I was on never talked, and didn't know anything about the other group." The culture of each group and how they choose to operate tend to silo the groups that could collaborate with one another. These formal processes (minutes and Roberts Rules of Order) (E4), or a consensus model (E12), or creating the decisions in more fluid in-the-moment manner (E14) can alienate rather than inspire.

Discussion and conclusion

The second generation of environmentalists, who are now in their older adult years, were asked to reflect across their life course to offer insights into their beginnings, how the historical events of their early adulthood affected their participation, and how they continued their environmental engagement into their older adult years in eastern Kansas. The environmentalists in this study were raised on farms or with an appreciation of the outdoors which provided the foundation to explore ideas through higher education and were influenced heavily by the social activism of their communities. They came of age in a time where attending meetings and gathering in groups was a productive method of community engagement, which creates a challenge for intergenerational participation. They threaded their environmental sensibilities through their professional, family, social, and community participation.

Those with children, while still involved in the organizations (who made special efforts to include them), struggled with trying to be a part of mainstream change (e.g., working for the EPA). Those without children maintained their engagements and relationships that evolved. While environmental organizations are often lacking in preparation and capacity to bring in older adults, we found an opposite problem, thus filling a major gap in the literature (Formosa, 2012; Pillemer et al., 2009). The older adults in this study are actively engaged with other older adults in environmental volunteering. Barriers to older adults' participation in environmental activities include: feeling that they lack sufficient expertise or knowledge about environmental issues, lack of awareness of opportunities to participate in these issues in their community, or finding these activities not as socially fulfilling as volunteering in their school or church (Pillemer et al., 2017). The participants found ways to naturally address these by providing the education and information, doing outreach across religious and civic organizations, establishing green teams in their churches, and meeting socially in their homes to plan advocacy and organizing activities. The participants serve as a model for engaging older adults in environmental engagement and volunteerism.

The ever-growing older adult population can be recruited and their abilities and talents can be utilized to protect the legacy of the earth for their grandchildren as well as their love of place. These older adults have lived and worked in this Kansas community and are willing to put their time and efforts towards preserving the places they care about (Bushway et al., 2011), thereby leaving a legacy for the next generations (Frumkin et al., 2012). Older adults who have aged in place may have a stronger attachment to their environment and may therefore be more likely to engage in environmental activities, to develop an "ecological identity" and recognize their own ability to maintain their local landscape (Bushway et al., 2011). The older adults indicated their sense of place through their connections to their family farms, raising their children in the same way, and their lifelong love of the outdoors.

This cohort experienced and was a part of huge battles over some incredibly difficult
events including the Vietnam War (which eventually ended), the Wolf Creek nuclear plant (eventually built), agitation for environmental legislation (the EPA, Clean Air and Water Acts) with highs and lows around those experiences. They were invested and saw collective success periodically. In thinking about some of the success their cohort had, one commented that today's generation feels, maybe, "What do you do as a college student for that? ... They feel it's completely intractable and they feel very disillusioned. They are more disillusioned, I think, about an environmental situation, than perhaps ever before" (E15). Environmental issues are often intangible with climate change being a big concept that manifests itself in a multitude of ways. People gather around a power plant opening or a prairie being plowed, but organizing around a large, intangible social and environmental issue can be daunting (Norgaard, 2011). The social work literature largely focuses on response to natural and environmental disasters (Dominelli, 2012; Gray, Coates, & Hetherington, 2012), which occur when concrete mobilization of resources and action are conducted. The older adults in this study serve as a model of steady and persistent engagement with environmental issues.

Bridging the gap across generations

The older adult participants are ordinary people whose work intersects with many macro social work values and practice skills in environmental justice efforts including: group work, community organizing, advocacy, education and lobbying, and influencing policy on their state and local levels. The organizations in this community have a large population of older adults who have created organizations, served on boards, and attended meetings across their life course. As a generation, they have aged with their participation and volunteerism and now have a different challenge of recruiting younger people to participate in their organizations. With regard to groups and organizations, a cultural shift in participation in and value of traditional groups occurred, even for the older adults themselves. The formal methods of meeting regularly in churches or community buildings using Roberts Rules of Order has created some disillusionment with the participants themselves while also hindering their efforts to recruit younger members. One model of intergenerational participation, such as Community Earth Councils, brings older adults and youth and/or young adults together to build community across generations and work on an environmental issue in their community (Utne, 2009). These types of models would help the older adults to recreate their work in a modern and inclusive manner that allows everyone to help shape the group or organization.

The environmentalists, both older and younger, need to build coalitions between environmental groups. Environmentalists from both age groups share similar environmental concerns (Steinig & Butts, 2009). The younger generations, such as the Millennials, have values of diversity and inclusion and, in this case, overcoming issues of ageism from both the older adult environmentalists towards the younger adults and vice versa is necessary to build a more intergenerational effort (Deloitte, 2014; National Association of Social Workers(NASW), 2017). Older adults are more likely to change their attitudes with new information and more likely to adopt perspectives of young people than vice versa (Frumkin et al., 2012). Environmental information needs to be directed towards older adults, because most of the education and outreach funding is directed towards children and shared in educational institutions (Johnson & Schwadel, 2018). Environmental justice activities should include program and development strategies that include an intergenerational framework (Steinig & Butts, 2009). Intergenerational participation in environmental activities also focuses on relationships as well as the tasks at hand. As evidenced by the older adults who found support and friendship, the intergenerational programs must privilege the relationship building as well as participating in meaningful work (Steinig & Butts, 2009).

The Millennial generation is also civically minded and believe in political engagement (Deloitte, 2014). Additionally, the recognition that the inspiration for participation originates in different cultural ways: the older adults were shaped by anti-war protests and civil rights activism. Younger generations today have lived the wars in the Middle East and were galvanized to action without similar positive outcomes compared to the anti-war protests for Vietnam, Civil Rights and women rights. However, they have developed new political campaign involvement, taken part in renewed feminist movement engagement through sexual assault awareness and the Women's March, and the sustained power of Black Lives Matter. Both of these generations' cohorts operate from the similar belief in social change through participation. These generations need a connector in order to build a bridge and appreciate the social justice values and practices in order to continue the environmental engagement in this community.

Finally, the older adults in this study reflected across their life course and identified key aspects of their development of an environmental conscious that galvanized their community involvement. They recognized that an inspirational teacher or professor ignited curiosity, developed their knowledge, and inspired their community engagement. As educators, it is our duty to include these topics in the social work curriculum and inspire future social workers to incorporate environmental social work into their practice as these issues will affect many marginalized and diverse groups, organizations, and communities throughout their careers.

Disclosure statement

No potential conflict of interest was reported by the authors.

ORCID

Paul Stock ⓘ http://orcid.org/0000-0002-1807-3895

References

Bengtson, V. L., Burgess, E. O., & Parrott, T. M. (1997). Theory, explanation, and a third generation of theoretical development in social gerontology. *The Journals of Gerontology Series B: Psychological Sciences and Social Sciences, 52*(2), S72–S88. doi:10.1093/geronb/52B.2.S72

Binstock, R., Sykes, K., & Reilly, S. (2009). Imagining the American community environmental services: A vision for environmentalists and elders. *Generations, 33*(4), 75–81.

Braun, V., & Clarke, V. (2006). Using thematic analysis in psychology. *Qualitative Research in Psychology, 3*(2), 77–101. doi:10.1191/1478088706qp063oa

Brulle, R. J. (2000). *Agency, democracy, and nature: The US environmental movement from a critical theory perspective.* Cambridge, MA: MIT Press.

Bushway, L. J., Dickinson, J. L., Stedman, R. C., Wagenet, L. P., & Weinstein, D. A. (2011). Benefits, motivations, and barriers related to environmental volunteerism for older adults: Developing a research agenda. *The International Journal of Aging and Human Development, 72*(3), 189–206. doi:10.2190/AG.72.3.b

Carson, R. (1962). *Silent spring.* New York, NY: Houghton Mifflin Harcourt.

Coen, C. H. (2001). *Selected chronology of political protests and events in Lawrence 1960-1973.* Retrieved from https://kuscholarworks.ku.edu/bitstream/handle/1808/20713/Coen_Lawrence_Political_Protests.pdf?sequence=1&isAllowed=y

Creswell, J. W. (2013). *Qualitative inquiry and research design: Choosing among five approaches.* (3rd ed.). Los Angeles, CA: Sage.

Deloitte. (2014). *Big demands and high expectations–The Deloitte millennial survey.* Retrieved from https://www2.deloitte.com/content/dam/Deloitte/global/Documents/About-Deloitte/gx-dttl-2014-millennial-survey-report.pdf

Dominelli, L. (2012). *Green social work: From environmental crises to environmental justice.* Cambridge, UK: Polity.

Dunlap, R. E., & Mertig, A. G. (2014). *American environmentalism: The US environmental movement, 1970-1990.* New York, NY: Taylor & Francis.

Elder, G. H., Johnson, M. K., & Crosnoe, R. (2003). The emergence and development of life course theory. In J. T. Mortimer & M. J. Shanahan (Eds.), *Handbook of the life course* (pp. 3–19). Boston, MA: Springer.

Formosa, M. (2012). Older persons and green volunteering: The missing link to sustainable future? In S. Rizzo (Ed.), *Green jobs from a small state perspective. Case studies from Malta* (pp. 33–43). Brussels, BEL: Green European Foundation.

Francis. (2015). *Laudato si': On care for our common home*. Retrieved from http://w2.vatican.va/content/dam/francesco/pdf/encyclicals/documents/papa-francesco_20150524_enciclica-laudato-si_en.pdf

Frumkin, H., Fried, L., & Moody, R. (2012). Aging, climate change, and legacy thinking. *American Journal of Public Health, 102*(8), 1434–1438. doi:10.2105/AJPH.2012.300663

Gottlieb, R. (2005). *Forcing the spring: The transformation of the American environmental movement*. Washington, D.C.: Island Press.

Gray, M., Coates, J., & Hetherington, T. (2012). Introduction. In M. Gray, J. Coates, & T. Hetherington (Eds.), *Environmental social work* (pp. 1–28). New York, NY: Routledge.

Johnson, E. W., & Frickel, S. (2011). Ecological threat and the founding of U.S. national environmental movement organizations, 1962–1998. *Social Problems, 58*(3), 305–329. doi:10.1525/sp.2011.58.3.305

Johnson, E. W., & Schwadel, P. (2018). It is not a cohort thing: Interrogating the relationship between age, cohort, and support for the environment. *Environment and Behavior*, 1–23. doi:10.1177/0013916518780483

Klein, N. (2015). *This changes everything: Capitalism vs. the climate*. New York, NY: Simon and Schuster.

Matthews, M. (2012). *Droppers: America's first hippie commune, Drop City*. Norman: University of Oklahoma Press.

Metz, C. (2010, April 21). 1970: Racial unrest sparked deadly violence. *Lawrence Journal World*. Retrieved from https://www2.ljworld.com/news/2010/apr/21/1970-racial-unrest-sparked-deadly-violence/

National Association of Social Workers (2017). *NASW Code of Ethics*. Retrieved from https://www.socialworkers.org/About/Ethics/Code-of-Ethics/Code-of-Ethics-English

Norgaard, K. M. (2011). *Living in denial: Climate change, emotions, and everyday life*. Cambridge, MA: MIT Press.

Pillemer, K., Wagenet, L., Goldman, D., Bushway, L., & Meador, R. (2009). Environmental volunteering in later life: Benefits and barriers. *Generations, 33*(4), 58–63.

Pillemer, K., Wells, N. M., Meador, R. H., Schultz, L., Henderson, C. R., & Cope, M. T. (2017). Engaging older adults in environmental volunteerism: The retirees in service to the environment program. *The Gerontologist, 57*(2), 367–375. doi:10.1093/geront/gnv693

Protest: Bleeding Kansas. (1970, May 4). *Time,18*(95), 25.

Ranney, D. (2002, July 16) Violence, racism marked era when police killed black teen. *Lawrence Journal World*. Retrieved from http://www2.ljworld.com/news/2002/jul/16/violence_racism_marked/

Steinig, S., & Butts, D. (2009). Generations going green: Intergenerational programs connecting young and old to improve our environment. *Generations, 33*(4), 64–69.

Taylor, D. E. (2000). The rise of the environmental justice paradigm: Injustice framing and the social construction of environmental discourses. *American Behavioral Scientist, 43*(4), 508–580.

Turner, F. (2010). *From counterculture to cyberculture: Stewart brand, the whole earth network, and the rise of digital utopianism*. Chicago: University of Chicago Press.

Utne, E. (2009). Community earth councils. *Generations, 33*(4), 95–96.

Preparing social workers for ecosocial work practice and community building

Meredith C. F. Powers, Cathryne Schmitz, and Micalagh Beckwith Moritz

ABSTRACT
In the context of the global ecological crisis, the profession of social work is increasingly shifting to embrace an ecosocial lens, recognizing the centrality of the ecological environment for human existence and the inextricable linkages of well-being for people and planet. Social work educators are contributing to this shift as leaders in the transformation of their home institutions and communities. We present examples within two models of education for ecosocial work, the infusion model and the integration model. Exemplars are based on the authors' expertise and contributions to ecosocial work education, community building, and ecosocial change, both locally and globally.

Evidence has established the fact of climate change (Intergovernmental Panel on Climate Change, 2018). The rapidity of the change has precipitated the global ecological crisis, which has led to a necessary response to mitigate and adapt to changes that support the earth and all the species that live here (Orr, 2016; Romm, 2016; Wallace-Wells, 2019). Individuals, governments, and organizations are taking action across the globe with a renewed sense of urgency. This action is seen on multiple fronts from the 2018 Special Report created by the IPCC, the annual United Nations Climate Summits, the 2019 report by the United States (US) National Aeronautics and Space Administration (NASA) and National Oceanic and Atmospheric Administration (NOAA) documenting the accelerated pace of climate change (National Aeronautics and Space Administration, 2019), and the increase in declarations of *climate emergency* by many cities and nations (Climate Emergency Declaration, n.d.).

The impact of climate change is dire for humans; as much of the earth becomes uninhabitable this century, life will become more precarious with increasing conflict over decreasing resources (Wallace-Wells, 2019). The consequences for humans, other species, and the earth itself is wide ranging and inclusive of mass migration, extinction of species, overpopulation, environmental racism, environmental injustice, lack of arable land, displacement due to ecological degradation, growing inequality, and increasing violent conflict over resources (Mason & Rigg, 2019; Powers, Schmitz, Nsonwu, & Mathew, 2018; Sloan, Joyner, Stakeman, & Schmitz, 2018; Sloan & Schmitz, 2019). The social, political, and economic human systems in which we work are dependent on the ecological environment (Schmitz, Matyók, James, & Sloan, 2013).

Social workers are increasingly recognizing the ecological crisis and becoming actively involved with responses, locally and globally (Besthorn, 2002; Jones, 2010; Jones, Powers, & Truell, 2018; Powers & Rinkel, 2018). Central to this professional response is the shift to embrace an ecosocial lens, or eco-centric paradigm, which recognizes the centrality of the ecological environment for human existence and the inextricable linkages of wellbeing for people and planet (Boetto, 2017; Powers & Rinkel, 2018). Ecosocial work *is* social work that has embraced this paradigmatic shift, from an anthropocentric focus to an eco-centric focus (Boetto, 2017). Thus, ecosocial work is not a niche for social work research and practice, rather a framework in which all social workers can operate (Powers & Rinkel, 2018). Ecosocial work honors an expanded understanding of person in environment, recognizing that the physical, ecological environment has major social impacts on communities, individuals, and families in those communities (Boetto, 2017; Powers, 2016).

Social work educators contribute to the profession's embrace of this paradigmatic shift by transforming their home institutions and communities through implicit (e.g., relationships, communication, normative practices) and explicit (e.g., policies, course curriculum) implementation of an ecosocial framework (Schmitz, Powers, Nesmith, & Forbes, 2017). Education for ecosocial work has been operationalized in two models, the *transformative approach* of infusing the ecosocial framework as the base for social work education and the integrating model for embedding, wherever possible, ecosocial concepts and materials into an existing curriculum which maintains its' anthropocentric framework (Boetto, 2017; Jones, 2018). Each model is explicated further in the sections below. Examples are presented for each model based on the authors' knowledge, experiences, and contributions to ecosocial work education, community building, and ecological change, both locally and globally. As background context, we first offer a brief exploration of what community means from an ecosocial lens and how transformational change has occurred through this lens in the example of the 'Green Belt Movement' (Maathai, 2003). This discussion further sets the stage for the urgency of preparing social workers for ecosocial work practice and community building as they join as leaders in addressing the ecological crisis.

Community and community building through the ecosocial lens

Making peace with the earth we make the world a place where we can be one with nature. We create and sustain environments where we can come back to ourselves, where we can return home, stand on solid ground, and be a true witness. (hooks, 2009, p. 120)

In this quote, bell hooks captures the strength of the connection to the earth at the personal, local, and communal level. This link highlights the ecosocial understanding of community as connection. Community and environmental sustainability depend on respect for and maintenance of the Earth's ecosystems, for the wellbeing of all life, including current and future generations.

Community, when engaging processes for bringing people together, holds the capacity to embrace growth. This "potential for change is often found in the common need for the development, access to, and control of local resources" (Sloan et al., 2018, p. 128). Often, for transformation to occur, it must be disruptive to power, as seen in the Green Belt Movement (Maathai, 2003). The Greenbelt Movement offers an exemplar of bringing the women of the community together around the need to rebuild the ecology and, with it, the relationships that enhance the empowerment of community (Maathai, 2006). The ecosocial lens is highlighted as the women come together, locally, around the very concrete task of germinating and planting trees (Maathai, 2006; Merton & Dater, 2008). Maathai, as a change leader, understood the need to build a movement through relationship. And, because she also understood the interconnection of marginalization, violence, and structural oppression, she spearheaded the process of empowering the community to learn and engage in political, economic, community, and civic change (Maathai, 2006; Merton & Dater, 2008; Sloan & Schmitz, 2019).

Maathai (2003) and hooks (2009) both bring forward the significance of connection to the land and to each other, which provides a place of belonging, a community (Block, 2009). It is through the development of collaborations that the capacity is created for rebuilding and supporting the development of local resources (Sloan et al., 2018). Climate change and environmental degradation impact the community beyond the personal to the communal. The need, therefore, exists to "move from the micro to the mega, building relationships, and community" (Sloan et al., p. 133). Communities have resources for healing that provide a framework for creating social, economic, political, and environmental change (Gamble, 2013; Gamble & Weil, 2010). According to Gamble and Weil (2010, p. 122), "neighborhood and community organizing takes place when people have face-to-face contact with each other, allowing them to feel connected to a place." The negative impacts and injustices related to climate change can be minimized when communities become sites for transformational action and change (McMichael, 2017; Powers et al., 2018). Collaborative community projects interconnect people creating possibilities for collective action in support of sustainable change (Orr, 2004) as a base for ecosocial practice.

The history of social work's commitment to community building and advocacy positions the profession as a leader in organizing for transformational change across disciplines. In times of high ecological and political risk, there is heavy responsibility calling for ecosocial work embedded in community. Never has there been a clearer link across human vulnerability, community risk, and the potential for resilience through ecosocial work and community building.

Education for ecosocial work practice

> Today we are faced with a challenge that calls for a shift in our thinking, so that humanity stops threatening its life-support system. We are called to assist the Earth to heal her wounds and, in the process, heal our own – indeed to embrace the whole of creation in all its diversity, beauty and wonder. (Taking Root, n.d.)

This quote by Wangari Maathai, incites us not only to action, but also to education that embraces the ecosocial lens. Social work educators are being challenged to transform our implicit and explicit curriculum to meet the need to educate the next generation for ecosocial justice (Bay, 2013; Hayward, Miller, & Shaw, 2012; Jones, 2010, 2018; Schmitz et al., 2017). Such education for ecosocial work is being operationalized in two models: (1) *transformative approach* of infusing an ecosocial lens across all aspects of the curriculum, and (2) embedding or integrating ecosocial concepts within existing social work curriculum (which is still situated in an anthropocentric lens) (Boetto, 2017; Jones, 2018). Both approaches are necessary to further ecosocial work education, and the integrating model may eventually lead to the infusion model. While we consider the first model of infusing a total shift to an ecosocial lens for a school's entire curriculum as ideal, we acknowledge this is not always possible.

Here, we present several examples, within these two models, to inspire other social work academics and students to initiate ecosocial education at their institutions and/or to elaborate the ongoing discussion at professional conferences and in the current literature. The complexity of living and practicing within the rapid pace of climate change encompasses a sense of urgency for ecosocial learning. As a community, the university campus becomes a site to explore and remediate environmental degradation, foster learning, and build leadership capacity (Whiteman & Powers, 2012). Our examples are based on practice experience as educators. They illuminate possible ways for engaging in multidisciplinary, multilevel curriculum, and university-based models for ecosocial work education.

Infusing a transformative approach to ecosocial work education

At the University of South Carolina College of Social Work (U of SC COSW), Powers (author 1) utilized the transformation approach to infusing the ecosocial framework (Boetto, 2017; Jones, 2018), in both implicit and explicit curriculum, across the policies, practices, and pedagogy of the College of Social Work (U of SC CoSW, 2014). This was made possible by supportive leadership within the College of Social Work and the university's campus-wide sustainability program, in which Powers was a doctoral student leader. As an ecosocial work educator, practitioner, and doctoral student leader, Powers cultivated these relationships creating formal and informal collaborations within the College and across campus with the university's sustainability staff and faculty, and the *Green Office* initiative.

Powers began by meeting with the Dean of the College, then working with students, faculty, and staff of the College to meet the standards of the university's *Green Office* initiative run by the sustainability program. This initiative also awarded Powers a small, internal grant to support the College's modifications and the establishment of new policies and practices needed to meet the *Green Office* standards (e.g., purchasing and placing recycling bins in each office; creating a policy for ordering supplies for events from local, sustainable vendors; posting sustainability tips in classrooms; and creating instructional materials such as videos). We began by coordinating campus recycling services and streamlining waste management within the College's offices and classrooms. In addition, we made multiple presentations for audiences of faculty, staff, students, and field instructors; we sent emails with information (i.e., green office tips, ways to consider ecosocial aspects in field settings, ways to embed ecosocial content into existing courses), and even created and disseminated a YouTube video, featuring Powers and the Dean of the College of Social Work (U of SC CoSW, 2013). Additionally, a series of workshops was developed and offered by Powers and other social workers for Continuing Education to community social workers, faculty, and students. Topics included: Roles for Social Workers in the Ecological Crisis, Putting the Environment in Person-and-Environment, Using Nature in Practice: Interventions using Wilderness Therapy, and Responsible Consumerism: Being Mindful of Social and Ecological Justice.

In addition, an *ecosocial tool kit* was also developed by Powers to engage interest in the community of educators within the College (including faculty, adjunct faculty, and field supervisors). This ecosocial tool kit consisted of a cover letter explaining the aim of the College of Social Work to shift to an ecosocial paradigm in all implicit and explicit curricula, offered key scholarly articles as examples, along with a list of other potential resources that could be useful. Individuals were invited to meet with Powers, for support as they shifted their paradigms to embrace an ecosocial lens, and as they infused it into their courses and field settings. Modifications sometimes included embedding or integrating ecosocial content, but this was always part of the larger transformative approach of infusing the ecosocial lens throughout the class/field setting, along with the entire College. Examples of this infusion (and integration) include, changing language in the course content description to reflect ecosocial values rather than anthropocentric values, adjusting assignments such as *client assessments* to include how the physical (i.e., built and natural) environments impact clients *and* how clients impact the environment (both positively and negatively). Readings that include ecosocial content were added and class lectures were adjusted to include ecosocial work content (e.g., when discussing food security, include community gardening programs; when discussing therapeutic interventions, include ecotherapy).

All of these efforts by Powers were focused on transforming the College of Social Work with the ecosocial lens, rather than merely adding ecosocial content as an additional learning competency for their already robust curricular goals. Each aspect of this transformation to the ecosocial lens was based on building community, first, within the College of Social Work uniting to earn the *Green Office* certification, infusing an ecosocial lens into the curriculum, and seeing themselves as part of the campus wide sustainability initiative; and, ultimately, strengthening the relationships between planet and people as they began to consider, through the ecosocial lens, their positive connections with nature, the potential for ecosocial healing, and their negative impacts on the ecological crisis and related injustices.

Integrating ecosocial concepts in social work education

Alternatively, some social work programs may not be ready to fully embrace the ecosocial lens and infuse it across the implicit and explicit curriculum. Though, support from leaders in traditional organizational structures helps tremendously in creating ecosocial transformation, individual faculty and/or student leaders have also been successful in initiating such changes, particularly higher education (Powers, 2016; Whiteman & Powers, 2012). Some social work educators are, thusly, approaching their programs through an integration model where ecosocial concepts are embedded, wherever possible, within the existing curriculum (Jones, 2018). For example, modifying existing courses to integrate environmental concerns or developing discrete courses focused on environmental justice, sustainability, and environmental oppression to add on to the existing curriculum (often as electives). In these courses, inter-and trans-disciplinary learning opportunities are also being created, making use of applied, community-based learning approaches, and global opportunities to recontextualize the ecological environment and locate social work opportunities within it.

Interdisciplinary course on environmental justice

The ecological crisis is multi-dimensional and global in its complexity (Schmitz et al., 2013). Addressing these concerns cuts across the natural and social sciences; the work in the natural sciences is more developed and focused than in the social sciences, but change cannot occur without addressing the human systems. The intimacy of the reliance of humans on the land and all ecology requires engaging students in interdisciplinary education in order to prepare them for practice in complex community and advocacy contexts.

One such course in this integration model was developed and implemented by Schmitz (author 2). It has been running at a mid-sized public university for eight years and has been further developed by both Powers and Schmitz during this time. A number of lessons were learned when trying to integrate this course into the social work curriculum. Of major significance was the title of the course. The course was not a draw for social science students until the title was changed to *Environmental Justice*. Students did not understand labels such as *green social work* or *sustainability*, which were interpreted as having a focus on business; but, they were drawn to the justice aspect of the revised title. While the course is taught through an ecosocial lens and from a broader *ecological justice* focus, the title remains more narrowly *environmental justice* as an easier entre into the typical students' current anthropocentric mindset. This focus has attracted graduate and undergraduate social work students along with students from other disciplines in the social, natural, and biological sciences, creating a rich, interdisciplinary learning environment.

Interestingly, some of the students entered the course not even knowing that there is an ecological crisis and without awareness of any potential solutions (e.g., corporate responsibility, reducing consumption patterns an waste streams, recycling), while other students came with a great deal of knowledge and experience. This student-body composition has proven fruitful with students learning not only from the instructor, but also from other students with varied educational and experiential backgrounds. Those with more knowledge became peer-educators, while also adding to their skills and knowledge. Course content in lectures, discussions, readings, and assignments cuts across disciplines and were designed to engage the broad range of experience and knowledge. Thus, the course falls in line with Education for Sustainability as the entire interdisciplinary course infuses the ecosocial lens (Jones, 2018).

Additionally, by exposing the students to these topics, especially those learning about them for the first time, they were able to realize that they may have been operating in an anthropocentric paradigm, and were exposed to the ecosocial lens, allowing them the opportunity to make their own paradigmatic shift, and/or changes in values and behavior changes that may impact their personal and professional lives (Jones, 2018). Introductory content was available for those students who needed this, and additional content allowed for greater exploration of topics for those more advanced. Additional support and resources were offered by the instructors, as needed, for either type of student. For example, students unfamiliar or less familiar to environmental issues were exposed to introductory topics such as local campus and municipal recycling information. While, some more advanced students in this course were invited to deepen their knowledge and expertise by coauthoring papers with Powers and Schmitz on topics they studied during their enrollment.

The course begins with exposure to the ecosocial lens and the complexity of the ecological crisis from climate change, to habitat loss and ecological degradation, specifically noting how these have the most destructive effect on vulnerable communities. Human political, economic, and social systems are increasingly destructive of local ecologies and wildlife, resulting in increasing conflict. Issues of environmental justice are quickly linked to social, political, and economic justice (see Schmitz et al., 2013 for further detail). Attention is paid to indigenous rights, decolonization, and environmental racism, along with the role of local voices in developing resilient community systems. Students learn about response systems across the globe such as ecosocial work with renewable energy in European countries or the use of herbal plants for medicinal purposes in Central America (Powers & Rinkel, 2018). As noted in the section above, Wangari Maathai and the Green Belt Movement (see Maathai, 2003; Merton & Dater, 2008) provide a strong example of change which connects environmental action to ecological change, community building, social and political oppression, and empowerment through civic engagement (Sloan & Schmitz, 2019).

Students learn multiple methods for engaging change that includes the link between individual empowerment and community building, critical education as a tool for change, the key role of relationship development, and the significance of change at the local level with the potential to shape political processes from this vantage point. Students are embedded in interdisciplinary teams that are engaged in exploring the ecological crisis and related issues of justice and potential ecosocial solutions. These teams, with support of the instructor, educate themselves on these issues, and then are responsible for educating the class; this way they all become teachers, as well as learners.

The context for ecosocial work is global, but systems of change are embedded in the local. Students in this course explore ways the natural environment is healing and engage with experiential educational opportunities within the context of community (i.e., campus community and beyond). For example, they volunteer with community agencies to investigate industrial and technical responses such as recycling, alternative energy, water rights, the risks of fracking and mountaintop removal, community gardening, tiny houses, animal assisted therapy, and habitat preservation. They learn and apply community building and advocacy skills in these community contexts.

Global education

As the world is becoming increasingly globalized, it is imperative that the field of social work increases its global focus (Mapp, 2008). Global learning can be integrated into campus curriculum at the local level. The global can be brought to life through the use of web-based exchanges and speakers, video exemplars, student projects and presentations, and experiential activities designed to expose students to the natural environment.

Students learn on multiple levels through global learning opportunities that expand their exposure to new regions, cultures, worldviews, and possibilities. Students might go for study abroad and incidentally learn about environmental concerns, solutions, and sustainability. They can learn through exposure to local responses to environmental pollution, recycling and reuse programs, and the use of trash to create a sustainable energy source. Not every student or curriculum, however, has the resources to take advantage of study abroad courses. There is value in global study aborad education for students; there is also value in learning from these programs to identify components that can be reproduced closer to home.

The Beckwith Moritz (author 3) offers here her experience as a social work educator in an intensive immersion curriculum offered in the Central American country of Belize. Some of the lessons learned in this example are related to the global component while others relate to ecological learning, local systems, and the role of community in resilience. This example falls within the integration model, as it is marketed as courses added on as electives or may count as core course requirements at a student's home institution, but does not itself offer full degree programs. However, the entire immersion curriculum once in Belize is within the infusion model (Boetto, 2017; Jones, 2018) as the campus itself and the curriculum, both implicit and explicit, are completely infused with the ecosocial lens.

The program in Belize (see website- http://www.creationcsp.org) has partnerships with multiple universities, individual professors, and organization, offering learning opportunities on multiple levels. The community where this program is located has rich ecological and cultural diversity, local involvement to support student learning, and an interdisciplinary teaching team and student body. It is an interdisciplinary curriculum, drawing faculty and students across disciplines, including social work. Belize is sparsely populated (around 330,000) and has the largest expanse of preserved land in Central America. It is a known destination for ecotourism due to its high levels of biodiversity; and the 17-acre, sustainable campus includes hiking trails and river access, providing students with experiential learning opportunities promoting eco literacy and a broad array of environmental education.

The program's partnership with many colleges, professors, and organizations, allows students to learn holistically, gaining an ecosocial perspective and understanding of their part in the interdisciplinary responses to the global ecological crisis. The pedagogy of the program involves an emphasis on experiential learning, exposing students to issues of justice (particularly ecological) through field trips paired with lectures, discussions, and critical reflection. Topics such as sustainable living, safety, cultural inclusion, and community involvement are embedded along with coursework on ecology, sustainability, and diversity. Each course is interdisciplinary as it elicits the perspectives of students who are from many different cultures and academic disciplines. While most courses are offered on the Belize campus, experiential learning is embedded through the incorporation of local excursions and speakers. Students learn firsthand about the impact of climate change on local farmers and ecosystems by visiting farms; they examine water quality in local streams to understand how runoff affects water sources, and therefore, nearby village communities and other habitats and species. They also spend time in a pristine rainforest, an ecosystem that includes rare birds, snakes, and plants, contributing to a greater understanding of the need to preserve forests and species. Marine Ecology is also offered. Each course and the campus itself provides students with visible connections to the ways humans contribute to conservation and destruction.

Meals on campus come from local food sources: the campus garden, the town market, a neighborhood dairy farm, and a women's cooperative that provides chicken for consumption. Through these practices, students learn to cook and eat locally and more sustainably–transferrable skills that can be taken back to their home countries. They experience the importance of minimizing waste and observe the environmental impact of individual and orgainzational choices. They see the need for advocacy and change on both micro and macro levels. Throughout their entire program, they are immersed in the significance of culture and respect for the local the ecosocial perspective and the need to center ecological and social justice. Exposure to other community players including local farms, Non-governmental Organizations (NGOs), and tourist offices also expands their learning.

Each of these components and opportunities could be adopted and/or modified for replication in non-study abroad contexts within local university communities. This exemplar of the Belize program, as an interesting combination of both the integration and infusion models, highlights components that enrich ecosocial learning – learning embedded in nature, connection to the land, community building among students, lessons from the local community, cross disciplinary learning, and connection to the wildlife and the loss of flora and fauna.

Discussion and conclusion

The ecological crisis is negatively reshaping the planet and increasing the threat for all forms of life inhabiting it. The impact of ecological destruction is inextricably linked to social, political, and economic injustices (Intergovernmental Panel on Climate Change, 2018). The daily lives of the individuals, families, organizations, and communities that social workers strive to serve are increasingly disrupted and strained as the devastating changes are coming faster than anticipated. This heightens the risks for the communities we serve, making it an urgent matter to promote ecosocial work within the profession at large and within our formal educational systems.

Formal educational structures, such as universities, can support integrated learning that incorporates implicit and explicit processes of knowledge development on campus and within the broader community (Whiteman & Powers, 2012). It is vital that social work faculty and students are a part of such learning processes, experiencing and understanding our relationships with each other and the natural world. Educational programs can increase global knowledge, embed interdisciplinary learning, highlight the ecosocial connections, and promote community as a site for practice in complex contexts. The complexity of the intersecting issues of the ecological crisis highlights the importance of multi-dimensional education. Environmental learning is not an isolated experience; it is intertwined with learning about social, political, and economic oppression. This learning includes exploring and disrupting implicit biases that support colonial practices and systemic oppression.

The two models, the infusion of a transformative ecosocial approach and the integration of ecosocial content (Boetto, 2017; Jones, 2018), both offer ways to operationalize changes to our social work pedagogical approaches. This paper further elaborated this discussion by offering exemplars for both models. Concrete approaches are suggested such as dedicated, interdisciplinary courses, study abroad experiences, and efforts to infuse an ecosocial lens across the curriculum. Experiential, classroom-based, local and global opportunities offered a wide range of contexts for tackling the complexity of the ecological crosos . The authors have found these models to be useful in transforming their home institutions and successful in expanding student knowledge about ecosocial work.

While the examples presented successes, more adjustments could be made to augment the impact. For instance, in the example of the infusion model in the College of Social Work, continual efforts are required to infuse the ecosocial lens as new leaders, faculty, staff, and students enter the organization and bring with them their own lenses, thereby influencing the community's lens (Powers, 2016). Indeed, creating a sustained shift to the ecosocial paradigm must not be based on any one champion, rather it needs to be situated firmly in community, partnerships, policies, practices, and pedagogy (Whiteman & Powers, 2012). Further, the interdisciplinary course on environmental justice and the study abroad program, could be used as stepping stones to infuse a transformative ecosocial lens into social work program(s) where such courses are offered. Additionally, the course title could be renamed *ecological justice* rather than *environmental justice,* and it could be made a mandatory course in that program rather than an elective.

Social work practitioners, educators, and students are increasingly engaged with environmental concerns and responses as they enter complex practice settings where they join communities and practitioners from other disciplines. Current and future social work professionals are essential leaders in the interdisciplinary response to the global ecological crisis. For example, ecosocial workers are joining with civic and governmental groups for community park renovation projects that enhance the possibility of people enjoying healthy connections with nature and each other. In such settings, the social worker, operating from an ecosocial lens, can help not only bring together and establish platforms for all voices to be heard, but can also be an advocate for ecological justice (e.g., how are the renovations impacting the whole ecosystem, not just looking at potential benefits for humans). Through embracing the ecosocial lens, such social work leaders, including the authors of this paper, have also developed interdisciplinary forums (e.g., books, Google, Facebook and Twitter groups) for collaboration, been instrumental in the integration of environmental justice as a competency for the Council on Social Work Education's (CSWE) Educational Program Standards of 2015, established a Committee on Environmental Justice for CSWE, and developed and established the International Federation of Social Workers (IFSW) Climate Justice Program. Such advocacy, community building, and civic engagement are key to the process of transformative ecosocial change.

Disclosure statement

No potential conflict of interest was reported by the authors.

References

Bay, U. (2013). Environmental social work. *Social Work Education: The International Journal, 32,* 1–2. doi:10.1080/02615479.2013.797655

Besthorn, F. H. (2002). Is it time for a new ecological approach to social work: What is the environment telling us? *The Spirituality and Social Work Forum, 9*(1), 2–5.

Block, P. (2009). *Community: The structure of belonging.* San Francisco, CA: Berrett-Koehler.

Boetto, H. (2017). A transformative eco-social model: Challenging modernist assumptions in social work. *British Journal of Social Work, 47*(1), 48–67.

Climate Emergency Declaration. (n.d.). *Call to declare a climate emergency.* Retrieved from https://climateemergencydeclaration.org/

Gamble, D. N. (2013). Well-being in a globalized world: Does social work know how to make it happen? *Journal of Social Work Education, 48*(4), 669–689. doi:10.5175/JSWE.2012.201100125

Gamble, D. N., & Weil, M. (2010). *Community practice skills: Local to global.* New York, NY: Columbia University Press.

Hayward, R. A., Miller, S. E., & Shaw, T. V. (2012). Social work education on the environment in contemporary curricula in the USA. In M. Grey, J. Coates, & T. Hetherington (Eds.), *Environmental social work* (pp. 246–259). New York, NY: Routledge.

Hooks, B. (2009). *Belonging: A culture of place.* New York, NY: Routledge.

Intergovernmental Panel on Climate Change. (2018). *Special report: Global warming of 1.5°C.* Retrieved from https://www.ipcc.ch/sr15/

Jones, D. N., Powers, M. C. F., & Truell, R. (2018). Global overview. In D. N. Jones (Ed.), *Global agenda for social work and social development: Third report. Promoting community and environmental sustainability* (pp. 1–50). Rheinfelden, Switzerland: IFSW.

Jones, P. (2010). Responding to the ecological crisis: Transformative ways for social work education. *Journal of Social Work Education, 46*(1), 67–84. doi:10.5175/JSWE.2010.200800073

Jones, P. (2018). Greening social work education: Transforming the curriculum in pursuit of eco-social justice. In L. Dominelli (Ed.), *The Routledge handbook of green social work* (pp. 558–568). New York, NY: Routledge.

Maathai, W. (2003, March). *The green belt movement: Sharing the approach and the experience.* New York, NY: Lantern Books.

Maathai, W. (2006). *Unbowed: A memoir.* New York, NY: Knopf.

Mapp, S. C. (2008). *Human rights and social justice in a global perspective: An introduction to international social work.* New York, NY: Oxford University Press.

Mason, L. R., & Rigg, J. (2019). Climate change, social justice: Making the case for community inclusion. In L. R. Mason & J. Rigg (Eds.), *People and climate change: Vulnerability, adaptation, and social justice* (pp. 3–19). New York, NY: Oxford University Press.

McMichael, P. (2017). *Development and social change.* Los Angeles, CA: Sage.

Merton, L., & Dater, A., (Producer and Director). (2008). *Taking root: The vision of Wangari Maathai [DVD].* Marlboor, VT, USA: Marlboro Productions.

National Aeronautics and Space Administration. (2019). *2018 fourth warmest year in continued warming trend, according to NASA, NOAA.* Retrieved from https://climate.nasa.gov/news/2841/2018-fourth-warmest-year-in-continued-warming-trend-according-to-nasa-noaa/

Orr, D. W. (2004). *Earth in mind: On education, environment, and the human prospect.* DC: Island Press.

Orr, D. W. (2016). *Dangerous years: Climate change, the long emergency and the way forward.* New Haven, CT: Yale University Press.

Powers, M., & Rinkel, M. (Eds.). (2018). *Social work promoting community and environmental sustainability: A workbook for social work practitioners and educators (Vol.2).* Rheinfelden, Switzerland: International Federation of Social Work (IFSW).

Powers, M. C. F. (2016). Transforming the profession: Social workers' expanding response to the ecological crisis. In A.-L. Matthies & K. Narhi (Eds.), *Ecosocial transition of societies: Contribution of social work and social policy (pp. 286–300).* London, UK: Routledge.

Powers, M. C. F., Schmitz, C. L., Nsonwu, C. Z., & Mathew, M. T. (2018). Environmental migration: Social work at the nexus of climate change and global migration. *Advances in Social Work, 18*(3), 1023–1040. doi:10.18060/21678

Romm, J. (2016). *Climate change: What everyone needs to know.* New York: Oxford University Press.

Schmitz, C. L., Matyók, T., James, C. D., & Sloan, L. M. (2013). Environmental sustainability: Educating social workers for interdisciplinary practice. In M. Gray, J. Coates, & T. Hetherington (Eds.), *Environmental social work* (pp. 260–279). New York, NY: Routledge.

Schmitz, C. L., Powers, M. C. F., Nesmith, A., & Forbes, R. (2017, October). *Environmental justice across the curriculum: 2015 EPAS and beyond.* Grand Challenges Teaching Institute accepted for presentation at Council on Social Work Education Annual Program Meeting, Dallas, TX.

Sloan, L. M., Joyner, M. C., Stakeman, C. J., & Schmitz, C. L. (2018). *Critical multiculturalism and intersectionality in a complex world.* New York, NY: Oxford University Press.

Sloan, L. M., & Schmitz, C. L. (2019). Environmental degradation: Communities forging a path forward. *Journal of Transdisciplinary Peace Praxis, 1*(1). https://jtpp.uk/

Taking Root. (n.d.). Words from Wangari: *Selected quotes from Taking Root.* Retrieved from https://takingrootfilm.com/the-film/words-from-wangari/

University of South Carolina College of Social Work. [USC CoSW]. (2013, December 4). *Seeking a big impact with a small footprint* [Video file]. Retrieved from https://www.youtube.com/watch?v=OdhAPrbC2go#t=35

University of South Carolina College of Social Work. [USC CoSW]. (2014, August 22). *Making a Big Impact with a Small Footprint: Infusing Ecological Consciousness into the College of Social Work at USC* [Video file]. Retrieved from https://www.youtube.com/watch?v=-9flGlhM6Og&feature=youtu.be

Wallace-Wells, D. (2019). *The uninhabitable earth: Life after warming.* New York, NY: Tim Duggan Publishing.

Whiteman, D., & Powers, M. C. F. (2012). Environmental leadership through campus project teams: Green structures for linking students, faculty, and staff. In D. Rigling Gallagher (Ed.), *Environmental leadership* (Vol. 1, pp. 459–467). Newbury Park, CA: SAGE Publications.

Integrating youth participation and ecosocial work: New possibilities to advance environmental and social justice

Tania Schusler, Amy Krings ⓘ, and Melissa Hernández

ABSTRACT
This article reveals possibilities to expand the role of youth within ecosocial work practice. The Where I Stand Youth Summit held in Chicago, Illinois, provided a safe space for young people to reflect upon their understanding of, and roles within, social and environmental justice movements. Drawing upon critical youth empowerment theory and participant observation, we note that youth shared experiences of oppression across unique social identities, while displaying authentic communication, acceptance, and desire for solidarity. Re-defining what knowledge matters, along with intention and self-restoration, also emerged as critical to building young people's agency and power to effect social change.

Climate change and environmental contamination disproportionately affect the health of marginalized groups, including racial and ethnic minorities and residents of divested communities (Mohai, Pellow, & Roberts, 2009; Roberts & Parks, 2006). Environmental hazards and a lack of access to environmental amenities are especially consequential for young people, because one's environment influences psychosocial and physical development (Evans, 2004, 2006; Markevych et al., 2014). These inequities – known as environmental injustice – reflect structural racism embedded in land use practices that disproportionately expose marginalized groups to toxins in their homes, schools and neighborhoods; limited enforcement of environmental and public health regulations; and land use decision-making processes that exclude vulnerable groups (Bullard, 1996; Cole & Foster, 2001). Among people disadvantaged by systemic racism and classism, concerns about environmental health impacts also are at risk of being discredited by media and public officials (Krings, Kornberg, & Lane, 2018).

Residents of affected communities advocate for environmental justice through campaigns that build local power and secure a fair distribution of environmental amenities (Bullard, 1993; Krings, Spencer, & Jimenez, 2013; Krings & Thomas, 2018). Social work that incorporates an ecosocial framework is well-suited to support these community-driven efforts. Understood to be emancipatory and political, ecosocial work calls upon social workers to act collectively with community members to support social and economic equality, human dignity, ecological sustainability, and collective wellbeing (Närhi & Matthies, 2018; Peeters, 2012). Thus, to effectively practice ecosocial work, social workers must understand the perceptions of people, including youth, who are already working for social and environmental justice. Without understanding the rich history of environmental justice organizing and perceptions of those already involved, social workers might miss possibilities for partnership or, worse, inadvertently perpetuate environmental injustices by silencing, tokenizing, or objectifying marginalized community members. Yet the perceptions of youth activists, and the role of youth participation within ecosocial work broadly, have received limited attention to date. A comprehensive review of social work literature addressing environmental topics (1991–2015) found no title nor abstract including the words "youth," "young people," or "children" (Krings, Victor, Mathias, & Perron, 2018a).

To begin to address this gap, this article examines the perspectives of youth who are actively working for environmental and social justice. Specifically, we report findings from the Where I Stand Youth Summit, a retreat held in 2018 in Chicago, Illinois. Drawing upon critical youth empowerment theory, we explore how youth and their adult mentors define social and environmental issues, consider opportunities for collaboration, and envision their own roles in enacting solutions. Our findings reveal new opportunities for ecosocial workers to support and strengthen youth participation within environmental justice movements.

Youth participation aligns with ecosocial work

Youth participation is a process of involving young people in the decisions that affect their lives (Checkoway & Gutiérrez, 2006). Hart (1997) describes forms of youth participation that vary in the degree to which young people are able to make decisions and effect change. Non-participation in the forms of manipulation, decoration, and tokenism appears to involve youth participants; however, adults retain decision-making authority. Models of real participation include consultation, social mobilization, children-in-charge, and shared decision-making. In these models, young people influence the institutions and decisions that affect their lives. Different forms of real youth participation are suitable to different contexts, cultures, and youths' varying interests and capabilities (Hart, 1997).

Critical youth empowerment expands upon this notion of participation by conceptualizing empowerment as a multi-level construct in which "individuals, families, organizations, and communities gain control and mastery, within the social, economic, and political contexts of their lives, in order to improve equity and quality of life" (Jennings, Parra-Medina, Hilfinger

Messias, & McLoughlin, 2006, p. 32). Critical youth empowerment includes six key dimensions:

- *A welcoming and safe environment* in which youth experience freedom to be themselves, express creativity, voice opinions in decision-making, and feel ownership.
- *Meaningful participation and engagement* characterized by opportunities for youth to contribute authentically as they learn and try new roles and skills.
- *Equitable power-sharing between youth and adults.* Youth are afforded leadership roles with actual power to influence organizational or community decision-making.
- *Engagement in critical reflection on interpersonal and sociopolitical processes.* Critical reflection enables understanding the structures, processes, social values, and practices that participants seek to alter.
- *Participation in sociopolitical processes in order to effect change.* Critical youth empowerment involves action to address unjust structures, processes, social values, and practices. For example, youth picking up litter provides a useful civic service; however, to be considered critical youth empowerment, youth would reflect upon and act to change the structures and processes that produce waste.
- *Integrated individual and community-level empowerment.* As youth develop "a critical awareness of processes, structures, social practices, norms, and images that affect them," they determine "how to live productively within those social spaces or, better yet, how to change them for the benefit of all" (Jennings et al., 2006, p. 50).

Critical youth empowerment, and youth participation more broadly, can benefit both youth and communities. Youth engagement can bolster participants' developmental assets (Schusler & Krasny, 2010) and their understanding of complex issues, including conservation and the environment (Ballard, Dixon, & Harris, 2017). Youth participation can also contribute to community and policy level change (Chawla, 2002; Sprague Martinez, Richards-Schuster, Teixeira, & Augsberger, 2018). Youth who collaborate with adults to improve local environments and communities also may exhibit personal transformation (Schusler, Krasny, Peters, & Decker, 2009).

Despite these benefits, supporting youth participation in decision-making and social change processes can be difficult. Barriers include perceptions held by some adults that youth lack capacity to be competent community builders or change agents (Finn & Checkoway, 1998). Such characterizations can be especially damaging in places like Chicago where youth and adults can internalize news coverage that focuses on crime and violence, absent reporting about the assets within their communities. Additionally, adults who hold authority and ultimate responsibility for actions within youth programs may resist sharing decision-making power, in part because of organizational cultures, norms, policies, and structures (Schusler, Krasny, & Decker, 2016; Zeldin, Camino, & Mook, 2005). Limited time for critical reflection by both youth and adults also can limit opportunities for growth and empowerment (Jennings et al., 2006).

Thus, a need exists for research that increases the understanding of contexts and mechanisms that support widespread youth participation (Richards-Schuster & Pritzker, 2015). This study examined how youth conceptualize their roles as agents of social change. Our findings rely on observational data collected during the Where I Stand Youth Summit, a two-and -a-half-day retreat for young people engaged in Chicago-based, youth-driven organizations working for social and environmental justice. The Where I Stand Youth Summit, particularly its embodiment of critical youth empowerment principles, provides guidance for ecosocial workers seeking to foster youth empowerment towards social and environmental justice.

Research methods

Research design

The research team included scholars of environmental sustainability (Schusler and Hernández) and social work (Krings) as well as the lead organizer of the Where I Stand Youth Summit (Anderson). The study's design and implementation reflect a participatory research process characterized by the equitable sharing of power between the academic and community-based team members in all methodological decisions (Checkoway & Gutiérrez, 2006). A memorandum of understanding between the team members outlined the research objective; specific roles and responsibilities; data access, usage, and secure storage; and the research budget. In designing the research, Anderson, who is also the director of Sacred Keepers Sustainability Lab (https://www.sacredkeepers.org), a Chicago-based organization that engages youth in consciousness-raising related to intersections of the environment, culture, justice, and wellbeing, shared input from her conversations with the Sacred Keepers Youth Council. This participatory design ensured that the research complemented and contributed to the Summit's aims. The team co-constructed the research question: how do youth and their mentors understand the interconnectedness of environmental justice and social justice, the role of collaboration in movement building, and their own roles in moving forward social change? The research team also agreed upon the data collection method of participant observation and collaborated in data analysis, as described later. The research was approved by the Institutional Review Board of Loyola University Chicago.

It may benefit the reader to know the positionality of the research team members. Anderson, the Summit's lead organizer, is an African-American woman whose relationships with youth, parents, youth organizations, educators, community organizers, and activists made the Summit possible.

Schusler and Krings are both white women and researchers at a private university in Chicago. Both have worked with youth as community practitioners, yet were largely outsiders in relation to the Summit's participants. Hernández is a Latina who, at the time of data collection, was an undergraduate student. Although considered a youth by some definitions, she was not from one of the participating youth groups; therefore, she had both insider and outsider status.

The research team selected participant observation as the data collection method because it positioned the researchers as co-learners, enabling them to listen deeply to the experiences and perceptions of youth as those unfolded in the context of the Summit. A fundamental distinction among observational strategies is the extent to which the observer also participates in the setting under study (Patton, 2002). Anderson co-facilitated the Summit with the Sacred Keepers Youth Council and the academic team members participated in the Summit to engage in learning and growing with the youth participants. During downtime, each observer wrote memos to document key themes. Data analyzed included field notes, memos, and event documents (e.g., recruitment materials, newsprint notes from the event, and identity crests created by the youth groups).

Participants and the summit

"Truth and justice seekers, it is time for us to gather to explore and connect our worlds, to deeply know how we best stand up in who we are, for one another, and for the healing of the planet," began a recruitment flyer for the Where I Stand Youth Summit. In addition to the Sacred Keepers Youth Council, Anderson recruited five youth groups to attend through her professional and personal networks using conversations, phone calls, e-mails, and flyers that described the Summit's purpose and format (Table 1). In all, twenty-three youth ages fourteen to nineteen participated along with eight adult mentors. These adult mentors included three youth group facilitators and five adults involved in the event's organization and sponsorship. During

Table 1. Youth-driven organizations participating in the Where I Stand Summit held in Chicago, Illinois in April 2018.

Organization	Social Change Focus
Bodhi Spiritual Center Teens	Encouraging unconditional love and spirituality
Chi-Nations Youth Council	*Raising awareness of cultural identity and promoting a healthy lifestyle through arts, activism, and education*
Sacred Keepers Youth Council	Engaging in environmental education and organizing service-learning projects that promote environmental justice and sustainability in Chicago and Kenya
Student Voice and Activism Fellowship	Conducting action research to improve conditions within Chicago Public Schools
Ujimaa Medics	Training people to provide first response care until paramedics arrive when shootings, asthma attacks, or other emergencies occur

the Summit, some participants specifically referred to their racial or ethnic identities as African-American, Latinx, Native, or mixed race. Youth and adult mentors came from neighborhoods throughout Chicago, a highly segregated city (Novara, Loury, & Khare, 2017), although most reported living in predominantly African-American or Latinx communities located on Chicago's south or west sides. For decades, public and private divestment has contributed to environmental injustices in these areas and they contain many of the city's most hazardous land uses (Pellow, 2004).

Consistent with the process of critical youth empowerment, the Summit was designed to create a safe place for youth participants to try out new roles and engage in critical refection about the structures, social practices, and images that affect them. Its design aimed to facilitate dialog while building connections between youth that would support their participation in socio-political processes for social and environmental justice (Table 1). Held in April 2018, the Summit lasted from Friday night until Sunday afternoon. Most participants lived, worked, socialized, and shared meals at the host site for the entire two and one-half days. Content included reflective discussions, skills-based workshops, community building hang outs, and self-care. Youth voices were front and center throughout, and all sessions, whether youth or adult-led, were facilitated by people of color.

At the start of the Summit, when all of the participants introduced themselves, Anderson introduced the academic researchers, vouched for their trustworthiness, described the research purpose, and explained that she and the research team gave careful consideration to acknowledge and reduce the power disparity that often exists between universities and local communities. In this way, the university researchers were described as co-learners rather than experts, and participants were provided the opportunity to ask questions, raise concerns, or offer suggestions. The research team did not promise confidentiality given that all interactions among participants occurred in group settings. The academic researchers did not have access to individually identifying data, unless participants shared it with the collective group.

Analysis

To analyze the data, the participant observers (Schusler, Krings, and Hernández) reviewed and discussed the field notes, documents, and artifacts. Each analyst inductively derived themes by coding and categorizing their own field notes to produce an analytic memo reflecting the research questions (Emerson, Fretz, & Shaw, 2011). They discussed their analyses face-to-face one week following the Summit. Although the initial organizational scheme of each analyst differed, they identified the same ideas, moments, and interactions as salient. They continued to compare and contrast their analyses through writing in a shared document in an iterative process of increasingly focused coding to arrive at the themes presented in the Findings below. At key decision points, the analysts deliberated about how to represent the data until reaching consensus.

The credibility of the findings was enhanced by the observers' diligence in taking rich, descriptively detailed notes that avoided inference, as well as by triangulating data sources and their analysis across the three academic researchers. Member checking of that analysis further increased the findings' credibility. Anderson and the Sacred Keepers Youth Council collectively reviewed an original draft of this manuscript, which led to two key changes. First, we strengthened emphasis on the sense of support and solidarity that participants acknowledged across their different communities, racial identities, and priorities for social change. Second, we explained how the academic researchers navigated their role as outsiders by participating in the Summit on equal footing with, not above or apart from, the youth.

Findings

In the subsections below, we describe themes that reflect the substantive essence of the Where I Stand Summit. We organize these themes by the three dimensions of the research question: (1) interconnectedness between environmental and social justice, (2) collaboration in movement building, and (3) youths' roles in creating social change. Although we present the themes as distinct conceptual units, the phenomena that they represent inevitably intersect.

Interconnectedness of environmental and social justice

Three threads emerged as key points of intersection across young people's experiences: unique and shared identities, place and land, and self-determination.

Unique and shared identities
Youth discussed struggles with marginalization specific to their racial and ethnic identity groups. Such marginalization took the forms of segregation; gentrification; gun-violence; cultural repression; tokenism in classrooms; misinformation in education that reinforces stereotypes; exclusion from decision-making over land-use; and lack of access to healthcare facilities, natural resources, and acceptable school infrastructure. Far from a "pity party," these dialogs seemed to validate and motivate youth in their activism for social justice. As some voiced their personal stories, they recognized shared experiences of injustice across their diverse struggles. For example, despite possessing different racial identities and engaging in social activism around different issues, multiple youth shared the experience of being labeled "radical" by adults: "When people of color try to make change, they are often viewed as radical, but really, we're just trying to live … . Society views something as radical when you're just trying to make sure you survive," explained a Native youth. An African American youth concurred, "I agree with that … . At

the end of the day nobody in here is hurting anybody. We're just trying to make places better for ourselves and others." These youth possessed unique individual identities and yet related to others through a shared identity as people of color in a society that promotes white privilege.

Place and land

"We're all related to the land; the only difference is that Indigenous people are on their ancestral lands," offered a Native mentor. The Native delegation explained that disconnecting people from the land is a tool of control by which colonizers disempower people of color. African American and Latinx youth identified connections between Natives' struggle to regain their rights to stolen ancestral lands and residents' efforts in their own neighborhoods to stay in their homes in the face of gentrification and/or deportation. The desire to influence decisions affecting the place one lives and the land to which one culturally connects arose as an important point of intersection across participants.

Self-determination

In discussions and skills-based workshops, participants deconstructed oppressive societal structures and sought to build young people's power towards realizing self-determination in their lands, lives, and communities: "Lots of people are talking recklessly about equity. We will define equity because we live inequity," emphasized a workshop facilitator. His words convey self-determination, or the right to influence decisions affecting oneself. He added that racial equity requires targeted investment in Black, Brown, and Indigenous communities to redress historical injustices.

Collaboration in movement building

One aim of the Summit was to enable youth to meet, learn about one another's work, and build relationships that could lead to future collaborations. We next describe three key facets of participants' interactions related to building cooperative relationships: authentic communication, loving acceptance, and solidarity.

Authentic communication

Young people exhibited a degree of authenticity uncommon in many adult conversations. They posed thoughtful questions and demonstrated vulnerability in sharing with one another challenging experiences and uncomfortable emotions. This authentic communication seemed to be enabled by the safe atmosphere created by Summit organizers and participants. Anderson opened the Summit by asking the youth to "be present" meaning:

not doing anything else while someone is talking besides being there and listening ... . Someone may be talking about what's breaking them and we need to show love and attention and that we care and that what they're going through matters.

A youth added that showing respect through being present also involves "not showing judgment" through facial expressions or body language as well as spoken language. Being present invokes self-awareness, attentiveness, and reciprocity. Being present contributed to a safe climate to be deeply authentic, which in turn provided a foundation for building collaborations.

Loving acceptance

The Summit's emphasis on acceptance of self and others also contributed to a safe atmosphere and encouraged relationship building. Youth collectively developed group agreements. Among these were, "Respect my space, voice, boundaries," "Acceptance/be open," and "Judgment free zone." These rules recognize that feeling accepted enables fuller participation. By the Summit's conclusion, acceptance – cemented with essential and unconditional love – seemed to permeate the space. One of the youth groups led a closing activity in which participants gave and received loving gestures, such as a hug or pat on the shoulder (or a non-physical sign for those preferring no touch). Reflecting on this activity, a youth with tears rolling down his cheeks expressed, "I don't usually cry in front of people. This shows my comfort being in this group. I had been feeling so broken," at which point others approached to affirm him. A mentor said, "Everything starts with love .... Take care of yourself and others' around you and the Earth, our home and sustenance ... .We can only be happy or live with love if we love our Earth and protect it so that it may protect us also."

Solidarity

An expressed desire for solidarity arose in part from youth recognizing connections between the injustices they experience:

> Black and Brown communities seem more apart than alike, but we go through similar issues. It's hard to be in solidarity when you're taught that your issues are different. We have been pulled apart so much ... .It's hard to care about others' issues when you're so focused on the ones in your own community.

Participants identified the city's segregation as a substantial barrier to achieving solidarity. Youth lack opportunities to visit other neighborhoods and face pressing issues (e.g., violence, public health, environmental quality, displacement through gentrification, and educational inequity) in their own communities: "If you're only seeing DAPL [Dakota Access Pipeline] or only seeing Black violence, it's hard to see how we can be in solidarity. That requires education." Hence, it is important for youth to come together to learn about each other's issues and how they can support one another: "We have to consciously be aware of working together not against each other."

Youths' roles in creating social change

Acknowledging their right to social and environmental justice, several of the youth described how they act to attain that justice. We next elaborate on how young people – with their mentors' support – build and apply power to create positive social change through youth agency, knowledge, intention, and self-restoration.

Youth agency

"Everyone has potential to create change," read a crest created by one of the youth organizations. Formal presentations given by youth about their activism illustrated that they not only exert their own agency but also work to build other people's capacity for changing problematic situations. One youth group raised funds to travel to Kenya and assisted the Maasai people in building a water tank and planting trees to aid reforestation. These youth described feeling rewarded by their ability to be of service while also learning from the Maasai's wisdom and respecting the Maasai's self-determination. Another youth described the emergency first response organization that she created to address the absence of trauma centers on Chicago's south side. She trains people to perform first response aid and they in turn train others, developing a circle of learning and care. In these and other examples, youth use their agency to acquire power, such as resources or knowledge, which they then share with others.

Knowledge

"The school system doesn't value what we learn outside of school, it's all about grades," said a youth. Whereas youth described schools as often rigid institutions that reinforce dominant standards of what knowledge is valued, many of the youth conceived of learning that takes place outside of schools (e.g. lived experiences, culture-specific collective memory, and activism and organizing work) as truly educational. Youth raised and critically examined questions like: what counts as knowledge? who is knowledge for? what knowledge is valuable? am I white washing myself to gain knowledge? The chasm between what counts as knowledge and what matters to youth is especially salient because youth recognized knowledge as essential to social change. For example, youth reconstructed a general expectation that education serves the purpose of an individual's upward mobility:

> School tells us 'we need more Black lawyers and doctors.' No, what we need is more kids to be aware [of social justice issues]. If you will be a doctor or lawyer, serve some sort of justice, build a hospital in the hood, make the hood better.

Added another:

> This [activism] work is preparing us to take on adult roles ... .We are seen as the best and brightest in our communities and outside voices are telling us we're gonna 'get out of the

hood.' No. That's your community. Go learn, and come back, and make it better. This work prepares us to be active in making our communities better.

Intention

The Summit encouraged young people's intentionality through reflective discussions and mindfulness practices designed to ground them within themselves. For instance, Anderson initiated a morning discussion by inquiring, "How do you greet the day?" She stressed that whether you wake up in a good or bad mood, the intentions you set affect how you experience that day. Being aware of one's energy and practices like focused breathing were infused throughout the Summit. For example, a dance movement therapist highlighted that our internal state affects what we bring to the external world. She asked everyone to take a soft gaze or close their eyes and mindfully scan each part of their body from the feet up to the head. This led into drawing, reflecting, and a collective activity involving expression through movement. Afterward, youth reported feeling relaxed and uplifted. This activity reinforced that through mindful, internal attention one can move through and exert agency in the external world.

Self-restoration

Mindfulness practices not only build intentionality; they can nurture the self-care required to sustain social change activism. Youth expressed deep satisfaction from their activism – "It doesn't feel like work. This is just how I live" – but also recognized that avoiding burnout requires caring for themselves: "The transitions between so many worlds that we're in exhausts us … . We're always playing the moderator, molding, adapting; our hands get tired …. How do we replenish?" Self-restoration – referred to by youth as "self-care," "healing," and "replenishing" – took multiple forms, including finding common ground in shared identities, practicing loving acceptance of self and others, and building solidarity, as described earlier.

Some youth perceived activism itself as restorative. For instance, the young person who developed the emergency first-response program described how her work helps her heal the wound caused by the loss of a childhood friend: "You can be wounded by a lot of things. By being active in your community, it's practicing self-care … [transforming] a traumatizing situation from fear to empowerment." Youths' roles as activists for social change intertwine with their need for care, healing, and personal replenishment, thereby sustaining their agency.

Potential relationships across themes

Because this research was not designed to examine cause-effect relationships, we cannot definitively discern associations among the phenomena observed during the Summit. Nonetheless, it is useful for identifying future research directions to consider how young people's insights about the interconnectedness of social and

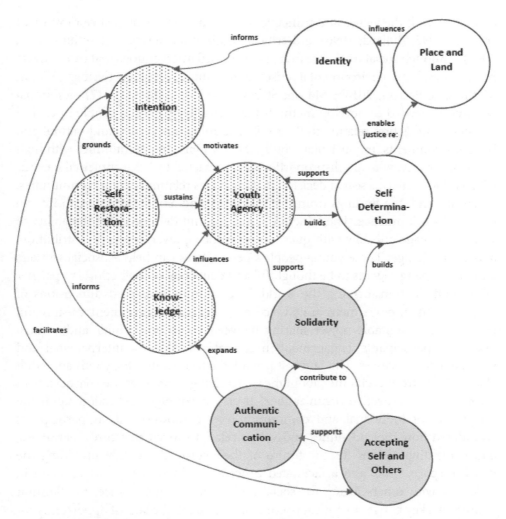

Figure 1. Concept map based upon key themes evident during the Where I Stand Youth Summit. This diagram illustrates how youth can build agency and solidarity towards self-determination related to social and environmental justice. Arrows indicate potential interactions between phenomena and suggest avenues for future research.

environmental justice relate to their perceptions of collaboration in movement building and their own roles in moving forward social change. Figure 1 suggests potential connections among the themes that emerged from participant's dialogs and interactions with one another during the Summit.

Discussion

Ecosocial work practice engages with community members to promote human dignity, ecological sustainability, and the empowerment and liberation of all people (Coates & Gray, 2012; Närhi & Matthies, 2018). In this way, ecosocial work can be understood as a form of anti-oppressive social work (Dominelli, 2002) that also is consistent with the values and principles of the environmental justice movement (Bryant, 1995; Bullard, 1996) and critical youth empowerment (Jennings et al., 2006). Although social work research has examined interventions that can mitigate harm caused by environmental crises and natural disasters (Krings, Victor, Mathias, & Perron, 2018b; Mason, Shires, Arwood, & Borst, 2017), additional research is needed to develop methods that proactively engage people in critical reflection and action relating to their self-determination, health, and natural and built environments. In particular, youth of color living in communities with high levels of poverty, who are disproportionately impacted by environmental hazards (Evans, 2004), merit a seat at decision making tables relating to their communities.

To this end, the findings from the Where I Stand Youth Summit can inform ecosocial work practice. The Where I Stand Summit demonstrated the ability of youth to engage critically with questions of justice, power, resource distribution, and social change. These young people's perspectives can help ecosocial workers and other change agents to be thoughtful and deliberate in their efforts to partner with youth in transforming the world. The Summit embodied dimensions of critical youth empowerment in its welcoming and safe environment, meaningful participation, equitable power-sharing between youth and adults, and – most notably – participants' engagement in critical reflection on interpersonal and sociopolitical processes. The Summit provided opportunities for youth and adult allies to learn from each other about the social change processes they participate in through their respective organizations. It also encouraged reflection upon the integration of individual and community-level empowerment, as participants considered how their identities and values relate to social structures, narratives, and competing visions for the future of their communities. By providing the physical space, time, and a facilitated process for discovering how to stand in solidarity with others acting for social and environmental justice, the Summit addressed a key barrier to critical youth empowerment: the lack of opportunity for critical reflection (Jennings et al., 2006). Indeed, Anderson and the Sacred Keepers Youth Council, in communication with other organizations, are planning for a future Summit of longer duration that will allow more time for individual and collective reflection to occur.

Conclusion

As social workers consider how the profession can contribute toward the United Nations' Sustainable Development Goals of ending poverty, protecting the planet, and ensuring prosperity for all (Jones & Truell, 2012), effective interventions must engage with the people affected by environmental impacts (Teixeira & Krings, 2015). The Where I Stand Youth Summit illustrates the potential for integrating youth participation into ecosocial work – fields that both view the participation of impacted groups as a right. The Summit offered the opportunity to understand how youth interpret (and re-interpret or re-write) society's dominant narratives and how they advocate for equity in the policies, institutions, and decisions affecting them. This research adds to a body of literature demonstrating the benefit – and perhaps necessity – of youth participation (Checkoway et al., 2003). Future research investigating youth participation within ecosocial work could examine the pathways indicated by the arrows in Figure 1, which suggest interactions between phenomena. For example, how does authentic communication contribute to knowledge and solidarity and, in turn, support youths' agency toward building power for self-determination in the decisions affecting their lives, lands, and communities? The answers to such questions can further inform ecosocial workers in facilitating critical youth empowerment.

Acknowledgments

We thank co-researcher Toni Anderson of Sacred Keepers Sustainability Lab for her vision and creativity designing the Where I Stand Youth Summit; the Sacred Keepers Youth Council, who co-led the Summit; and the other participating youth groups: Bodhi Spiritual Center Teens, Chi-Nations Youth Council, Student Voice and Activism Fellowship, and Ujimaa Medics. We also thank those who led workshops or otherwise contributed: Alliance for the Great Lakes, Monimia Macbeth of Creative Passages, Jhmira Alexander of 29Eleven Consulting, Toni'Mono Monix, Seva Gandhi and Samantha Sainsbury of the Institute of Cultural Affairs, Stacy Gibson of Transform the Collective, Kels the Yogi, Olatunji Oboi Reed of Equiticity, and Kenisha Jamison of Waist Ware Circles. A Faculty Fellowship Award from Loyola University Chicago's Center for the Human Rights of Children provided funding for this research.

Disclosure statement

No potential conflict of interest was reported by the authors.

Funding

This work was supported by the Loyola University Chicago Center for the Human Rights of Children [Faculty Fellowship 2017-2018];

ORCID

Amy Krings ⓘ http://orcid.org/0000-0001-5499-5101

References

Ballard, H. L., Dixon, C. G. H., & Harris, E. M. (2017). Youth-focused citizen science: Examining the role of environmental science learning and agency for conservation. *Biological Conservation, 208,* 65–75. doi:10.1016/j.biocon.2016.05.024

Bryant, B. (Ed.). (1995). *Environmental justice: Issues, policies, and solutions.* Washington, DC: Island Press.

Bullard, R. D. (1993). *Confronting environmental racism: Voices from the grassroots.* Cambridge, MA: South End Press.

Bullard, R. D. (1996). Environmental justice: It's more than waste facility siting. *Social Science Quarterly, 77*(3), 493–499.

Chawla, L. (Ed.). (2002). *Growing up in an urbanising world.* London, England: Earthscan.

Checkoway, B., & Gutiérrez, L. (2006). Youth participation and community change. *Journal of Community Practice, 14*(1–2), 1–9. doi:10.1300/J125v14n01_01

Checkoway, B., Richards-Schuster, K., Abdullah, S., Aragon, M., Facio, E., Figueroa, L., ... White, A. (2003). Young people as competent citizens. *Community Development Journal, 38*(4), 298–309. doi:10.1093/cdj/38.4.298

Coates, J., & Gray, M. (2012). The environment and social work: An overview and introduction. *International Journal of Social Welfare, 21*(3), 230–238. doi:10.1111/j.1468-2397.2011.00851.x

Cole, L. W., & Foster, S. R. (2001). *From the ground up: Environmental racism and the rise of the environmental justice movement.* New York: New York University Press.

Dominelli, L. (2002). *Anti-oppressive social work theory and practice.* New York, NY: Palgrave Macmillan.

Emerson, R., Fretz, R., & Shaw, L. (2011). *Writing ethnographic fieldnotes* (2nd ed., Chicago guides to writing, editing, and publishing). Chicago, IL: The University of Chicago Press.

Evans, G. W. (2004). The environment of childhood poverty. *American Psychologist, 59*(2), 77–92. doi:10.1037/0003-066X.59.2.77

Evans, G. W. (2006). Child development and the physical environment. *Annual Review of Psychology, 57,* 423–451. doi:10.1146/annurev.psych.57.102904.190057

Finn, J. L., & Checkoway, B. (1998). Young people as competent community builders: A challenge to social work. *Social Work, 43*(4), 335–345. doi:10.1093/sw/43.4.335

Hart, R. A. (1997). *Children's participation: The theory and practice of involving young citizens in community development and environmental care.* London, England: Earthscan.

Jennings, L. B., Parra-Medina, D. M., Hilfinger Messias, D. K., & McLoughlin, K. (2006). Toward a critical social theory of youth empowerment. *Journal of Community Practice, 14* (1/2), 31–55. doi:10.1300/J125v14n01_03

Jones, D. N., & Truell, R. (2012). The global agenda for social work and social development: A place to link together and be effective in a globalized world. *International Social Work, 55*(4), 454–472. doi:10.1177/0020872812440587

Krings, A., Kornberg, D., & Lane, E. (2018). Organizing under austerity: How residents' concerns became the Flint water crisis. *Critical Sociology, 45*(4–5), 583–597. doi:10.1177/0896920518757053

Krings, A., Spencer, M. S., & Jimenez, K. (2013). Organizing for environmental justice: From bridges to taro patches. In S. Dutta & C. Ramanathan (Eds.), *Governance, development, and social work* (pp. 186–200). London, England: Routledge. doi:10.4324/9780203796009

Krings, A., & Thomas, H. (2018). Integrating green social work and the U.S. environmental justice movement: An introduction to community benefits agreements. In L. Dominelli (Ed.), *The Routledge handbook of green social work* (pp. 397–406). New York, NY: Routledge. doi:10.4324/9781315183213

Krings, A., Victor, B., Mathias, J., & Perron, B. (2018a). *Environmental social work in the disciplinary literature, 1991–2015.* Unpublished raw data.

Krings, A., Victor, B., Mathias, J., & Perron, B. (2018b). Environmental social work in the disciplinary literature, 1991 – 2015. *International Social Work.* doi:10.1177/0020872818788397

Markevych, I., Tiesler, C. M., Fuertes, E., Romanos, M., Dadvand, P., Nieuwenhuijsen, M. J., & Heinrich, J. (2014). Access to urban green spaces and behavioural problems in children:

Results from the GINIplus and LISAplus studies. *Environment International, 71,* 29–35. doi:10.1016/j.envint.2014.06.002

Mason, L. R., Shires, M. K., Arwood, C., & Borst, A. (2017). Social work research and global environmental change. *Journal of the Society for Social Work and Research, 8*(4), 645–672. doi:10.1086/694789

Mohai, P., Pellow, D., & Roberts, J. T. (2009). Environmental justice. *Annual Review of Environment and Resources, 34,* 405–430. doi:10.1146/annurev-environ-082508-094348

Närhi, K., & Matthies, A. L. (2018). The ecosocial approach in social work as a framework for structural social work. *International Social Work. 61,* 490-502. doi: 10.1177/0020872816644663

Novara, M., Loury, A., & Khare, A. (2017). *The cost of segregation.* Chicago, IL: Metropolitan Planning Council.

Patton, M. Q. (2002). *Qualitative research and evaluation methods* (3rd ed.). Thousand Oaks, CA: Sage Publications.

Peeters, J. (2012). The place of social work in sustainable development: Towards ecosocial practice. *International Journal of Social Welfare, 21*(3), 287–298. doi:10.1111/j.1468-2397.2011.00856.x

Pellow, D. N. (2004). *Garbage wars: The struggle for environmental justice in Chicago.* Cambridge, MA: MIT Press.

Richards-Schuster, K., & Pritzker, S. (2015). Strengthening youth participation in civic engagement: Applying the Convention on the Rights of the Child to social work practice. *Children and Youth Services Review, 57,* 90–97. doi:10.1016/j.childyouth.2015.07.013

Roberts, J. T., & Parks, B. (2006). *A climate of injustice: Global inequality, north-south politics, and climate policy.* Cambridge, MA: MIT Press.

Schusler, T. M., & Krasny, M. E. (2010). Environmental action as context for youth development. *Journal of Environmental Education, 41*(4), 208–223. doi:10.1080/00958960903479803

Schusler, T. M., Krasny, M. E., & Decker, D. J. (2016). The autonomy-authority duality in shared decision-making with youth. *Environmental Education Research, 23,* 533–552. doi:10.1080/13504622.2016.1144174

Schusler, T. M., Krasny, M. E., Peters, S. J., & Decker, D. J. (2009). Developing citizens and communities through youth environmental action. *Environmental Education Research, 15* (1), 111–127. doi:10.1080/13504620802710581

Sprague Martinez, L., Richards-Schuster, K., Teixeira, S., & Augsberger, A. (2018). The power of prevention and youth voice: A strategy for social work to ensure youths' healthy development. *Social Work, 63*(2), 135–143. doi:10.1093/sw/swx059

Teixeira, S., & Krings, A. (2015). Sustainable social work: An environmental justice framework for social work education. *Social Work Education: The International Journal, 34*(5), 513–527. doi:10.1080/02615479.2015.1063601

Zeldin, S., Camino, L., & Mook, C. (2005). The adoption of innovation in youth organizations: creating the conditions for youth–adult partnerships. *Journal of Community Psychology, 33*(1), 121–135. doi:10.1002/jcop.20044

Social work students' perspective on environmental justice: Gaps and challenges for preparing students

Jessica L. Decker Sparks, Katie Massey Combs, and Jennifer Yu ⓘ

ABSTRACT
The integration of environmental justice into social work education, research, and practice has grown substantially in the past decade. However, social workers still report feeling unprepared to address these challenges with their clients and communities. To understand the disconnect between education about and application of environmental justice principles, semi-structured qualitative interviews were conducted with graduate social work students (n = 14). Findings suggest this disconnect is catalyzed, in part, by the environment's meta nature and a lack of facilitated education on the dynamic feedbacks between the physical environment and social justice issues. Implications for social work educators are discussed.

In the 1990s, the social work profession concertedly began expanding its definition of environment beyond social and built environments to also include the natural environment in response to Earth's ecological changes (e.g., global warming, pollution disparities, and desertification) (National Association of Social Workers [NASW] Delegate Assembly, 2003). In recent years, interest in integrating the natural environment into social work teaching, practice, and research has grown in the United States with the creation of the Council on Social Work Education's (CSWE) Committee on Environmental Justice; the Society for Social Work and Research's Changing Urban and Global Environments special interest group; and the American Academy of Social Work and Social Welfare's Create Social Responses to a Changing Environment Grand Challenge (n.d.). In addition, CSWE's (2015) educational policy and accreditation standards (EPAS) included environmental justice (EJ)[1] as a core competency (three) and as a component of competency five, policy engagement. There has also been a steady increase in EJ research (Bexell, Decker Sparks, Tejada, & Rechkemmer, 2019), including an influx in manuscripts conceptualizing how to integrate the natural environment into social work curricula through foundational perspectives such as person-in-environment (e.g., Gray & Coates, 2015; Philip & Resich, 2015; Teixeira & Krings, 2015).

EJ's growth throughout social work education, research, and practice in the United States is in response to client needs. Nesmith and Smyth's (2015) survey of social work practitioners in a Midwestern state found almost three-quarters of respondents worked with a client experiencing an environmental injustice – when vulnerable populations "'bear a disproportionate share of the negative environmental consequences resulting from industrial, governmental and commercial operations or policies'" (U. S. Environmental Protection Agency, 2018). The environmental injustices experienced by social work clients in the United States are diverse and include, but are not limited to, disproportional exposure to and impacts from climate change (e.g., displacement of Alaska Native communities from sea-level rise); natural disasters (e.g., Hurricane Katrina's unbalanced impacts on low-income, black communities); and pollution and environmental toxins (e.g., low-income communities of color experiencing higher rates of asthma, Flint water crisis) (Kemp & Palinkas, 2015). Specific injustices vary by region, identity (e.g., gender, race), and socioeconomic status (Dominelli, 2013; Drolet & Sampson, 2014), with low-income communities and persons of color "hit first and worst" (Faber & Krieg, 2002).

Despite EJ's relevance, surveyed social work practitioners reported feeling unprepared and powerless to address clients' environmental issues due to a lack of resources, training, and education (Nesmith & Smyth, 2015). Grise-Owens, Miller, and Owens (2014) hypothesized the lack of appropriate education may be further perpetuated by traditional social work paradigms, which emphasize micro-, mezzo-, and macro-practice and often lack recognition of the interdependencies between social work concerns on a micro scale and global problems. These paradigms may also not be sufficiently complex to engage the meta purview needed to address environmental challenges. Defined as "'the global social aspects that both overarch and interact with macro, mezzo, and micro practice,'" Grise-Owens et al. (2014, p. 47) argued that a meta-practice for social work is necessary due to societal transformations from increasing global interdependence. Without a framework for meta-practice, educators may risk creating a sense of powerlessness, where a problem seems too large to be within one's knowledge scope and skills.

However, these conclusions remain theoretical, as a paucity of studies exploring why social workers feel unprepared to address environmental challenges exists. As such, this exploratory study aimed to obtain an in-depth and nuanced understanding of the gaps and challenges inhibiting social work practitioners by seeking to better comprehend the lived experiences of sampled social work students who are immersed in social work training and education. Interviewing social work master's-level students also provides insight into any shifts in curriculum or education related to the recent EPAS requirements and broader societal attention to environmental issues since Miller and Hayward's (2014) study noted social work students' increasing interest in learning about and integrating EJ into their post-schooling practice

Methods

Two researchers conducted semi-structured, phenomological interviews with 14 students from seven MSW programs in the United States from July to December 2016 to understand how social work students experience EJ in their curricula. Sample size was consistent with recommendations for achieving a saturation of themes in qualitative, phenomenological studies (Creswell, 2013). Non-probability, maximum variation sampling was used to obtain a sample that was geographically, racially, and ethnically diverse, and represented private and public, and practice and research-oriented (i.e., absence or presence of a doctoral program) programs. Table 1 displays participant demographics and their MSW program characteristics. Participants were racially diverse with over half (n = 8) identifying as a person of color, in comparison to the 50.8% of MSW students nationally who identify as White (non-Hispanic). Though this sample was largely female (85.7%), it was consistent with national social work student demographics, which reported 85.3% of full-time students and 85.1% of part-time students identifying as female in 2017 (Council on Social Work Education [CSWE], 2017). Both research-oriented programs and programs in the Rocky Mountain region were overrepresented compared to national statistics (CSWE, 2017).

Table 1. Participant demographics and MSW program characteristics, N = 14.

Characteristic	% (n)/M (SD)
Race	
White/Caucasian	42.9% (6)
Black	14.3% (2)
Latina	14.3% (2)
Native American or	14.3% (2)
Arab	7.1% (1)
Asian-Indian	7.1% (1)
Gender	
Female	85.7% (12)
Male	7.1% (1)
Transgender	7.1% (1)
MSW Program Characteristics	
Type	42.9% (6)
Private	57.1% (8)
Public	42.9% (6)
Research versus Practice oriented	
Research-oriented	64.3% (9)
Practice-oriented	35.7% (5)
Region	
Northeast	14.3% (2)
Mid-Atlantic	21.4% (3)
Midwest	14.3% (2)
West	14.3% (2)
Rocky Mountain	35.7% (5)

Recruitment occurred electronically through listservs of various graduate schools of social work, and through program coordinators or social work faculty members who circulated the recruitment email at their respective universities. Students emailed the researchers to indicate interest, and an interview was then scheduled. Participants were emailed a consent form prior to the interview, and the interviewer received verbal consent before conducting the interview. Participant inclusion criteria was the completion of one semester of a MSW program. MSW programs were selected over bachelor programs since the master's degree is considered the profession's terminal degree for practice. Interviews took place over phone and lasted between 25 to 45 minutes. Both interviewers had advanced training in qualitative methods. All participants received a $15 Amazon e-gift card at the interview's completion. The authors' university-based Institutional Review Board approved the study protocol.

A semi-structured interview guide was used to facilitate interviews. Participant insights and experiences largely directed the interview; however, interviews discussed three main topics: 1) understanding of EJ, 2) EJ's relevance to social work, and 3) barriers to addressing EJ. Example questions included: "'What does environmental justice mean to you?'" (topic 1); "'Can you describe social work issues included in environmental justice?'" (topic 2); and "'Do you feel prepared to address environmental justice in your placement? Why or why not?'" (topic 3). Interviews were recorded, transcribed, and analyzed in Dedoose using an inductive, iterative coding process that reduced content to themes and codes through three cycles (Saldaña, 2013). Two researchers independently coded the data using descriptive and process coding (first-cycle), emotion and value coding (second-cycle), and focus and pattern coding (third-cycle) (Saldaña, 2013). Focus coding used a codebook generated from first and second-cycle codes with inter-rater agreement assessed at 93.8%.

Results

Relevant, but unprepared

Of the 14 student participants, 13 (92.8%) reported EJ being relevant to social work. Though the sampled students overwhelmingly felt that EJ was relevant to social work, only five students (35.7%) disclosed feeling prepared in any capacity to address these issues in their practice, and two of these five participants characterized their preparedness as limited. Participant 7 described, "feeling confident in my ability to recognize EJ. But I guess with my lack of experience with it, I don't think I have a hand directly in it to make a difference, single-handedly." Another participant described only feeling prepared to address the policy aspects of environmental injustices. These were also the only five participants who received EJ content in their MSW program, though three of the five (60%) reported content only from a singular social policy course, and two of the three students were from the same program. Of those who received EJ content in more than one course, one (participant 5) was completing a dual degree program and received all EJ content through their public health program.

Student willingness to take ownership of their education also highlighted the lack of EJ content in MSW coursework. Per participant 12, classroom discussions about EJ were depicted as being "student-led" and as noted by multiple participants, students were engaging with EJ content through their own initiative by selecting EJ-focused topics for individual and group assignments. Participant 3 stated that if they wanted content on EJ, "I feel like I have to go out on my own and find out." And as detailed by participant 6, instructors were supportive when students selected EJ focused topics, "but there are certain students who I'll share that I did that, and they'll be like oh I would have totally done the same thing if that was an opportunity."

Barriers in connecting EJ to social work and social work clients

Beyond a lack of exposure to EJ content through instructor-facilitated learning (e.g., readings, coursework, internships), sampled students described an inability to connect the environment to social work clients. Three subthemes arose regarding barriers in connecting EJ to social work clients including: 1) being overwhelmed by the environment's abstract nature and magnitude, 2) personal detachment from the environment and environmental injustices, and 3) lack of understanding of dynamic feedback loops between environment and people.

Though having a strong sense of its relevancy, participants simultaneously described EJ as an elusive concept and "abstract thing" (participant 1) with an expansive reach, "I've been thinking on a very, very small scale in terms of community as opposed to a bigger, like environmental seems like such a bigger word than community." As detailed by participant 6, "the environment is present in every situation even though it's not. It may not necessarily be visible. It's probably operating or connected to that issue in some way, shape, or form." This magnitude and pervasiveness was described as so "broad" that it was overwhelming (participants 7 and 11). Some participants expressed concern this difficulty was also experienced by social work instructors, causing instructors to "exclude" and "overlook" the relationship between other social justice issues and EJ (participant 3). "The professors ... may not see like these overarching systemic issues' connections" [to more micro issues] (participant 2). Participant 13 suggested educators "might hesitate bringing that [environmental health] discussion to class because it doesn't seem like it's an instant fix or something that we can do within the next month." Because of this lack of educator-facilitated learning, when attempting to describe environmental injustices, students (e.g., participants 1 and 2) often conflated the built, physical, and natural environments or their definition was limited to geographical barriers impeding access to services.

Participants also expressed that their personal disconnect from the environment and environmental injustices was a barrier to understanding EJ and addressing environmental issues in their practice, particularly since participants' perceptions were that many students select a subfield within social work because of a personal connection to the issue. Students articulated that education about EJ was even more imperative because they lack the experiences themselves "to normalize" clients' situations: "It [EJ education] would help me explain and connect to these individuals because I do not have these experiences personally" (participant 1). And indeed, at the conclusion of interviews, when researchers further explained and defined environmental justice to participants, the students further engaged in the discussion by applying the person-in-environment perspective and ecological model (e.g., participant 3) to environmental injustices.

Though participants confidently described environmentalism, they could not expand upon it to identify links between environment and people. For example, participant 1 explained, "In my mind environmental justice was protecting the Earth itself, not in how it affected people." Similarly, participant 4 described environmental justice as, "making sure people are taking care of the environment and treating it decently and not doing any harm ... I honestly wouldn't even have considered race, ethnicity."

Discussion

Among this sample of master's students, few indicated their MSW education equipped them to address EJ or exposed them to facilitated learning on EJ, which parallels Miller and Hayward's (2014) and Nesmith and Smyth's (2015) findings. Though substantial attention has been drawn to EJ within social work in the United States through the Grand Challenges, EPAS changes, and calls to action, these results suggest social work education and training has not fully adapted to incorporate these topics, and that the problem of being unprepared to address environmental injustices is entrenched throughout the profession.

Students had difficulty contextualizing the environment's role in their practice, particularly in clinical settings. This disconnect was driven by the environment's magnitude, detachment from the environment and environmental injustices, and a lack of understanding of feedback loops between the natural environment and people. Ultimately, these themes underscore the continued divide between social work's micro-macro gap. Further, EJ is an intersectional issue compounded by racial, reproductive, and socio-economic inequities. If social workers are unable to apply EJ frameworks to their practice, then they will be unable to critically examine how environmental inequities intersect with other social issues.

While students' attempts to self-educate on EJ issues can be perceived as a strength to begin building an EJ movement within the profession, it is also problematic. Due to the macro, and potentially even meta elements of the environment's interactions with vulnerable populations, mitigating environmental injustices will require a transdisciplinary approach. However, if the profession continues to rely on a small fragment of self-selecting students and practitioners to self-educate, the field is in danger of lacking an expertize readily identifiable by other disciplinary professionals and being excluded by innovative, transdisciplinary teams. Further, without formal and holistic education facilitated by social work educators – particularly in systems thinking linking micro and mezzo systems to the more abstract environment – students and practitioners, and their interventions, risk overlooking negative feedback loops that perpetuate unintended, and often harmful, consequences.

Students' inability to connect the environment to social work clients has numerous implications for the ongoing and imperative implementation of EPAS competency three. Tools for integrating the natural environment into psychosocial assessments must be taught in foundational clinical social work courses. For example, questions about pollution and environmental toxins for clients experiencing repeat health concerns or questions about flooding and fire risks integrated into the housing components of assessments. Since EJ emphasizes eliminating systemic environmental inequities related to race/ethnicity, gender, and abilities, content is also relevant to foundational multicultural classes and course content using a power, privilege, and oppression lens. Macro focused students (including students in foundational social work with community courses and courses exploring human behavior in the social environment) should also be encouraged to apply new paradigms, theories, and frameworks such as social-ecological systems and One Health to their focus areas and to consider how these frameworks can complement and expand upon existing social work perspectives.

Resources are available to aid educators in developing content to integrate EJ into social work curricula. There are social work specific resources developed by the NASW (e.g., Social Work Speaks), CSWE Committee on Environmental Justice, Katherine A. Kendall Institute for International Social Work Education (e.g., their compilation of effective syllabi) and social work scholars (e.g., Beltrán, Hacker, & Begun, 2016 among others), as well as textbooks (e.g., Dominelli's (2012) Green Social Work: From Environmental Crisis to Environmental Justice). In addition, other complementary disciplines may serve as knowledge sources for social work – such as public health, environmental education, and environmental psychology. Since many clinical faculty maintain licensure, integration of EJ concepts into their curriculum and practice should also be offered in professional development activities such as continuing education.

Master's programs are also continuously undergoing curriculum reviews in preparation for accreditation. Therefore, administrators also have a role in identifying gaps as well as links and connections between EJ and other courses throughout the curriculum to aid educators that may lack the capacity for integration. If administrators or curriculum leads feel underprepared for this task, other faculty from both within and outside a program should be used in consultation. Educators also need to be cognizant of providing students with concrete strategies for addressing environmental injustices to prevent a sense of overwhelming helplessness that leads to inaction. Due to the students' expressed personal detachment from environmental injustices, experiential courses in diverse settings (e.g., urban, rural, domestic, and international) experiencing environmental injustices would be beneficial. These courses may then generate further interest, which could be addressed by internships with environmentally-focused agencies. To truly imbue EJ's transdisciplinary nature to social work students, the capacity for social work students to engage in classes and problem-solving oriented projects with students from other disciplinary backgrounds is essential. It is likely that elective courses outside social work will be needed to fill this gap (Miller & Hayward, 2014). However, social work faculty should provide support integrating key social work values into course content through facilitated learning.

Limitations related to this exploratory study should be noted. Though we targeted a diverse range of universities, this study used a non-probability sampling and included a relatively small number of participants who likely opted to participate due to interest in the topic. It is possible the current study contains results that summarize perspectives of a few students who are the most interested in EJ. While participants often reflected on other social work experiences unrelated to their current program (e.g., their undergraduate experiences if they had earned a BSW), their knowledge remained school-specific. Thus, these results are not generalizable to social work students at large, but rather provide preliminary emergent themes that can inform initial classroom responses while also providing a base of understanding for the future investigation that is necessary to refine and tailor classroom approaches. It is also possible students felt a need to present their beliefs in ways they believe the researcher saw as "correct." While interviewers underwent extensive training in ethical research and interviewing, and placed emphasis on establishing rapport, such limitations are nearly impossible to completely eliminate.

Conclusion

As Earth's ecological changes continue and increase in severity and frequency, so too will the disproportionate environmental impacts on social work clients. Meanwhile, social work students and practitioners in the United States continue to report a sense of unpreparedness when faced with clients experiencing environmental injustices. This study found that few and inconsistent opportunities for facilitated learning on EJ in social work training and education exist. Additionally, a key to effective training on EJ may be to connect social work approaches to the grandiose nature of these environmental problems, which interact with other social justice issues across micro, mezzo, and macro scales. As the CSWE has mandated the integration of EJ into social work curricula, there may be a need for a paradigm shift within the profession that incorporates a meta-practice, as first postulated by Grise-Owens et al. (2014), into existing approaches to identify the interconnections between social issues long considered under social work's expertize and emerging threats to equitable and sustainable development.

Note

1. CSWE adopted the United States Environmental Protection Agency's definition of environmental justice from the 1994 EJ executive order, "'the fair treatment and meaningful involvement of all people regardless of race, color, national origin, or income with respect to the development, implementation and enforcement of environmental laws, regulations and policies'" (2018), For the purpose of this study, we have used the same definition, but recognize that there is a lack of a universally agreed upon definition within the field of social work.

Disclosure statement

No potential conflict of interest was reported by the authors.

Funding

This work was supported by the University of Denver's Interdisciplinary Research Incubator for the Study of (In)Equality (IRISE) under a graduate student research grant.

ORCID

Jennifer Yu ⓘ http://orcid.org/0000-0002-4176-6825

References

American Academy of Social Work and Social Welfare. (n.d.). *Grand challenges for social work*. Retrieved from http://grandchallengesforsocialwork.org

Beltrán, R., Hacker, A., & Begun, S. (2016). Environmental justice is a social justice issue: Incorporating environmental justice into social work practice curricula. *Journal of Social Work Education*, *52*(4), 493–502. doi:10.1080/10437797.2016.1215277

Bexell, S. M., Decker Sparks, J. L., Tejada, J., & Rechkemmer, A. (2019). An analysis of inclusion gaps in sustainable development themes: Findings from a review of recent social work literature. *International Social Work*, *62*(2), 864–876. doi:10.1177/0020872818755860

Council on Social Work Education. (2017). *Annual statistics on social work education in the United States 2017*. Alexandria, VA: CSWE. Retrieved from https://www.cswe.org/Research-Statistics/Research-Briefs-and-Publications/CSWE_2017_annual_survey_ report-FINAL.aspx

Council on Social Work Education Commission on Educational Policy and the CSWE Commission on Accreditation. (2015). *2015 educational policy and accreditation standards for baccalaureate and master's social work programs*. Alexandria, VA: CSWE. Retrieved from https://cswe.org/getattachment/Accreditation/Standards-and-Policies/2015-EPAS/2015EPASandGlossary.pdf.aspx

Creswell, J. W. (2013). *Qualitative inquiry & research design: Choosing among five approaches* (3rd ed.). Thousand Oaks, CA: SAGE Publications.

Dominelli, L. (2012). *Green social work: from environmental crises to environmental justice. cambridge, uk & malden.* MA: Polity Press.

Dominelli, L. (2013). Mind the gap: Built infrastructures, sustainable caring relations, and resilient communities in extreme weather events. *Australian Social Work*, *66*(2), 204–217. doi:10.1080/0312407X.2012.708764

Drolet, J. L., & Sampson, T. (2014). Addressing climate change from a social development approach: Small cities and rural communities' adaptation and response to climate change in British Columbia, Canada. *International Social Work*, *60*(1), 61–73. doi:10.1177/0020872814539984

Faber, D. R., & Krieg, E. J. (2002). Unequal exposure to ecological hazards: Environmental injustices in the commonwealth of Massachusetts. *Environmental Health Perspectives*, *110* (supp2), 277–288. doi:10.1289/ehp.02110s2277

Gray, M., & Coates, J. (2015). Changing gears: Shifting to an environmental perspective in social work education. *Social Work Education*, *34*(5), 502–512. doi:10.1080/02615479.2015.1065807

Grise-Owens, E., Miller, J., & Owens, L. (2014). Responding to global shifts: Meta-practiceas a relevant social work paradigm. *Journal of Teaching in Social Work*, *34*(1), 46–59. doi:10.1080/08841233.2013.866614

Kemp, S. P., & Palinkas, L. A. (with Wong, M., Wagner, K., Mason, L. R., Chi, I., Nurius, P., Floersch, J., & Rechkemmer, A.). (2015). *Strengthening the social response to the human impacts of environmental change* (Grand Challenges for Social Work Initiative Working Paper No. 5). Cleveland, OH: American Academy of Social Work and Social Welfare. Retrieved from http://grandchallengesforsocialwork.org/wp-content/uploads/2015/12/WP5-with-cover.pdf

Miller, S. E., & Hayward, R. A. (2014). Social work education's role in addressing people and a planet at risk. *Social Work Education*, *33*(3), 280–295. doi:10.1080/02615479.2013.805192

National Association of Social Workers Delegate Assembly. (2003). Environmental policy. In *Social work speaks: NASW policy statements* (6th ed., pp. 116–123). Silver Spring, MD: NASW.

Nesmith, A., & Smyth, N. (2015). Environmental justice and social work education: Social workers' professional perspectives. *Social Work Education*, *34*(5), 484–501. doi:10.1080/02615479.2015.1063600

Philip, D., & Resich, M. (2015). Rethinking social work's interpretation of 'environmental justice': From local to global. *Social Work Education*, *34*(5), 471–483. doi:10.1080/02615479.2015.1063602

Saldaña, J. (2013). *The coding manual for qualitative researchers* (2nd ed.). Thousand Oaks, CA: Sage Publications.

Teixeira, S., & Krings, A. (2015). Sustainable social work: An environmental justice framework for social work education. *Social Work Education, 34*(5), 513–527. doi:10.1080/02615479.2015.1063601

U. S. Environmental Protection Agency. (2018, November 17). *Environmental justice*. Retrieved from https://www.epa.gov/environmentaljustice/

Nature and social work pedagogy: How U.S. social work educators are integrating issues of the natural environment into their teaching

Jon Hudson ⓘ

ABSTRACT
The article presents a study of how U.S. social work educators are including discussion, exercises, readings, and other pedagogical approaches to the natural environment into their classrooms. The findings are part of a larger, naturalistic study that gathered data using a semi-structured interview format. The three major themes that emerged were human behavior theory, ecological and environmental justice, and environmental sustainability. The participants are introducing issues of the natural environment using varied pedagogical techniques including readings, in-class discussions and exercises, service learning, assignments, including written and practical work, research, self-awareness exercises, and class facilitation. Questions for further investigation of social work and the natural environment are included.

The negative physical and mental health effects of environmental degradation are disproportionately borne by those who identify as Black, and Hispanic or Latinx, those living with poverty, those with less education, women, and children (Bullard, Mohai, Saha, & Wright, 2008). This dynamic of intersecting environmental degradation and social injustice is known variously as environmental racism or environmental injustice (Bullard et al., 2008; Commission on Racial Justice, 1987). The inextricable link between people and nature is such that addressing issues of the natural environment is imperative for the social work profession (Dominelli, 2012). This begins with educating social work students about why it is important to focus social work practice on environmental issues and not only on the effects environmental degradation has on humans (Hayward, Miller, & Shaw, 2013). Social work is charged with advocating and intervening for change on the part of people and elements in the environment with which we are interconnected, interrelated, and interdependent (Besthorn, 2007; Coates, 2003; Gray & Coates, 2012). This holistic worldview is the basis for integrating an expansive person-in-environment perspective in practice, which incorporates "discussions of the natural environment, ideas of habitat destruction, chemical contamination, environmental racism, environmental justice, and sustainability" (National Association of Social Workers [NASW], 2009, p. 124). "The natural environment is thought to consist of the geosphere, hydrosphere, atmosphere, biosphere, and noosphere. The first of these alludes to facets of the soil, water, air, and biological species which impact human survivability" (Besthorn, 1997, p. 8).

For nearly twenty-five years a committed group of social work scholars have been focused on the implications of the human interconnection with natural environment for social work (Berger, 1995; Berger & Kelly, 1993; Besthorn, 1997; Besthorn & Hudson, 2018; Coates, 2003; Coates & Gray, 2011; Hoff & McNutt, 1994; Rogge, 1996a; Zapf, 2009). However, this work has been primarily theoretical and exhortative. There were no studies regarding what information is reaching students. This study begins the process of addressing and filling that gap in the social work literature. Therefore, the over-arching research question is: How are social work educators in the United States (U.S.) introducing issues of the natural environment relevant to social work into their teaching?

Literature review

Benjamin Chavez, former head of the National Association for the Advancement of Colored People (NAACP), coined the term "environmental justice" in 1987 (Grossman, 1994). Chavez released the first study that showed people living in poverty and those who identify as Black, and Hispanic or Latinx were more likely to live near an existing source of toxic waste (Commission on Racial Justice, 1987). The issue of exposure to toxic waste has also been studied by several social work scholars including Streeter and Gonsalvez (1994); Hoff and McNutt (1994); Hoff and Rogge (1996); Rogge (1993, 1994, 1996a, 1996b); Rogge and Combs-Orme (2003); Rogge, Davis, Maddox, and Jackson (2005). These studies emphasized the disproportionate exposure to industrial toxic waste related to race and presented a compelling argument for environmental justice as a social work issue. Together they show that economically and politically marginalized populations suffer negative health effects such as increased incidence of birth defects, neurologic disorders, lung cancer, hypertension, heart disease, and pulmonary disorders, associated with exposure to industrial toxins at a significantly higher rate than the general population.

Low and Gleeson (1998) were the first to use the term *ecological justice* to describe the concept of extending the principle of justice to the entire ecosphere, thus applying the principle of justice to the natural environment.

In accord with ecological justice it has been suggested that social work go beyond simply extending the principle of environmental justice to humans.

As we currently understand it, "environmental justice is an extension of the distributional and utilitarian aspects of modern Western ideas of social justice" (Besthorn, 2013, p. 35). Besthorn goes on to critique social work's efforts at environmental justice as commendable and necessary in addressing the systematic oppression extant in the dumping and storage of industrial toxic waste. However, he suggests that a radical equalitarian model of justice is necessary if the ecosystem and humans are to thrive, indeed to survive. "[A]ll species, human and non-human alike, are entitled to a just and equal claim to existence that ensures their well-being and enduring ability to thrive" (p. 38). He referred to this model of justice as, "… the proper and necessary framework for social work as it moves into the troubled waters of a world on the edge of environmental and economic collapse" (p. 21).

Proponents of ecological justice do not seek to supplant the justice needs of humans where the social or natural environments are concerned. "[W] here environmental justice focuses on the needs and risks of humans in the physical environment, ecological justice focuses on the needs and risks of nature and how humans fit in it" (Miller, Hayward, & Shaw, 2012, p. 271).

The inextricable relationship between humans and the ecosphere makes the concept of justice for social work complex. Social work scholars have suggested professional and academic responses that range from addressing the negative impacts of environmental degradation on humans, to beginning to consider our professional responsibility to the non-human world (Drolet, 2015; Gray & Coates, 2012). The term *non-human world* has been defined in the social work literature as referring to "issues concerned with climate change, global warming, environmental degradation, pollution, chemical contamination, sustainable agriculture, disaster management, pet therapy, wilderness protection" (Gray & Coates, 2012, p. 239). Others use the term *non-human* in reference to indirect social work practice with these, and other, natural environmental issues (Erickson, 2018).

These researchers have suggested that social work's emphasis on person-in-environment and social justice make the profession especially well-suited for intervening in issues of exposure to industrial toxic waste and the negative impacts of environmental degradation on marginalized peoples and they have carried on the discussion of environmental justice as a social work issue resulting in a growing body of research on the topic.

Nature and social work theory

The origins of social work's person-in-environment perspective can be traced to the earliest days of the Charity Organization Societies and the Settlement House Movements (Trattner, 1999). As the drive to professionalize social work began in the early 20th century this focus narrowed to practice with individuals and their fit with the *social* environment (Austin, 1983; Hudson,

2014). However, there was never a policy decision made to narrow the definition of the environment in social work's person-in-environment perspective to the social environment (Besthorn, 1997). In the 20th century scholars began to conceptualize theory and practice more broadly (Besthorn, 1997; Weick, 1981). In particular, this refocusing has been on social work pedagogy regarding the conceptualization of core theories such as general systems (von Bertalanffy, 1969), dynamic systems and theories often associated with dynamic systems because of shared theoretical concepts such as boundaries, interdependent, interconnected sub-systems, and the tendency for change on part of the system to affect the entire system. A partial list of these theories includes ecology, eco-systems, deep ecology, and eco-feminism (Robbins, Chatterjee, Canda, & Leibowitz, 2019). All are about living systems and not social (human made) systems.

Ecofeminism and deep ecology have a great deal in common. Both emphasize "the interdependency between human beings and the total planetary ecology." They also share a focus on personal awareness of the interconnectedness of all gives rise to moral imperatives for nonviolence and compassion toward all beings" (Robbins et al., 2019, p. 45). However, ecofeminism goes further, examining the social context of the oppression of both women and nature as a product of patriarchy (Merchant, 2003).

During social work's process of professionalization, in the second half of the twentieth century, programs of social work education taught theories such as ecology and the eco-systems perspective that concerned the natural environment but neglected those aspects that concerned nature. Instead students learned only about the frameworks and over all dynamics as they applied to human created social systems (Besthorn, 1997; Coates, 2003). Coates went on to suggested that in response to social and ecological justice crises, programs of social work education should begin teaching theories that emphasize nature, (e. g., ecology, eco-systems, eco-feminism, and deep ecology), as they were originally conceived.

Methods

This study includes in-depth semi-structured interviews with 16 educators from programs of social work education from 14 states. Of these there was a purposive sample of 11 who had conducted and published research on social work and the natural environment and a snowball sample of five who had not published but who did integrate issues of the natural environment into their teaching. They teach across the social work curriculum at the BSW and MSW levels.

The participant pool was made up of four who identified as male and twelve who identified as female. Three participants identified as being non-White. Six participants had over twenty years of experience as social work educators, three had over five years, and six had less than five years. Their ages ranged from 36 to 85 years of age (the age was not available for one of the participants); the mean age was 50 years. The group included one retired professor, one university administrator, ten pre-tenure status educators, and four post-tenure status educators.

The purpose of the study was to determine how U.S. social work educators are introducing issues of the natural environment into their teaching.

Interviews and analysis

Participants were asked to describe their personal relationships with the natural environment; speak to why they believe the natural environment is an important issue for social work; characterize the central mission of social work and how the natural environment might expand our current understanding of our mission, and describe specific methods and techniques they use to introduce the natural environment into their teaching.

Atlas ti® qualitative data analysis software was used for data management. Each interview transcript was assigned a file number in order to protect the identity of the participants and an alias was assigned to each for the purpose of this report. The constant comparative method was used for data collection and analysis (Lincoln & Guba, 1985).

Each participant was invited to submit course syllabi for review at the time of their interview. Six of the participants (37.5 percent) supplied syllabi for eleven courses.

Research questions

The overarching question guiding this study was: How are U.S. social work educators introducing issues of the natural environment (e.g. ideas of habitat destruction, chemical contamination, environmental racism, environmental justice, and sustainability) into their teaching?

Subsidiary questions

- How were social work educators preparing students to address the non-human aspects of the current environmental crisis (e.g. ideas of habitat destruction, chemical contamination, sustainability, bio-diversity, wilderness protection) in social work?
- What were their perspectives on the significance of introducing issues of the natural environment into social work education for the fundamental mission of the social work profession?

Trustworthiness

Research consultants gave feedback on the preliminary themes regarding how social work educators are integrating issues of the natural environment into their teaching. The consultants were two senior social work faculty from a research-one university in the mid-western United States. Research one universities offer doctoral degrees in at least 20 disciplines and demand a very high level of research activities from faculty. One consultant is male one is female; both have conducted qualitative research for over 20 years each and both have extensive experience teaching qualitative inquiry at the PhD level.

Member checks were conducted throughout the interviewing process and comprehensive member checks were conducted after the preliminary data analysis was complete. As a form of data triangulation course syllabi served to support data gathered in participant interviews. The use of these strategies with interview participants and research consultants helped expand, add to, and refine codes thereby creating trustworthiness and supporting the credibility of the study (Lincoln & Guba, 1985).

Findings

The participants discussed content and techniques they use to introduce issues of the natural environment into their teaching (i.e., social work practice, research, policy, or human behavior theory courses). This discussion of findings includes the three themes that emerged from the interviews including, the introduction of nature in human behavior theory classes; ecological and environmental justice, and sustainability. See Table 1 below for a summary of the main findings. These themes are part of a larger study and are mostly deductive. They came about largely in response to direct questions in the interview process.

Human behavior theory

Participants shared that theory classes were the appropriate place to introduce issues of the natural environment. They also shared that social work has

Table 1. Main themes.

Theme	# Participants	Definition
Ecological justice	11	Extending the principle of Justice to the natural environment
Environmental justice	5	Impact of environmental Degradation on marginalized Populations
Introduce nature in HBSE	6	The appropriate place to introduce nature in the social work curriculum is in HBSE courses
Sustainability	16	Environmental sustainability Is very important for soci work

been neglecting the natural environment in foundational theories for years. Miller et al. (2012) stated, " ... the 'environment' for social work was a human-centered 'world' where the focus was the 'social environment' in which human beings functioned" (p.71). Coates (2003) suggested that for many years social work educators have removed nature from theories and attended only to ways in which the person interacted with the social environment. He encouraged social work educators to begin re-introducing nature when we teach these theories and concepts.

Four of the participants spoke of teaching theoretical frameworks and concepts to include nature. For example, David indicated that HBSE (Human Behavior in the Social Environment) is a good place to introduce students to issues of the natural environment.

> I think the most natural place for this often times is in HBSE where we're exposing students to the theoretical foundations of the profession and all the person-in-environment vernacular and so it's a kind of a natural place to introduce some discussion about well what do we mean by environment ... ?

Leann reintroduces aspects of nature into theories that are traditionally thought of as integral to social work and integrates them into practice by re-designing some basic practice techniques. She has added aspects of nature to eco-maps and gen-o-grams, which are supported by ecological and dynamic systems theories, to make assessment more comprehensive.

> I think [environment] does mean the natural environment. But ... social work has limited it. Our gen-o-grams and our eco-maps are all about the social systems that they're [clients] involved in. You don't normally see one[s] that includes ... their interactions with nature or what their natural environment is like.

In-class exercises may be used to help students learn how to integrate theory into practice or to help them concretize theoretical concepts. Marlene developed an in-class group exercise that helps students conceptualize dynamic systems using common items; many of them waste, to represent components of a dynamic system for her HBSE course.

> I get some bags and things and throw all kinds of random stuff into the bags and then clipped some of them shut and [some] partially open to do a kind of metaphorical model, open systems, closed systems ... I also put in a couple of social work books ... I'd say these are the concepts from systems theory that I want you to try to locate in this stuff. I want you to try to craft some kind of narrative about this – what you believe – identify your system, supra system [and so on] and come up with some sort of narrative and then think about boundaries, think about all of these things. Think about the system, the crises and how you define it.

Supplemental readings help students to see the practical side of theory. Reading about the specific threats to children when toxic chemicals are introduced into their environment can emphasize why it is important for social work to address environmental issues. Maggie and her colleagues use a supplemental reading in HBSE classes to help students learn about issues of the natural environment.

> I know we've got two or three colleagues [in] both of our ... location[s] and a distance learning education function and there are faculty in at least two of those programs who are using Terry Combs-Orme's (Rogge & Combs-Orme, 2003), *Kids and Chemicals* article in their HBSE classes.

Theorists who publish on social work and the natural environment have suggested that social work is uniquely placed to address issues of environmental and ecological justice. The reason is not because educators and practitioners are constantly coming up with new innovations for how to address the current environmental crisis but because they know we can rely on the same professional skills to address these issues that have defined our profession for over a century.

This section indicates that this group of educators is not trying to reinvent social work education regarding the natural environment. They are doing what works and integrating the theoretical work on social work and the natural environment that has been established over two and a half decades. They are finding the appropriate place to introduce nature, in HBSE. Theoretical frameworks and concepts that we already teach are a good fit with social work practice in environmental and ecological justice. Basic pedagogical techniques we have long used in social work education are well adapted for inclusion of issues of the natural environment. If social work is uniquely placed to address environmental and ecological justice it is only because it impacts populations already living on the margins of society.

Ecological and environmental justice

Issues of ecological and environmental justice emerged as one of the dominant themes in the study. At some point in their interviews all the participants described one or both of these concepts. The research cited above indicates that the negative impact of environmental degradation on human populations is a social justice issue. That would suggest that addressing environmental justice is within social work's professional mandate.

Tom introduces students to the *National Environmental Policy Act* (, NEPA, 1969 2014 and the NASW (2009)*Environment Policy* in his social policy course as a way to help them understand the relevance of the natural environment for social work.

> I'll talk about the National Environmental Policy Act and some other issues tied into child and family policy. You have to look at direct connections between the importance of this to our populations and why as social work practitioners it's in

their best interest to understand this because … it's in our interest to understand how the environment impacts our populations.

Rita specifies a week during the semester of her foundation level MSW course as environmental justice week. Students are assigned to select an environmental justice issue, research the issue, and facilitate a class on that issue.

> I teach a first semester course for MSW students – it's Social, Economic and Political Environment … it's one out of five weeks where students are facilitating most of the class and the students take on an issue – homelessness, immigration, whatever it might be, and so one of those is environmental justice.

Theoretical frameworks, such as ecology and eco-systems, lead us to an understanding of humans and nature as one, irreducible system. For many of the participants that means an ecological approach to social work's justice mission is appropriate.

Marlene said environmental justice is a good place to start but that the profession has a responsibility to address the "bidirectional aspects" of the human/nature relationship. She teaches about both.

> One of the ways to … invite folks … who are not as inclined to see the relationship between social work and the natural environment … is from the standpoint of environmental justice … From my standpoint … that's a good place to start … [B]ut in my opinion it doesn't go philosophically far enough. I think about … ecological justice, not only the impacts upon humans, but the impacts [of humans] upon the … rest of the world … We do actually have to think about the bidirectional aspects of that relationship.

Regina also voiced her concern that the social work profession in the U.S. seems to be approaching the natural environment hesitantly, as if it is important that we not get *too* involved. She described a part of the philosophy behind her teaching this way.

> The idea [is] that … social workers would work … on human well-being and social justice issues and … broader ecological justice kind of issues. We would do that in ways that are preventative as well as reactive and in ways that are holistic and interdisciplinary. We would work with and on behalf of those who are vulnerable and marginalized and oppressed by whatever structural influences keep them in those positions.

One important way educators are beginning to integrate an expanded concept of justice that includes both the ecological and environmental justice is to develop field placements and service-learning opportunities. Donna developed a service-learning experience focused on ecological justice, working with non-human clients, a form of indirect practice. In her class students were required to contribute six hours of service learning at a local environmental organization. For example, one group chose to serve at an animal sanctuary where they helped rescue and rehabilitate injured animals and released them back into the wild.

Marlene developed an environmental justice service-learning opportunity in which students help improve local school children's access to nutritious foods. She partnered with other departments at her university and a number of local elementary schools in her community to focus on food security.

> I created this ... service learning program that brought social work students together with horticulture students ... and ... students who are majoring in food and nutrition ... and I collaborate[d] with these people ... in a local elementary school ... growing and working with school gardens.

Sustainability

Sustainability refers to how well we live within the confines of what we call natural resource renewability. In systems terms it means "balancing the needs of the parts with the needs of the whole" (Coates, 2003, p. 70). Two sub-themes emerged from the discussion of sustainability including sustainability and social work practice and the justice issues involved with food systems.

Maggie's focused elective emphasizes sustainability as social work practice. She has developed a course that is specifically designed to help students integrate social work knowledge and skills and bring them to bear on environmental sustainability and a number of issues related to it. The course description states "[s]tudents review and apply conceptual frameworks, such as those based on human rights, social development, and sustainable development, to a range of global social problems."

> I teach a class called Environment and Sustainability in Social Work Practices. It's a dedicated class and the topic really is environmental issues and the interface of that and being a social worker and practicing as a social worker.

Marvin teaches in a social work program that has integrated an assignment into their curriculum that he described as a "final communities project, like a thesis project." The assignment requires the student to reflect on the values of the program that focus on locally produced food and on "pulling more and more away from eating industrialized food on campus.

... [W]e spend a lot of time talking about how important the natural environment is for us in terms of ... our own gathering, and our hunting and our own fishing and how we teach for sustainability."

Katherine's focused service learning elective connects food systems with social and environmental justice. Students study the justice implications of local, organic food systems by volunteering to work for an organic farm owned and operated by a local Oneida Nation.

> This course is designed to increase the cultural competency of students entering social work or other helping professions. In addition to readings, written

assignments, and class discussion, students will contribute time to the class service partnership with [the organic farm], a program of the Oneida Community Integrated Food System.

Most communities give attention to economic sustainability, which can be their life-blood. These participants, however, are concerned that economic sustainability can be at odds with environmental and ecological sustainability. Participants discussed teaching about the concept of sustainability itself as the need for humans to live in harmony with the natural environment – being mindful to not outstrip the natural resources and acknowledging the intrinsic value of nature.

Discussion

In a naturalistic study the job of the researcher is to conceptualize an over-arching research question and then allow the participants to answer that question (Lincoln & Guba, 1985). In answering how educators are introducing issues of the natural environment into their teaching, the participants acknowledged that there are theoretical innovations regarding the natural environment and that innovations represent change. They also acknowledged that where there is change there is often resistance. There was no research hypothesis regarding how educators are integrating issues of the natural environment into their teaching. The answer, however, is gratifying both in terms of pedagogical techniques and implications for practice. They are using techniques that have been used for many years in higher education and they are recommending that students be taught to bring existing social work professional knowledge and skills to bear in this area of practice.

Overall the participants in this study believe that HBSE courses are the appropriate place in curricula to introduce issues of the natural environment; that social work must address both ecological and environmental justice issues, and that environmental sustainability is an important issue for the social work profession.

Implications for practice

The sources of environmental injustice are many and relate to populations that social work has served for many years. As such it is one more social issue that negatively impacts the lives of many who are already living on the margins of society. Addressing environmental justice, then, is a matter of bringing the skills of the social work profession to bear on the issue.

Social Workers must reconceptualize resource networks to align with a more ecological approach to practice that accounts not only for social but natural resources. In doing so workers must consider the fit between clients at all levels of practice and the environment in its most complete meaning, social, physical, and natural. When making assessments they must keep demographics as well as local environmental issues in mind and make environmental assessments standard practice. Some questions may include: Where does your client live? Is there industrial activity in or near their neighborhood? What kind of industry? How long has it been there? Is it still active? What is the source of their water? Has it ever been tested? Is there a natural water source in or near the neighborhood (a stream or river)? Do they know anything about it? Do they use it for anything (recreation or dietary supplementation)? Students should also consider nature when conducting strengths assessments. Question may include: Are there recreational and/or green spaces available for respite and relaxation in your neighborhood? Do they utilize those spaces? Do they have pets or service animals? This is, of course, not a comprehensive list of questions. Many of the same questions may be pertinent for both urban and rural social workers due to the presence of manufacturing, mining, and industrial farming and ranching in those areas.

The emphasis on ecological justice raises the possibility of the need to develop practicum placements in non-traditional areas, such as city or university offices of sustainability and administrative offices of environmental advocacy groups, such as The Sierra Club, The Nature Conservancy, or National Parks. The development of these placements will lead to new professional opportunities for social workers.

Practitioners addressing environmental issues will need to adjust interventions as they do when they work with any specific population or issue. But in general, they will likely be social work interventions at all levels of practice including clinical treatment and case management services, advocacy for services, sound policy, and access to resources and services.

Implications for research

One of the major findings of the study is that eleven of the sixteen participants indicated that an ecological justice approach to social work education and practice is appropriate. Qualitative studies tend to focus on smaller numbers of participants and explore question with them deeply. However, even given the relatively small number, the percentage of those participants who use this approach is remarkable, roughly 80 percent. A larger study focusing on whether social work educators utilize an environmental or ecological justice approach in social work would provide feedback for national organizations, (NASW and CSWE), regarding the state if the art in social work pedagogy. Some participants suggested that, while they have made some important changes, social work's professional bodies, CSWE and NASW, might be overcautious in their approach to addressing issues of the natural environment. If social work educators differ significantly from CSWE and NASW in the way they are conceptualizing the environment that could help the national organizations to broaden their definition of environment to include nature as well.

Much of the social work research and literature on the natural environment comes from scholars from countries such as Canada, Australia, Britain, and Finland (Dominelli, 2012; Gray, Coates, & Hetherington, 2013; Matthies, Närhi, & Ward, 2003). A study that compares how educators from those, and other, countries are introducing issues of the natural environment into their teaching could prove beneficial. This could broaden and deepen our understanding of the natural environment for social work education by adding cross-cultural perspectives (Hudson, 2014, p. 184).

Limitations

This group of participants was selected using purposive sampling. This is the norm with many qualitative methodologies and the process was made as transparent as possible in the methods section. Given that there were significant resource and time limitations on the study the participant group was not as diverse as one might like. The demographic description shows some cultural and sex and gender diversity; however, it should be acknowledged that, with more resources, a more diverse group could have been assembled. Also, some cultural and ethnic demographics have been withheld in order to protect participant confidentiality.

Conclusion

Social work scholars, dating back to the mid 1980s have called for a re-visioning of social justice placing it at the nexus of human and natural environmental systems. It has taken decades of work on their part to construct a body of professional evidence on social work and the natural environment. That body of work has successfully expanded social work theory in such a way that they have led us, not to a radical shift, but a return to our historical roots to deal with a crisis many believe is the most serious humankind has ever faced (Besthorn & Meyer, 2010; Coates, 2005; Dominelli, 2011; Hasbach, 2014). Until recently the literature on nature and social work has been theoretical and exhortative. This study has taken us beyond that dynamic and begun a conversation about how social work educators are integrating the work of those scholars into their teaching. What we have learned indicates that they are using many time- tested pedagogical techniques to adapt the theoretical, practice, research, and policy aspects around issues of the natural environment for social work in their classes. This study indicates that they are assigning readings on social work and the natural environment from the theoretical and research-based writings and from outside of the social work literature. They are assigning written work that requires students to research, reflect upon, and write about the natural environment for social work. They also use visual aids such as documentary videos and representative models to help students conceptualize the interconnection between human and natural systems. In order to deepen and add experience to students' learning, educators are also designing features of field education that incorporate the natural environment into their classes in the form on service learning requirements. Most importantly, they are going beyond the environmental justice dynamic and teaching about the concept of ecological justice, practicing the principle of justice with the environment in its own right.

They have shared readings, lessons, curriculum development, service learning, and other innovations to show that social work is well positioned to integrate issues of both environmental and ecological justice as dimensions of our professional practice at all levels. There are serious, far-reaching environmental issues that need social work's attention such as exposure to toxic waste, the negative impacts of industrial exposure to harmful materials born by marginalized populations in their jobs, and the systematic negative impact of environmental degradation born by those in under-developed places around the world. This work bears further investigation beyond a single study. We must be certain we are continuing to expand upon this issue in social work education in the U.S. and advocating at the level of educational policy to make that possible. We must also begin to inquire into the ways this issue is being integrated into social work professional practice in the field at all levels and in the appropriate domains.

Disclosure statement

No potential conflict of interest was reported by the author.

ORCID

Jon Hudson http://orcid.org/0000-0003-3930-7790

References

Austin, D. M. (1983). The Flexner myth and the history of social work. *Social Service Review*, *57*(3), 357–377. doi:10.1086/644113

Berger, R. M. (1995). Habitat destruction syndrome. *Social Work*, *40*(4), 441–443. doi:10.1093/sw/40.4.441

Berger, R. M., & Kelly, J. J. (1993). Social work in the ecological crisis. *Social Work*, *38*(5), 521–526. doi:10.1093/sw/38.5.521

Besthorn, F. H. (1997). *Reconceptualizing social work's person-in-environment perspective: Explorations in radical environmental thought* (Doctoral dissertation). ProQuest Dissertation Publishing. (9811571)

Besthorn, F. H. (2007). En-voicing the world: Social construction and essentialism in natural discourse – How social work fits in. In S. Witkin & D. Saleebey (Eds.), *Social work dialogues: Transforming the canon in inquiry, practice, and education* (pp. 167–202). Alexandria, VA: CSWE Press.

Besthorn, F. H. (2013). Radical equalitarian ecological justice: A social work call to action. In M. Gray, J. Coates, & T. Hetherington (Eds.), *Environmental social work* (pp. 31–45). New York, NY: Routledge.

Besthorn, F. H., & Hudson, J. (2018). The spiritual dimensions of ecosocial work in the context of global climate change. In B.Hudson (Ed), *The spiritual dimensions of ecosocial work in the context of global climate change* NY: Routledge. (pp. 338-346: spirituality and social work. New York. doi:10.4324/9781315679853

Besthorn, F. H., & Meyer, E. E. (2010). Environmentally displaced persons: Broadening social work's helping imperative. *Critical Social Work, 11*(3), 123–138.

Bullard, R. D., Mohai, P., Saha, R., & Wright, B. (2008). Toxic waste and race at twenty: Why race still matters after all of these years. *Environmental Law, 38*(2), 371–411.

Coates, J. (2003). *Ecology and social work: Toward a new paradigm.* Halifax, Canada: Fernwood Publishing.

Coates, J. (2005). The environmental crisis: Implications for social work. *Journal of Progressive Human Services, 16*(1), 25–49. doi:10.13000/J059v16n01_3

Coates, J., & Gray, M. (2011). The environment and social work: An overview and introduction. *International Journal of Social Welfare, 21*, 1–9. doi:10.1111/j.1468-2397.2011.00851.x

Commission on Racial Justice. (1987). *Toxic waste and race in the United States: A national report on the racial and socio-economic characteristics of communities with hazardous waste sites.* New York, NY: United Church of Christ.

Dominelli, L. (2011). Climate change: Social workers' roles and contributions to policy debates and interventions. *International Journal of Social Welfare, 20*, 430–438. doi:10.1111/j.1468-2397.2011.00795.x

Dominelli, L. (2012). *Green social work: From environmental crisis to environmental justice.* Malden, MA: Polity Press.

Drolet, J. (2015). Editorial. *International Social Work, 58*(3), 351–354. doi:10.0020/872814561402

Erickson, C. L. (2018). *Environmental justice as social work practice.* New York, NY: Oxford University Press.

Gray, M., & Coates, J. (2012). Environmental ethics for social work: Social work's responsibility to the non-human world. *International Journal of Social Welfare, 21*(3), 239–247. doi:10.1111/j.1468-2397.2011.00852.x

Gray, M., Coates, J., & Hetherington, T. (2013). *Environmental social work.* New York, NY: Routledge.

Grossman, K. (1994). The people of color environmental summit. In R. Bullard (Ed.), *Unequal protection: Environmental justice and communities of color* (pp. 272–297). San Francisco, CA: Sierra Club Books.

Hasbach, P. H. (2014). Therapy in the face of climate change. *Ecopsychology, 7*(4), 205–210. doi:10.1089/eco.2015.0018

Hayward, R. A., Miller, S. E., & Shaw, T. V. (2013). Social work education on the environment in contemporary curricula in the USA. In M. Gray, J. Coates, & T. Hetherington (Eds.), *Environmental social work* (pp. 246–259). New York, NY: Routledge.

Hoff, M. D., & McNutt, J. G. (1994). *The global environmental crisis: Implications for social welfare and social work*. Brookfield, VT: Ashgate.

Hoff, M. D., & Rogge, M. E. (1996). Everything that rises must converge: Developing a social work response to environmental injustice. *Journal of Progressive Human Services, 7*, 41–57. doi:10.1300/j059v07n01_04

Hudson, J. (2014). *The natural environment in social work education* (Doctoral dissertation). ProQuest Dissertation Publishing. (3641717)

Lincoln, Y. S., & Guba, E. G. (1985). *Naturalistic inquiry*. Thousand Oaks, CA: SAGE Publications.

Low, N., & Gleeson, B. (1998). *Justice, society, and nature: An exploration of political ecology*. New York, NY: Routledge.

Matthies, A., Närhi, K., & Ward, D. (2003). *The eco-social approach in social work*. Jyväskylä. Finland: SoPhi.

Merchant, C. (2003). *Reinventing Eden: The fate of nature in western culture*. New York, NY: Routledge.

Miller, S. E., Hayward, A., & Shaw, T. V. (2012). Environmental shifts for social work: A principles approach. *International Journal of Social Welfare, 21*, 270–277. doi:10.1111/j.1468-2397.2011.00848.x

National Association of Social Workers. (2009). *Social work speaks: National association of social workers policy statements*. Washington DC: NASW Press.

Robbins, S. P., Chatterjee, P., Canda, E. R., & Leibowitz, G. S. (2019). *Contemporary human behavior theory: A critical perspective for social work practice*. Upper Saddle River, NJ.: Pearson Education.

Rogge, M. E. (1993). Social work, disenfranchised communities, and the natural environment: Field education opportunities. *Journal of Social Work Education, 29*, 111–120. doi:10.1080/10437797.1993.10778803

Rogge, M. E. (1994). Environmental justice: Social welfare and toxic waste. In M. Hoff & J. McNutt (Eds.), *The global environmental crisis: Implications for social welfare and social work* (pp. 53–74). Brookfield, VT: Avebury.

Rogge, M. E. (1996a). Social vulnerability to toxic risk. *Journal of Social Service Research, 22*, 109–129. doi:10.1300/j079v22n01_07

Rogge, M. E. (1996b). *Social vulnerability to toxic risk from commercial and industrial chemical releases* (Doctoral dissertation). ProQuest Dissertation Publishing. (9704447).

Rogge, M. E., & Combs-Orme, T. (2003). Protecting children from toxic exposure: Social work and U.S. social welfare policy. *Social Work, 48*, 439–450. http://dx.doi.org.www.remote.uwosh.edu/sw/48.4.439

Rogge, M. E., Davis, K., Maddox, D., & Jackson, M. (2005). Leveraging environmental, social, and economic justice at Chattanooga Creek: A case study. *Journal of Community Practice, 13*(3), 33–53. doi:10.1300/J125v13n03_03

Streeter, C. L., & Gonsalvez, J. (1994). Social justice issues and the environmental movement in America: A new challenge for social workers. *Journal of Applied Social Sciences, 18*(2), 209–216.

Trattner, W. I. (1999). *From poor law to welfare state: A history of social welfare in America*. New York, NY: The Free Press.

U. S. Environmental Protection Agency. (2014). *National environmental policy act*. Retrieved from www.epa.gov/compliance/nepa

von Bertalanffy, L. (1969). *General systems theory: Foundations, development, applications*. New York, NY: George Braziller Inc.

Weick, A. (1981). Reframing the person-in-environment perspective. *Social Work, 26*(2), 140–145. doi:10.1093/sw/26.2.140

Zapf, M. K. (2009). *Social work and the environment: Understanding people and place*. Toronto, Canada: Canadian Scholars' Press Inc.

Index

Agyeman, J. 225
air pollution 121, 125–8
Alaska Native communities 103, 140, 279
Alberini, A. 136
Alfred, T. 83
Alliance of Small Island States (AOSIS) 63–4
American Academy of Social Work and Social
  Welfare (AASWSW) 48
American Farmworkers Union 233
AmeriCorps 146
Anderson, Toni 265, 266, 272
Andersson, H. 164
Ando, A. W. 146
Andorra 65
anthropocentrism 1
anthropogenic disturbances 2–3, 30–2, 38, 39,
  42, 43
anti-capitalistic movement 23–4
anti-colonial movement 23–4
anti-colonial practice 90–2
anti-nuke protests 239
Association for Community Organization and
  Social Action (ACOSA) 1
Asthma and Allergy Foundation of America,
  2018 120–1
ATLAS-ti V.8.2 33–4, 292, 293
Audubon Society 233, 239, 241
Australia 64, 83, 301
Austria 69

back-to-the-land movement 240
backyard GI programs 135, 137, 145, 146, 148
Bailey, W. T. 137
Balram, S. 158
Baltic Sea 34, 37, 38
Baltimore Neighborhood Indicators Alliance–
  Jacob France Institute (BNIA-JFI) 152
Banco Popular's Social Innovation and
  Collaboration Community 50
*Basel Convention on the Control of
  Transboundary Movements of Hazardous
  Wastes and their Disposal* 175
Begravningskassa 35
Belgium 5
Bell, Finn McLafferty 3
Beltrán, Ramona 4
Billiot, Shanondora 4

biodiversity depletion 3
Black Detroiters 89
Black Lives Matter 245
Black Power 233
blue revolution 15, 24
BNIA-JFI 152, 158–9
Boddy, J. 85
Boetto, H. 130
Bönaböckling 36
Bönan (a fishing community in Sweden)
  30, 32–3; coastal fishing community 34–7;
  community resilience and community
  capital 39–41; map of 35; social work in
  community practice 41–2; structural and
  ecosocial changes 37–9
Boudet, H. S. 207, 211, 212
Bouilly, Emanuelle 21
Bristow, Ann 4
Britain 301
Brooks, C. 118
Brown, Danica 4
Brown, Freddie Mae 130
Bullard, R. D. 222
Burger, J. 15
Bygdeföreningen 39

Canada 64, 83, 190, 301
Canadian Association of Social Workers
  (CASW) 80
Cape Verde 11
Care Model 218
Carolina 221
Carson, R. 233
Carter, A. V. 207, 212
Centers for Disease Control and Prevention
  (CDC) 127
Charity Organization Societies and the
  Settlement House Movements 291
Chernobyl nuclear disaster 36, 38
Chicago 264, 271
China 65
Choctaw Nation of Oklahoma (CNO) 108
civic mobilization 207–12; analytical
  framework 207; civic capacity 208–10;
  economic hardships 211; experience with
  prior land-use issues 211; level of threat
  and perceived risk 207–8; LNG project 212;

political opportunity 210–11; Western Maryland 212
Civil Rights 221, 233, 239, 245
client assessments 252–3
Climate Action Plan, 2012 152
climate change 1–4, 11, 82–4, 92, 93, 105, 121, 128, 134, 163, 217, 226, 262, 279
climate emergency 248
climate gap 128
coal mining 212
coastal community 2–3, 29, 30, 32, 33, 36, 41, 42
Coates, J. 117, 295
Cohen-Callow, Amy 4
collective survival strategies (CSS) 80, 82, 85–90, 92
colonialism 2, 3, 4, 14, 15, 80, 82–5, 87, 90, 91, 99–101
colonization 7, 80, 82, 84, 85, 89, 91, 92, 97, 101, 105
Colorado 240
Combs, Katie Massey 6
Combs-Orme, T. 290
common heritage of (hu)mankind (CHM) 64
community-based organizations (CBOs) 146, 151, 154–5, 160, 163–4, 166
community-based participatory research (CBPR) 153, 195–6
community building 55, 183, 244, 249–51, 255, 257, 259, 264, 267
community capitals 31, 42
community development 192, 193, 226
community engagement 135, 243, 245–6
community organizing 2–4, 48, 171–3, 184, 219, 221, 225, 244, 250
community resilience 3, 30–4, 39–43, 49, 55, 81, 82, 85–6, 163
Community Technology Center (CTC) 171–3, 175–83, 186; characteristics of **178**; descriptive information **180**; organizational functions and subfunctions **181**
Comstock Lode 190
Comstock Mining Incorporated (CMI) 195–9, 201–2; negotiations 200
Cornell National Social Survey 234
corporate social responsibility (CSR) 193, 194
Council on Social Work Education (CSWE) 5, 259, 278, 280, 284, 286, 286n1, 300–1
Coyne, C. 50
critical youth empowerment 263–5, 267, 274, 275
Crosnoe, R. 235

Dakota Access Pipeline (DAPL) 100–1, 270
Dauber, M. L. 49
Dave, J. 128
Davis, K. 290
Decker-Sparks, Jessica L. 6
deforestation 217
Denmark 34, 38
Dennis, Mary Kate 3, 5

desertification 3, 278
Detroit Black Community Food Security Network (DBCFSN) 225
Detroit Digital Justice Coalition, 2009 175
Devil's Gate 198
Díaz, Alejandro Silva 3
digital divide 174, 175
digital justice 171, 173–5
dioxins 36
disaster response 48–50, 52, 55, 81
disproportionate burdens 63–4
Dominelli, L. 17, 117, 284
Don't Frack Maryland (DFMD) Coalition 208, 210
Dragićević, S. 158
Drop City 240

eco-centric paradigm 249
ecological injustices 3–4
ecological justice 1, 5–7, 252, 258, 259, 290–2, 294, 296, 297, 300, 302
ecological social work 17
Economic and Social Council (ECOSOC) 65, 66, 68, *68*, 70
economic equity 72–3
ecosocial change 2–3
ecosocial lens 259
ecosocial problems 16–17
ecosocial tool kit 252
ecosocial transition projects 225
ecosocial work 2–6, 30, 31, 43, 48–9, 55, 79–81, 84–5, 87, 117, 121, 122, 129–30, 147, 191, 203, 216–17, 219–20, 224, 228, 249, 251, 273, 274; concepts 253; education 251; environmental justice 253–5; and fracking 206–7; global education 255–7; transformative approach 251–3
educational policy and accreditation standards (EPAS) 278, 283, 284
egg alumni 237
Egypt 69
Ekenga, Christine C. 4
Elder, G. H. 235
Ellzey, J. L. 137
#EnAcción initiative 52
Energy Transfer Partners 100–1
Environmental Alliance for Senior Involvement 234
environmental amenities 262
environmental degradation 3
environmental injustice 248–9, 262, 279, 283, 299
environmentalism 130, 233–5, 240
environmental justice (EJ) 1, 5, 171, 173–4, 229n1, 254, 258, 262, 265, 271, 278–83, 285, 290, 296–8, 302; and social work clients 282–3
Environmental Protection Agency (EPA) 194, 198, 233
environmental racism 248–9

INDEX

environmental social work 17, 217, 232
environmental sustainability 16, 84, 110, 250, 265, 298, 299
equitable development 286
Eritrea 65
e-Stewards 174
Estonia 34
European Union (EU) 3, 15, 22, 24, 36, 39, 64
eutrophication 3
Evans, John 107
e-waste (electronic waste) 40, 172–9, **180**, 183, 184
the expedition of hope 23
extinction of species 248–9

Fabbre, Vanessa D. 4
Facebook 52, 139
Federal Emergency Management Agency (FEMA) 47, 54, 55
feminism 233
Fernandez, Angela 4
Field, C. B. 15
Finland 5, 34, 36, 38, 301
fishing communities 3, 12, 13, 19–25, 30, 34–7, 39, 42
Flint Water Crisis 220, 222–4, 279
Food and Agriculture Organization (FAO) 11, 18, 59, 73n1
Food & Water Watch and Chesapeake Climate Action Network 208
Fort Berthold Reservation 100
fracking 5, 206–7, 210–13, 255; and ecosocial work 206–7
France 65
franchise activis 176
Free Geek model 176
Freitas, L. P. 146
fresh water scarcity 217
Friends of Puerto Rico 50
Functional Community Organization (FCO) 171–3, 175–7, 182, 184–6
Fundación Ángel Ramos 50
Fundación Comunitaria de PR 50
Fusco, L. M. 207, 212

Gagné, S. A. 147
Gamble, D. N. 250
Garrett County Farm Bureau 211
Gästrikland 36
geographical communities 2–3
Geographic Information System (GIS) 208
Germany 5, 34
getting onboard 16
Ghana 69, 193
Gilbert, D. J. 137
Gleeson, B. 290
globalization 38, 82, 172
Global Ocean Commission (GOC) 63
global social work 16–17
Global Social Work Statement of Ethical Principles (GSWSEP) 24

global warming 278
glocalization 29, 31, 41, 172, 186
Gonsalvez, J. 290
The Graduate (film) 237–8
Gray, M. 16, 85, 117
Green Belt Movement 249, 250, 255
green capitalism 15
green infrastructure (GI) 4, 35, 135–8, 140, 142; awareness of 142, 143; Backyard 136–7; dependent variables 140; familiarity **143**; independent variables 140–1; interest 143–5, **144–5**
Green Office 252, 253
Greenpeace 18, 23, 239
green revolution 15
green social work 48
Green Space 130, 134–6, 152–4, 158, 161, 300
greenwashing 7
Grieser, J. M. 137
Grise-Owens, E. 279, 286
gross domestic product (GDP) 65, *66–8*, 69, *69*
Grube, L. 50

Hardin, Garrett 15
Hart, R. A. 263
Hayward, R. A. 3, 279, 283
Heinsch, M. 129
Held, M. L. 137
Hernández, Melissa 6, 266
High Seas Alliance (HSA) 61, 72
Hilltop community 155; demographic and descriptive information for survey respondents **156**; study period *161*
Hilltop Improvement Association (HIA) 152–3
Hilmers, A. 128
Hilmers, D. C. 128
Hirvilammi, T. 5
Hoff, M. D. 290
Holmgren, M. 164
Hopkins, Karen M. 4
Hudson, J. 6
Human Behavior in the Social Environment (HBSE) 295–6, 299
human behavior theory 294–6
human rights 72–3

illegal migrants 20
illegal, unreported and unregulated (IUU) fishing 62
India 5, 220, 224–6
indigenism 90
Indigenist Stress Coping model 108
Indigenous communities 101, 269
Indigenous Knowledge (IK) 80, 85, 90–2, 98, 99, 103, 109
Indigenous people 93, 101–2, 105, 110
Indigenous social work 90
industrial pollution 217
Information and Communications Technologies (ICTs) 174, 181
information poverty 175

Inter-American Tropical Tuna Commission (IATTC) 63
inter-disciplinary education 254
intergenerational participation 242–3
Intergovernmental Panel on Climate Change (IPCC) 86, 248
International Association of Schools of Social Work (IASSW) 16
International Council on Social Welfare (ICSW) 16
International Court of Justice (ICJ) 65, 67, *67*
International Federation of Social Workers (IFSW) 5, 16, 259
International Institute for Sustainable Development (IISD) 63
International Monetary Fund (IMF) 14, 15, 17
international non-governmental organizations (INGOs) 23
international social work 16, 23–5
Intersectionality-Based Policy Analysis (IBPA) 3, 59, 64, 65
Israel 83
Italy 5
Izlar, Joel 4

Jackson, M. 224, 290
Jamaica 68
Japan 62, 64
jappi 225
Jarden, K. M. 137
Jefferson, A. J. 137
Johnson, M. K. 235
Journal of Community Practice 1

Kang, Joonmo 4
Kansas community 243–4
Katrina, Hurricane 279
Kemp, S. P. 97, 118, 218, 227
Kerala 224
Klein, Naomi 14
Klomp, R. W. 31
Knoxville 138, *139*
Korea 69
Krieger, N. 102
Krings, Amy 3, 6, 266
Kvam, August 4

La Plata Lake dam 51
Latinx communities 267
Latvia 34, 36
Laudato Si: On care for our common home (Francis) 232
Lavoie, C. 3
Least Developed Countries (LDCs) 61, 63, 67, 68, 70, 71, 74n2
legacy of colonialism 3–4
Lemke, J. 50
Liberia 11
Libya 65
Life Below Water 18, 61
life course theory 235

liquefied natural gas (LNG) project 207, 211, 212
Lithuania 34
local community 11, 12, 21, 22, 24, 31, 40, 41, 49, 192
Loh, P. 225
Low, N. 290

Maathai, Wangari 87, 250, 251, 255
Maddox, D. 290
Marcellus Shale region 206
Maria, Hurricane 47–50
Maryland 206, *209*
mass migration 248–9
Master of Social Work based in Indigenous Knowledges (MSW-IK) 90
Mathias, J. 224
Matthies, A.-L. 5, 118, 225
Mattocks, Nicole 4
Mayring, P. 13
McAdam, D. 207, 211–12
McGurty, E. M. 221
McNutt, J. G. 290
Mentes Puertorriqueñas en Acción, Inc. (MPA) 50, 52–4
Metropolitan St. Louis Sewer District (MSD) 124
Meyer, Megan 4
Middlebay community 155, 164; demographic and descriptive information for survey respondents **157**
Middlebay Development Organization (MDO) 152–3
Midwest 280
millennial generation 245
Miller, J. 279
Miller, S. E. 279, 283, 295
mining community 194
mining industry 191
Mitchell, Felicia M. 4
Mohai, P. 222
Monaco 65
Morello-Frosch, R. 128
Moritz, Beckwith 256
Morris, Zachary 3
MSW programs 280, **280**, 281, 282
Mullaly, R. 86
mutual care 17
Myanmar 69

Närhi, K. 5, 118, 225
National Aeronautics and Space Administration (NASA) 248
National Association for the Advancement of Colored People (NAACP) 290
National Association of Social Workers (NASW) 80, 245, 278, 284, 290, 300–1
National Environmental Policy Act (NEPA) 296
national jurisdiction 60, 61
National Oceanic and Atmospheric Administration (NOAA) 248
National Parks 300

national social work 16, 23–5, 280, 284
Nature Conservancy 300
neighborhood environmental issues 121
neoliberal capitalism 2–3
neoliberal globalization 29
neoliberalism 15–17, 29
neo-liberalization 1
Nesmith, A. 279, 283
Nevada Division of Environmental Protection (NDEP) 190–1
Nevex Gold Company 195
Newburn, D. A. 136
New Community Organizing 172, 184
non-governmental Organizations (NGOs) 12, 17, 18, 21, 22, 55, 257
non-human world 291
Non-profit Industrial Complex 183
non-profit organization 195–6
Norgaard, R. B. 15
Norrlandet.se functions 39–41
North Korea 65
Norway 38, 69

Ostrom, E. 15
over-consumerism 1
Overfishing, Social Problems and Ecosocial Sustainability in Senegalese Fishing Communities (Jönsson) 3
overpopulation 248–9
Owens, L. 279

Pacific Small Island Developing States (PSIDS) 64
Palinkas, L. A. 97
Paris Climate Agreement 130
Pastor, M. 128
Peabody Energy Company 100
pedagogy 5–6
Peeters, J. 117
persistent organic pollutants (POPs) 36
Peru 69
Petts, J. 118
Pfefferbaum, R. L. 31
place-based education 104, 108
Poland 34
Policansky, D. 15
policy advocacy 226, 227
pollution disparities 278
polychlorinated biphenyl (PCB) 220–1
Port of Gävle 34, 39
Powell, Kathleen H. 4
Precht, Francis L. 4
Preparing Social Workers for Ecosocial Practice and Community Change 6
preppers 87–8
progressive political campaigns 239
Puerto Rico 47–8, 50, 51, 55
Puerto Rico Aqueduct and Sewer Authority (PRASA) 51

QualCoder 179
Quizar, J. 88

racism 4, 102, 121–4, 126–30, 220–2, 249, 255, 262, 289–90
Rambaree, Komalsingh 3
Ramos, Yamirelis Otero 3
Ramsay, S. 85
regional fisheries management organizations (RFMOs) 61–3, 71
resilience 79, 81–2, 106
Responses and resistance 13
Rhea, L. 137
Rogge, M. E. 290
Roy, A. H. 137
Russia 34, 62, 65

Sacred Ecology 98, 99
Sacred Keepers Sustainability Lab 265
Sacred Keepers Youth Council 265, 266, 268, 274
Sadd, J. 128
Sage-grouse 194
Saha, R. 222
San Marino 65
Schmitz, Cathryne 254
Schusler, Tania 6, 266
Secretariat 65, 66
self-determination 6, 86, 88, 90, 91, 268, 269, 271, 273, 274, 275
Senegal 7, 11–14, 19, 20; fishing communities 21–4; social work 17–18
Settlement House movement 217–18
settler-colonialism 82–4, 99–100
Sharpe, C. 83
Shepard, B. 172, 184
Shonkoff, S. B. 128
Shuster, W. 137
Sierra Club 233, 239, 241, 300
Sierra Leone 11
Silent Spring 233
Silver City 194–9, 201, 202
Sjöberg, Stefan 3
slow violence 117
Small Island Developing States (SIDS) 61, 63, 66, 67, 69–71, 74n2
Smyth, N. 279, 283
social action 1, 171–2
social capital 40, 49, 137, 152, 153, 160
social change 1–3, 16, 23, 30–1, 85, 86, 90–1, 138, 172, 173, 175–6, 179, 182, 213, 225, 228, 232, 235, 245, 264, 265, **266**, 268, 274; intention 272; knowledge 271–2; self-restoration 272; youth agency 271
Social Determinants of Health (SDOH) 153
social development 72–3
social-ecological crisis 117
social justice 6, 15, 16, 23, 24, 59, 61, 72–3, 97, 118, 129, 138, 174, 175, 225, 245, 257, 263, 265, 268, 271, 282, 286, 291, 296, 297, 301; place and land 269; self-determination 269; unique and shared identities 268–9
social license to operate (SLO) 192, 193, 197, 201

social mobilization 42
social work 4, 16–17, 24, 48, 49, 97, *103*, 110, 216, 249, 258–9, 262–3, 289, 294
social work education 98, 104, 107, 147, 249, 253, 278, 280, 283, 284, 292, 293, 296, 300; global education 255–7; inter-and trans-disciplinary learning 253; interdisciplinary course on environmental justice 253–5
Social Work Speaks 284
socioecological system 136
socioeconomic status (SES) 49, 51
sociotechnical system 136
solidarity economy movements 225
Sorqvist, P. 164
South Pacific Regional Fisheries Management Organization (SPRFMO) 63
sovereign equality 65
Spain 38
Stamm, I. 5
Standing Rock Sioux Reservation 100
St. Louis: African Americans 123–4; environmental injustice 124–7; Public Schools 127; violence and racism 122–4
Stockholm Resilience Centre 31
Stock, Paul 5
Storr, V. H. 50
Streeter, C. L. 290
street science 223, 226
sushi 59
sustainability 298–9
sustainable community development 2, 41
Sustainable Development Goals (SDGs) 1–2, 6, 15–16, 23–5, 45, 58, 62, 66, 70, 191, 216, 218, 219, 274, 286
Sweden 3, 7, 30, 32, 34, 36, 38, 39, 43, 69
Swedish Research Council, 2018 33
Switzerland 64
Syria 65

Tayouga, S. J. 147
Tennessee 138, *139*
thematic saturation 197
Tierney, K. 81, 82, 85, 86
Toxic Wastes and Race in the United States 221
Traditional Ecological Knowledge (TEK) 98, 99, 105, 110
traditional solidarity 17, 18, 22
The Tragedy of the Commons 15
TreeBaltimore 158–9
Trinidad 240
Trusteeship Council 65
trustworthiness 294
Trygghetsboende 40
Turunen, Päivi 3

unconventional natural gas development (UNGD) 206
UN General Assembly (UNGA) 65–7, 69, *69*, 70
United Church of Christ (UCC) 221
United Kingdom (UK) 5, 65

United Nations (UN) 1–2, 59, 60, 63, 65, 70, 73, 191
United Nations Convention on the Law of the Sea (UNCLOS) 58, 59, 64, 71–3; current policy responses 63–4; current representations of the problem 61–2; differential impacts 62–3; high seas policy 60–1
United Nations Development Programme (UNDP) 11
United Nations Environmental Programme (UNEP) 174
United States (US) 5, 62, 64, 65, 83, 99, 122–3, 137, 190, 220, 248, 278, 280, 290, 294
University of Maryland School of Social Work (UMSSW) 152
University of South Carolina College of Social Work (U of SC COSW) 251–2
UN Security Council (UNSC) 65, *66*, 67–9
UN Straddling Fish Stocks Agreement (UNFSA) 61, 71
urban flooding 134–5
urbanization 82, 163
U.S. Environmental Protection Agency, 2018 135

Venezuela 65, 68
Vietnam War 239, 244
Villa Calma community 51, 52
Villa del Sol 51, 52
VISTA programs 146

Wadsworth, Nancy 107
Walsh-Dilley, M. 89
Ward Transformer Company 220
water 2–3
water scarcity 235
Webb, S. 16
Weil, M. 185, 250
West Africa 14, 18, 20, 23, 24
Western and Central Pacific Fisheries Commission (WCPFC) 71
Western Maryland Fracking Fight, 2017 207
Where I Stand Youth Summit 264–6, **266**, 268, *273*, 274
White, M. M. 225
Whole Earth News 240
Whyte, K. P. 82–4, 86
Willett, Jennifer 4
World Bank 14, 15, 17, 65, 70
World Health Organization 153, 154
World War II 17, 30, 36, 38, 233, 237, 238
Wright, B. 222

Yappallí project 109
Young, L. B. 137
youth voice 267
Yu, Jennifer 6

zeitgeist–national and local movements, 1960 and 1970 236–7, 239–41